Stress & Health

SECOND EDITION

Phillip L. Rice

Stress and Health

SECOND EDITION

Stress and Health
SECOND EDITION

Phillip L. Rice
MOORHEAD STATE UNIVERSITY

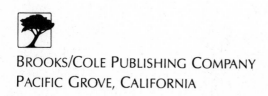

BROOKS/COLE PUBLISHING COMPANY
PACIFIC GROVE, CALIFORNIA

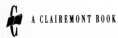 A CLAIREMONT BOOK

Brooks/Cole Publishing Company
A Division of Wadsworth, Inc.

Printed in the United States of America

10 9 8 7 6 5 4 3 2

Library of Congress Cataloging-in-Publication Data
Rice, Phillip L., [date]
    Stress and health / Phillip L. Rice. — 2nd ed.
        p. cm.
    Includes bibliographical references and index.
    ISBN 0-534-17280-6
    1. Stress (Psychology) 2. Medicine, Psychosomatic.   I. Title.
    [DNLM: 1. Stress, Psychological.   WM 172 R497s]
BF575.S75R53 1992
155.9'042—dc20
DNLM/DLC   91-36428
for Library of Congress   CIP

Sponsoring Editor: CLAIRE VERDUIN
Editorial Assistant: GAY C. BOND
Production Editor: MARJORIE Z. SANDERS
Manuscript Editor: LAURIE VAUGHN
Permissions Editor: MARIE DuBOIS
Interior Design: VERNON T. BOES
Cover Design: ROY R. NEUHAUS
Art Coordinator: LISA TORRI
Interior Illustration: SCIENTIFIC ILLUSTRATORS
Part Opening Illustration: ROY R. NEUHAUS
Photo Editor: RUTH MINERVA
Typesetting: BOOKENDS TYPESETTING
Printing and Binding: THE MAPLE-VAIL BOOK MFG. GROUP

To Ruth, my quiet strength,
and
to Rene, Michelle, and Sean, my inspiration.

PREFACE

The years that have passed since publication of the first edition of *Stress and Health* have been exceptionally productive years for stress research. We have good reason to be excited by many breakthroughs, including those in the fascinating but complex area of stress and immunocompetence. Still, many conceptual and methodological problems remain. These problems suggest that we maintain an attitude of guarded optimism mixed with a healthy dose of skepticism. There is much reason for hope yet much to be done.

The changes incorporated in this second edition reflect important developments in research and theory. They also reflect changes in my thinking about what is important in a text on stress and health. New challenges to existing stress models, including the cognitive-transactional model, have arisen. I review these criticisms in Chapter 1. New material on the systems model is also included. The systems model is the historical and logical progenitor of the biopsychosocial model, a model that is receiving widespread attention in health psychology and behavior medicine. I will not dwell here on that clumsy, albeit descriptive, label for what still is a systems approach.

In response to suggestions by several users of the first edition, I have added a complete new chapter (Chapter 2) on research methods in stress and health. This material provides a base for understanding research studies presented later in the text. It introduces the reader to several problems in research design that require critical thinking whether one is a research designer or a consumer. It provides examples of specific types of design in order to help students see more clearly how a particular design may be applied to a specific research question. Further, I introduce the terminology and procedures of epidemiological research. This approach is not typically taught in traditional courses on behavioral science research. Health researchers use epidemiological procedures extensively to answer questions about the relationships between lifestyle and disease and between therapeutic interventions and improved health. As such, the importance of epidemiological procedures cannot be overlooked or minimized. Finally, Chapter 2 introduces the student to a new analytic procedure called *meta-analysis*. This new technique quantitatively analyzes a group of similar studies to discover trends and resolve discrepancies.

I have added a new chapter on coping (Chapter 10) to lead into discussion of specific coping skills. This chapter grapples with issues in defining coping and then presents a theoretical model of coping. It also presents several analyses that suggest specific types of coping to use for certain situations.

The chapter on cognitive processes has been substantially rewritten to include more material on the Health Belief Model. It also includes conceptual notions deriving from Seligman's revised model of helplessness, which is called the *attribution model*. Many research studies have begun to examine how cognitive attributions may influence the course of illness.

Continuing research on the Type A behavior pattern has narrowed the focus of attention to a toxic core of anger. The development of this line of thinking is chronicled here in both logical and empirical detail. Research on the relationship between specific types of personality and vulnerability to particular types of disease led Friedman and Booth-Kewley (1987)* to postulate a general "disease-prone personality." The critical thinking and methodology that led to this notion is also detailed.

The chapter on family process reflects increased attention to cognitive models and systems models of family stress. These models should not be viewed as antagonistic nor redundant. Instead, they focus on different levels of analysis of the same problem. Ultimately they may be merged into a single explanatory theory for the personal, interpersonal, and social processes that malfunction or are distorted in family stress.

The material on social stress has been revised, and the chapter on victimization has been drastically shortened and combined with the chapter on social stress. I continue to think that victimization is an important issue for stress research, and recent work in this area reinforces this view. Nonetheless, so much new material has been added to this book that a decision had to be made about what might be cut with least damage to its integrity. The chapters on job stress and environmental stress have been updated but otherwise retain much the same structure as in the first edition.

As noted earlier, a new chapter on coping introduces the section on coping skills. The previous two chapters on relaxation have been condensed to one chapter and the verbatim relaxation instructions moved to an appendix. More recent theoretical and empirical information has been added to these skills chapters, but their structure remains much the same. Perhaps the most substantive changes occurred in the nutrition and exercise chapter. These changes are based on nationally formulated health goals and refinements in information about the relationships between diet and wellness and between exercise and wellness.

As with the first edition, *Stress and Health* is intended to be an introductory text for a variety of psychology, health, and education courses. It is, I believe, more rigorous than the first edition, without, I hope, being more difficult. Still, I have no illusions that the book will meet all preconceived notions about stress texts. It is not a how-to manual in the strictest sense, though the skills chapters

---

*Friedman, H. S., & Booth-Kewley, S. (1987). The "disease-prone personality: A meta-analytic view of the construct." *American Psychologist, 42,* 539–555.

will provide a motivated reader with most of what is necessary to develop a base of coping skills. Neither is it a compendium of research and theory. The field is simply too expansive and the body of literature too immense for any single book to make that kind of claim. Still, this book has filled niches that I did not initially expect to fill.

I am grateful to those who, while teaching from the first edition, provided feedback about where and how they were using it. It is gratifying to know the range of course objectives and student needs that have been met. It has made the job of revising easier, although decisions on what to include and what to exclude were still painful.

TO THE INSTRUCTOR

If time permits using the entire book, the course will provide a fair balance between the principles and the practice of coping and wellness. If time does not permit covering all the topics in the book, some choices obviously must be made based on the needs of the typical student and the objectives of the course.

The book has been organized to permit the instructor to teach either a *principles syllabus* or an *applied syllabus*. The principles syllabus covers major content areas of stress and health. The chapters that are intended to serve this focus include Chapters 1 through 10 and Chapter 15, which cover the following topics:

Chapter 1: Stress Concepts, Theories, and Models
Chapter 2: Stress Research
Chapter 3: The Cognitive Stress System
Chapter 4: Personality and Stress
Chapter 5: The Physiology of Stress
Chapter 6: Stress in the Family
Chapter 7: Job Stress
Chapter 8: Social Sources of Stress
Chapter 9: Environmental Stress
Chapter 10: Coping Strategies
Chapter 15: Behavioral Health Strategies

The applied syllabus covers the major techniques that enable an individual to cope more effectively with stress, eliminate high-risk behaviors, and maintain better total health. The chapters that serve this purpose are Chapters 1, 6, 7, and 10 through 15. These chapters cover many topics and techniques central to self-help–type programs, as indicated by this list of topics:

Chapter 1: Stress Concepts, Theories, and Models
Chapter 6: Stress in the Family
Chapter 7: Job Stress
Chapter 10: Coping Strategies
Chapter 11: Progressive Muscle Relaxation
Chapter 12: Cognitive and Imagery Techniques

An instructor's manual with test-item file is available. The test-item file is also available on computer disk in ASCII format.

ACKNOWLEDGMENTS

As noted earlier, I am grateful to the instructors who have forwarded suggestions for making this a better text; some reviewers examined the manuscript for the first edition and others the manuscript for the second edition: Dan Canete, Sioux Falls College; Gary Felsten, Clarkson University; Jeffrey E. Harris, West Chester University; Frederick G. Lopez, Michigan State University; Gunter Reiss, Loma Linda University; and Fred E. Stickle, Western Kentucky University. Your comments have proven very useful in a number of ways. I have continued to benefit from the support, patience, and encouragement of my family, friends, and colleagues. My children would have preferred that I put off writing another book until they graduated from college, but they understood my need to pursue this and vocally have encouraged my efforts. For my part, I have found new ways of managing time to be with them while still maintaining a semblance of schedule.

My research assistants, Tessa Taylor and Tiffany Krumm, put in many hours and miles between my office and the library to obtain the many books and articles that became the database for this book. I am most grateful to Claire Verduin for her continued support of this work. I am also grateful for the efforts of all the great people at Brooks/Cole, who take the tedium out of the many minutiae. To Marjorie Sanders, production editor, a special thanks for managing the many technical details that helped to make this book a better work. Laurie Vaughn has provided exceptional help in copy editing, catching even small details that might have slipped through. Thanks to Marie DuBois, who managed the many details of permissions, and to Ruth Minerva for her assistance in obtaining needed photographs. I am also grateful to Lisa Torri, who managed the line art, and to Roy Neuhaus for the cover and interior graphics. Thanks again to all of you.

Phillip L. Rice

BRIEF CONTENTS

CONTENTS

CHAPTER 4

Personality and Stress:
Traits, Types, and Biotypes   85

CHAPTER 5

The Physiology of Stress:
The Brain, Body, and Immune Systems   116

PART THREE

SOCIAL SYSTEMS AND STRESS   147

CHAPTER 6

Stress in the Family:
Adjustment, Conflict, and Disruption   149

CHAPTER 7

Job Stress:
Dissatisfaction, Burnout, and Obsolescence   180

CHAPTER 8

Social Sources of Stress: Social Changes,
Technological Changes, and Life-Changes   210

CHAPTER 11

Progressive Muscle Relaxation: Premises and Process   286

CHAPTER 12

Cognitive and Imagery Techniques: Autogenics, Desensitization, and Stress Inoculation   308

APPENDIX
Relaxation Instructions   406

Stress and Health

SECOND EDITION

PART ONE

THEORY AND RESEARCH: THE BACKGROUND

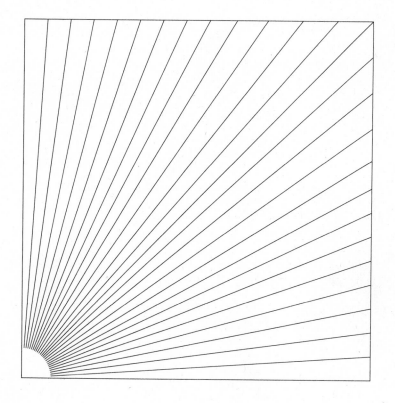

Stress Concepts, Theories, and Models

The concept of stress is somewhat like the illusive concept of love: everyone knows what the term means, but no two people would define it the same way. Commonsense definitions, dictionary definitions, and formal scientific definitions all point in the same general direction but continue along different paths. Hans Selye, the grand master of stress research and theory, said that "stress, like relativity, is a scientific concept which has suffered from the mixed blessing of being too well known and too little understood" (1980, p. 127).

Our first task in this chapter, therefore, will be to impose some order on the confusing array of stress terms. Then we will review major theories of stress that have evolved in the last few years. This will lay the foundation for an indepth study of stress sources in later chapters.

COMMON SENSE AND NOT-SO-COMMON DEFINITIONS OF STRESS

When most people talk about stress, it is usually in terms of pressure they are feeling from something happening around them or to them. Students talk about being under stress because of poor exam performance or an impending deadline for a major paper. Parents talk about the strain of raising teenagers and the financial burdens of running a household. Teachers talk about the pressure of maintaining professional currency while still managing to keep on top of duties connected with classroom teaching. Doctors, nurses, and lawyers talk about meeting the endless demands of their patients and clients.

In each case, it is obvious that several other terms could be substituted easily for the term **stress.** Two such terms, **pressure** and **strain,** were already substituted in the preceding paragraph without any forewarning. Most readers probably would not notice anything unusual about the substitutions. Yet *Webster's New Twentieth Century Dictionary* uses precisely those two terms in its definition of stress. The definition that appears in *Webster's* is "strain; pressure;

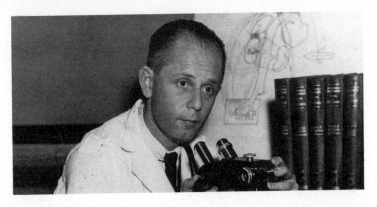

Hans Selye, the grand master of stress research and discoverer of the General Adaptation Syndrome
SOURCE: UPI/Bettmann.

especially, . . . force exerted upon a body, that tends to strain or deform its shape."
This variation in terminology suggests that stress wears many masks.

Stress or Distress: The Negative View

Many people use *stress* and **distress** as though they are interchangeable terms. Perhaps this is because common sense suggests that stress is something bad. To avoid this dilemma, Selye introduced the terms *distress* and **eustress.** According to Selye (1974), distress is "damaging or unplesant stress" (p. 31). Expressed in these terms, stress is much the same as a state of anxiety, fear, worry, or agitation. The core of the psychological experience is negative, painful, something to be avoided.

Stress or Eustress: The Positive View

Pleasurable, satisfying experiences come from what Selye (1979) calls *eustress*. Participation in a wedding ceremony, anticipation of competing in a major sports event, and performing in a theatrical production are examples of eustress. This is positive stress. We even hear of the "joy of stress," a phrase some use to emphasize the good that can come from stress (Hanson, 1986).

Eustress heightens awareness, increases mental alertness, and often leads to superior cognitive and behavioral performance. Eustress may supply the arousing motivation for one individual to create a work of art, another an urgently needed medicine, another a scientific theory. It is, in other words, challenge, stress to be sought out and used as an ally for personal and professional growth.

The relationship between arousing stress and performance is not a simple one, though. The **Yerkes-Dodson Law** was the first attempt to summarize this relationship (Yerkes & Dodson, 1908). The law states that, *up to a point,* perfor-

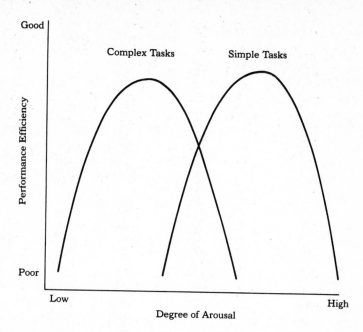

FIGURE 1-1
Effects of amount of stress or arousal on efficiency of performance

mance will increase as arousal increases. Performance is best when arousal is optimum (not maximum). Beyond the optimal level of arousal, performance begins to deteriorate. A graphic illustration of this relation appears in Figure 1-1.

With exceptionally high levels of tension, performance may be as bad as when a person is not aroused at all. Compare the performance efficiency of someone about to fall asleep because of fatigue or boredom with the performance efficiency of someone who is hysterical. Both are generally inefficient and nonproductive.

People perform best with at least some pressure. Too little stress is just as bad as too much. *The aim of stress management, then, is not to eliminate stress entirely but to control it so an optimal level of arousal is present.* Selye (1974) said that "Complete freedom from stress is death" (p. 32). It is extreme, disorganizing stress that we want to avoid.

FORMAL DEFINITIONS OF STRESS

Walter Cannon (1932), a noted Harvard physiologist, probably introduced stress terminology to the scientific community. Cannon contributed the idea of **homeostasis,** the tendency of organisms to maintain a stable internal environment. Cannon also investigated mechanisms of emergency preparedness, the fight-or-flight response. He showed that this response involves a complex interaction between sympathetic nervous system arousal and hormonal secretions from the adrenal glands. Still, the key to Cannon's use of the term *stress* may have been his observation that organisms tend to "bounce back" or "resist" deforming influences from external forces (Hinkle, 1974). In other words, the organism tries to maintain balance when it is confronted with stress. This use of the term is still evident, although new uses of the term have also appeared.

In contemporary scientific literature, *stress* has at least three distinct meanings. First, stress may refer to any event or environmental stimulus that causes a person to feel tense or aroused. In this sense, stress is *external* to the person.

Second, stress may refer to a subjective response. In this sense, stress is the *internal* mental state of tension or arousal. It is the interpretive, emotive, defensive, and coping processes occurring inside a person. Such processes may promote growth and maturity. They also may produce mental strain. The particular outcome depends on factors that will be explained later in the cognitive model of stress.

Finally, stress may be the body's *physical reaction* to demand or damaging intrusions. This is the sense in which both Cannon and Selye used the term. Demand promotes a natural arousal of the body to a higher level of activity. The function of these physical reactions is probably to support behavioral and psychological efforts at coping (Baum, 1990). Recent evidence suggests that repeated exposure to arousing stressors may lead to **physiological toughness.** Dienstbier (1989) defines physiological toughness as increased capacity for responding to stress plus increased resistance to the potential physical damage that stress can produce.[1] Conditions of chronic stress, though, may bring about negative states, including exhaustion, disease, and death.

Stress as External Cause

When speaking of stress as an external stimulus, it is more appropriate to talk of **stressors.** The concept of stressors is similar to the notion of force in engineering. An engineer might calculate the force exerted by cars on a bridge or the pressure of wind against a skyscraper. The demands we experience daily are the forces that wear on us: too much work, too little money, too many creditors, the arrival of a baby, the excitement of a new job, and so on. These are stressors, not stress. Just as the bridge must withstand the load of cars and trucks, we must have some means of meeting or resisting the pressure of external stressors. We do this through coping strategies or defensive reactions.[2]

Stress as Psychological Resistance and Tension

Cognitive processes, such as problem solving, planning, decision making, and cognitive restructuring are positive methods for resisting stress. Rationalization, denial, and fantasy are cognitive processes that people usually consider negative.

[1]Chapter 5 will elaborate on this idea.
[2]I will discuss coping strategies in Chapter 10.

Yet research suggests that negative coping strategies may help people through the early stages of traumatic stress[3] (Matheny, Aycock, Pugh, Curlette, & Silva-Cannella, 1986).

Even when resistance is effective, cognitive side effects are likely to occur during periods of stress. You can respond outwardly to stress passively or actively. But the mental processes involved in meeting external demands are in some sense always active, energy-consuming, and tension-producing.[4] Emotional reactions are likely to be more volatile, marked by increased irritability, explosiveness, and displacement of anger and frustration (Berkowitz, 1990). Perceptual processes involved in interpreting external stimuli may be distorted. Situations previously treated as humorous or nonthreatening become ominous and threatening. The rational planning and decision-making processes may deteriorate or fail to function at all.

Although the focus is on internal states, people still use a variety of physical terms to report their personal batting average against stress. They may talk about being on the verge of a physical or emotional collapse, or they may suggest that they are ready to snap or break. When cognitive, physical, and behavioral coping resources have been taxed to the limit, they may say things like, "This is beyond me," or "I just can't take this (pressure) anymore." Some may even reach a point where they say, "I just feel like giving up." These are signs of the cracks in the defensive armor, reflections of the *strain* that accumulates while enduring stress.

Just as the term *stressor* refers to forces bearing on a person, *strain* refers to the effect of that pressure within the person. According to Selye (1974), though, strain occurs whether the stressor is pleasant or unpleasant. All that "counts is the intensity of the demand for readjustment or adaptation" (pp. 28–29). Whether it is distress or eustress, the demand on coping resources is the same. Further, whether strain fosters growth through challenge or is detrimental to physical and mental health depends on personal appraisals of demands and resources (Lazarus & Launier, 1978). This notion will be discussed in more detail later.

Stress as Bodily Defenses

The third definition of stress emphasizes the global biological reaction to stress. Selye (1974) stated that *"Stress is not merely nervous tension"* (p. 30). Stress is *"the nonspecific response of the body to any demand made upon it"* (p. 27). Three body systems control this nonspecific response: the neural (*H*ypothalamus), glandular (*P*ituitary and adrenal), and hormonal (*A*drenaline, among others) reactions to stressors. In stress physiology, this three-part system has a

---

[3]See Chapters 3 and 10 for more detail.
[4]Tension should be taken here in the most neutral sense of the term—that is, simply "aroused and straining." When you get involved in a TV murder mystery, you may actively try to figure out who did it. You are in a state of mental tension. This does not necessarily mean extreme strain, such as a rope stretched to the breaking point.

name, the HPA complex. Selye rarely dealt with the psychosocial side of stress; this is now thought to be a weakness in his theory. In response to Selye, then, we also would say that *stress is not just physical arousal.*

To summarize, a stressor is an external force. Strain is the wear and tear that result from resisting pressure. In this view, the stressor is the cause and strain is the combined psychological and physiological effect. When the term *stress* or *strain* occurs without qualification, then, think of this combined psychological and physiological arousal.

DISTINGUISHING STRESS FROM OTHER EMOTIVE STATES

Several related terms appear frequently in discussions of stress, sometimes almost as though they are interchangeable. These include **anxiety, conflict, frustration,** and **hassles.** Some clarification of their usage in stress literature may be helpful.

Anxiety

Anxiety generally refers to "a specific, unpleasurable state of tension which indicates the presence of some danger to the organism" (Budzynski & Peffer, 1980, p. 413). The most serious anxiety reactions are panic attacks. These attacks involve a "sudden onset of intense apprehension, fear, or terror. Often there is a feeling of impending doom" (American Psychiatric Association, 1987, p. 236).

Anxiety differs from fear in that anxiety is a general state of apprehension, and fear has a specific object. A person is afraid of spiders or snakes or heights, for example. Anxiety, on the other hand, does not seem related to anything in particular, at least, not that the person can point to directly.

Distinguishing anxiety from stress, though, is nearly impossible. In one entire volume devoted to the topic, the authors never distinguish between stress and anxiety (Kutash, Schlesinger, & Associates, 1980). Thus, stress and anxiety can both refer to the subjective psychological result of environmental pressure.

Conflict

Competition between two goals results in conflict. The fact that conflict can produce ulcers in rats (Sawrey & Weiss, 1956) is another indicator that negative emotion has the potential to harmfully influence health. There are three types of conflict (Lewin, 1948; Miller, 1944). **Approach-approach conflicts** occur when two equally desirable goals compete and only one goal can be obtained. For example, a high school graduate applies to two equally attractive universities. Upon admission to both, she may go through some degree of conflict before making a decision. Choosing whether to buy a new car or a new boat also may entail conflict when only one can be purchased.

Avoidance-avoidance conflicts occur when two goals have equally unattractive values. The choice of having to either rake the leaves or wash all the windows in the house illustrates this type of conflict. Deciding whether to study for an important exam or go to the library and work on a term paper that is due could also raise this type of conflict.

Approach-avoidance conflicts exist when the same goal has both positive and negative features. Marriage provides permanence and stability in one's primary intimate relationship, a sense of teamwork and sharing, and the prospect of family. It also may contain negatives such as the perception of loss of freedom and independence, overwhelming responsibility, and an uncertain yet seemingly irreversible commitment to one person. Most of life's day-to-day pressures are probably of an approach-avoidance variety.

Frustration

When some barrier comes between a person and the attainment of a goal, frustration occurs. The student who works hard to get into medical school may be frustrated by earning poor grades on the entrance exams. Someone who wants to begin a small business but cannot save enough money to get started experiences frustration. Similarly, the person who wants to impress a boss or a potential lover but finds someone else constantly interfering will likely feel frustration.

One possible, though not inevitable, outcome of frustration is aggression. Berkowitz (1990) provided evidence that a primary negative emotion, such as frustration, works through a sequence of body-arousal and cognitive attributions to increase the likelihood of aggression. The person wanting to start the business may decide to steal the money. The person thwarted in an attempt to impress the boss or lover may become verbally or physically aggressive toward the person who interferes.

Hamilton (1979) believed that anxiety "is the major and most fundamental source of strain in the person" (p. 86). He also suggested that "the greater the load from these sources [conflict, frustration, and anxiety], the greater the number and the severity of the stressors and the farther the movement towards a limit of 'stress' tolerance" (p. 80).

Hassles

Recently, Richard Lazarus suggested we should substitute the term *hassles* for the frequently used and oft-abused *stress*. In everyday conversation, *hassles* conveys the sense that pressures are piling up ("I don't need this hassle") or that someone is pressing too hard ("Don't hasle me"). More formally, hassles are "the irritating, frustrating, *distressing* demands that in some degree characterize everyday transactions with the environment [italics added]" (Kanner, Coyne, Schaefer, & Lazarus, 1981, p. 3). Parallel to Selye's eustress, there are also *uplifts,* positive experiences such as loving relationships, finishing a job, and being healthy.

Hassles are less intense than catastrophic types of stress, but they are persistent, nagging thorns in the flesh. The types of events used to illustrate hassles come from everyday life. They include losing the car keys, bills piling up with no end in sight, constant interruptions, not enough time for leisure, and the shoelace that breaks when you're in a hurry. In comparing hassles with life changes such as divorce or death of a spouse, Lazarus and his colleagues showed that hassles and illness are more strongly related than life changes and illness. This finding has been confirmed cross-culturally as well (Nakano, 1989).

IN SICKNESS AND IN HEALTH: HEALTH STATUS AND SOCIAL ROLES

A major concern today is the nature of the relationship between stress and health. To consider this connection, we must ask some basic questions. What does it mean to be sick or diseased? When one displays illness behavior, is that the same as sickness? Is health the opposite of being sick? How do health behaviors relate to being healthy? These terms—disease, health, illness behavior, and health behavior—are discussed briefly in this section.

Disease and Sickness

Disease refers to a physical condition that results from a body malfunction. It may be due to a breakdown in a body organ or a malfunction in one of the body's systems. Disease is most often explained by the germ model; that is, a toxic microorganism invades the body, causing alterations in body tissue leading to observable symptoms of distress. Sickness and illness are equivalent terms that refer to a state of suffering from a disease.

Illness Behavior

Symptoms are the first visible signs of disease. When they appear, you probably run through an internal check that evaluates and attaches meaning to the symptoms. In the process, you form a plan of action that may involve family members and a trip to the doctor's office.

Upon reaching the clinic, you complain about your discomfort and describe your symptoms. You seek medical remedies and signs of support from medical staff, family, and friends. This process—evaluating symptoms, seeking medical help to bring relief, and seeking support from family—is the core of **illness behavior** (Mechanic, 1966).

Illness behavior can occur with or without physical indicators of disease. It is appropriate when a medical diagnosis or obvious symptoms (such as vomiting) occur. It is deviant, or at least frowned on, when it occurs in the absence of a diagnosed illness. Thus, *disease* refers to a physical condition of the body, while *illness behavior* defines a social role with expectations for both the sick and the healer (Parsons, 1951).

An important characteristic of illness behavior is that it often brings **secondary gains,** rewards or benefits obtained through the sick role. These gains include increased sympathy and attention, special favors such as being waited on, and release from duty such as school or work.

When conducting research on stress and health, we must not confuse the social role of illness behavior (including unverified reports of sickness) with physical disease. This could lead to the erroneous conclusion that stress causes disease, when it may only increase people's tendency to engage in illness behavior.

Health: The Opposite of Sickness?

We could define **health** as the absence of disease. Most people, though, would easily recognize the weakness in this definition. One can be free of disease but still not enjoy a full, wholesome, satisfying life. Health entails quality valuations of physical and mental vigor. The World Health Organization defined health as "a state of complete physical, mental, and social well-being and not merely the absence of disease or infirmity" (cited in Seeman, 1989, p. 1100). On the physical side, it means that the person enjoys a robust life with the energy needed to engage in satisfying pursuits and explorations of the environment. Simultaneously, the healthy person enjoys emotional fulfillment and self-esteem, both signs of positive mental health. Finally, social well-being is shown by the formation of close personal relationships.

Health Behavior

Kasl and Cobb (1966) defined **health behavior** as activity undertaken, by a person who believes himself or herself to be healthy, for the purpose of preventing disease. It is estimated that 50% of premature deaths are a result of lifestyle risks and that lifestyle contributes 54% of the variability to cardiovascular disease (Institute of Medicine, 1979; Wilson, 1989). Health behavior may include reducing or eliminating high-risk behaviors such as smoking or poor diet. The person also may adopt positive behaviors such as regular exercise. Finally, health behavior may involve adhering to a distasteful though necessary medical regimen.

BUILDING THEORIES: THE EXPLANATORY STORIES OF SCIENCE

Many theories have been developed to explain what stress is, how it works, and how it relates to health. Though the term *theory* sounds very formal, theories are really the explanatory stories of science. Theories summarize a body of data. They provide an organized, coherent picture of some part of nature or some aspect of human behavior. When a theory can generate new, testable hypotheses that fill more gaps in our knowledge, the theory is powerful. Theories are never fully verified; some leap of inference is always made between the theory and the data that support it. Finally, theories are never complete. They evolve and change as new data accumulate and new techniques allow more sophisticated tests of relevant hypotheses.

Some theories, such as Selye's physiological theory, attempt to explain the way the body responds to stress. Psychological theories attempt to understand the way in which personality, expectations, and interpretations turn a personal or social event into a situation of stress. They try to build plausible explanations of the way behavior changes because of stress. Further, psychological theories try to explain how coping behaviors may reduce the impact or prevent the reappearance of stress. Social theories provide explanations of stress based more on group conflict and the unequal distribution of power and wealth. Holistic health theories espouse a set of social and personal values based on the idea that body and mind must be treated in unified fashion. Finally, systems theory attempts to explain how organisms engage in self-regulation even when embedded in more complex self-regulating systems.

Table 1-1 has been prepared to aid the reader in the rest of the chapter. This table summarizes the key features, plus strengths and weaknesses, of the major theories. It may be helpful to refer to the table periodically while reading.

VARIETIES OF BIOLOGICAL STRESS THEORIES

While many biological theories of stress exist, only two such theories will be discussed here. The first is Hans Selye's (1974, 1979) **General Adaptation Syndrome;** the second is genetic-constitutional theory.

The General Adaptation Syndrome

Selye's theory may be summarized in four general statements:

1. All biological organisms have an innate drive to maintain a state of internal balance, or equilibrium. The process that maintains an internal balance is homeostasis. As it turns out, maintaining homeostasis is a lifelong task.
2. Stressors, such as germs or excessive work demands, disturb internal equilibrium. The body responds to any stressor, whether pleasant or unpleasant, with a nonspecific physiological arousal. This reaction is defensive and self-protective.
3. Adjustment to stress occurs in stages. The time course and progress through the stages depends on how successful the resistance is in relation to the intensity and duration of the stressor.

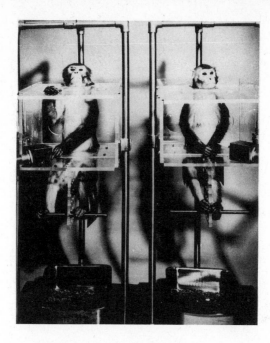

Executive monkeys with responsibility to press a lever to avoid shock for themselves and their yoked-control partners
SOURCE: Used with permission of Walter Reed Army Institute of Research (WRAIR), Washington, D.C. (1955).

4. The organism has a finite reserve of adaptive energy. When depleted, the organism lacks the ability to cope with continued stress, and death may follow.

The pioneer research program that led to this theory was already under way in the 1950s and 1960s. Selye (1956) observed laboratory animals subjected to stressors such as those encountered in learning a difficult task. The animals reacted with signs of physical stress, up to and including acute traumatic ulcers of the stomach and subsequent death.

Many studies supported Selye's conclusions, but one study will be discussed in detail—the classic executive monkey study (Brady, Porter, Conrad, & Mason, 1958). This study illustrates some of the complexities of designing research to provide unequivocal answers to important questions. It will show, further, how other explanations may be proposed and tested.

In the Brady study, four pairs of monkeys learned how to press a lever to avoid a punishing shock. Each monkey in the pair faced a completely different situation. The executive monkey could engage in an avoidance response that would prevent the punishment from being delivered to both himself and his yoked-control partner, who could do nothing to avoid the shocks. The partner's safety and comfort depended solely on the alertness and decision process of the executive monkey.

TABLE 1-1
Comparison of Key Features of Stress Models

Stress model	Definition of stress	Source(s) of stress	Model's strengtbs	Model's weaknesses
General Adaptation Syndrome	Nonspecific demand on body—disturbs body equilibrium	Various environmental pressures—chronic—depletes energy reserves	Empirically derived and extensively tested	Extreme biological emphasis Treats good and bad stressors the same way Ignores cognitive-social factors in stress
Diathesis-stress model	No specific definition provided	Mismatch between biological endowment and environmental stressors	Interaction model Gives equal weight to internal and external factors	Indirect evidence rather than direct tests Difficult to give terms operational reference
Psychodynamic theory	Defined primarily by reference to anxiety	Signals of danger and intrapsychic conflict	Uses few constructs with great power Intuitive appeal	Inadequate in scope Little or no consideration of biological or social factors Difficult to test
Learning theory	Faulty conditioning causing conditional emotional responses	Presence of any conditional stimuli and/or reinforcing stimuli	Empirically derived Clear operational definitions for basic terms and procedures Attempted explanation of related coping actions	Scope is limited Largely ignores any biological factors Limited use of social-context factors Ignores or denies importance of cognitive process

Transactional theory	Relationship between demand and coping sources	Real or perceived psychosocial pressures	Compatible with both the biological and social models	Criticized for its circularity
			Large and growing body of supporting evidence	Some constructs not well-defined
				Does not explicitly suggest how the mind influences body process
Social stress theory	Pressures to conform or adapt to social systems/norms	Social conflict and coercion	Incorporates many plausible social factors related to stress	Very broad and ill-defined
		Social change and living conditions		Difficult to give terms operational reference
		Lack of access to resources		Ignores biological variables
				Ignores individual differences
Control theory	Disturbance between reference (normal) value and comparator value in feedback loop	Any data that produce disequilibrium in the system	Has potential to include all the different systems that influence stress reactions	Difficult to operationalize and test
Holistic health theory	No specific definition provided	Implies that stress results from failure to treat the person as a functional whole	Scope is global	Not a formal theory
			Tacit acceptance of interaction between biological, psychological, and social factors	Lacking in formal operational definitions
				Lacking in specific supporting research

The outcome of this story has been widely publicized. The four executive monkeys charged with the responsibility to act developed ulcers and died. The four monkeys with no responsibility suffered no ill effects. It seemed that the demands of work, the responsibility placed on the *executives,* produced the stress and, ultimately, death.[5]

A major flaw in the procedure, however, was not as widely publicized. That flaw had to do with a simple principle of experimental design: the monkeys were not randomly assigned to be executives or controls. Instead, when the monkeys first received shocks, the first member of the pair to respond became the executive, and the other one became the yoked-control member. It is possible that the monkeys who responded first were more emotional or hyperreactive. This, in turn, suggests that physiological differences existed between the pairs, such as increased autonomic reactivity and gastric motility. If so, the executive monkeys would be more susceptible to ulcers because of preexisting differences in temperament and constitution. This biological explanation would be as acceptable under the circumstances as the responsibility explanation.

The responsibility explanation became even less acceptable when subsequent studies did not replicate Brady's findings (Weiss, 1968, 1971). Indeed, most subsequent findings are in direct opposition to Brady's. That is, helpless animals generally develop more ulcers than controlling animals (Wiener, 1961). Control theory suggests that organisms generally fare better under threat when they have some response available that will be instrumental in dealing with the threat. What might account for this discrepancy?

One possible explanation concerns the type of control the executives had. In the Brady study, the executives lacked feedback about success. Fisher (1988) argued that such control is more stressful and may have contributed to the outcome of this study. This brief excursion into a classic study should alert the reader to the importance of sound research design. It should also encourage an attitude of healthy skepticism and critical analysis of the details and published interpretations of research.

Selye's research program led him to propose the existence of a three-stage process called the General Adaptation Syndrome, or GAS (Figure 1-2). The syndrome can be summarized as follows.

1. **Alarm Reaction.** The alarm reaction occurs at the first appearance of a stressor. For a short period, the body has a lower than normal level of resistance. Short-term increases in gastrointestinal disturbances and elevated blood pressure may result. Then the body quickly marshals defensive resources and makes self-protective adjustments. If the defensive reactions are successful, the alarm subsides and the body returns to normal activity. Most short-term stresses are resolved in this phase. Such short-term stress may be called an *acute* stress reaction.

2. Stage of **Resistance.** If stress continues because of factors outside the organism's control or because the first reaction did not remove the emergency,

---

[5]Investigators attempting to follow up on Brady's executive monkey study made an interesting discovery. They found that it was while off duty—in other words, the vacation time, that the ulcers developed in the executive monkeys, not during the working time.

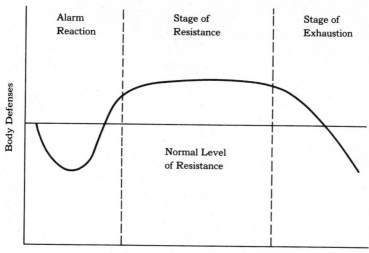

FIGURE 1-2
Reaction to stress varies with duration of the stressor
SOURCE: Selye (1956).

the body will call for full-scale mobilization. The problem is that the body has to expend many resources to win this war, which generally results in decreased resistance over time. In addition, more serious physical symptoms, such as ulcers or atherosclerosis, may develop. These physical symptoms may reduce resistance even more.

3. Stage of **Exhaustion.** If the stressor is unusually severe or drawn out, the body further depletes or exhausts its reserves of energy. Resistance breaks down altogether, and death may follow shortly thereafter (Selye, 1980).

Influential as Selye's theory has been, its narrowness is not compatible with current views of stress. One major weakness is that it does not encompass the psychosocial factors of critical importance to understanding human stress. It does not address the cognitive processes that influence when demand becomes challenge or when demand becomes threat. Further, it does not consider the selection of strategies to combat stress or the effectiveness of coping strategies.

Genetic-Constitutional Theories

The ability to resist stress depends on the coping strategies applied in the face of a current emergency. In addition, several factors related to individual genetic history, called **predisposing factors,** affect resistance. They influence resistance through preset organ weaknesses, by increasing risk for diseases, or by setting response sensitivities (irritability). Predisposing factors may be likened to threshold or tolerance factors.

Genetic-constitutional research attempts to establish a link between genetic makeup (genotype) and some physical characteristic (phenotype) that lowers the person's general ability to resist stress. Genetic factors may reduce resistance in several ways. Genetic makeup influences balance in the autonomic nervous system, the fight-or-flight emergency reaction system. General temperament is also genetically determined in part. **Temperament,** a very broad term, refers to three differences in initial response patterns. First, activity levels vary on a continuum from active to passive. Second, emotional responses range from pleasant to unpleasant. Finally, reactivity to stimuli varies from hypersensitive to hyposensitive (Fuller & Thompson, 1978).

Genes also control the codes for the structure and function of organs and body systems. Of most importance to stress resistance are the kidneys, the cardiovascular system (risks for coronary, high blood pressure, arteriosclerosis), the digestive system (risks for stomach and duodenal ulcers), and the nervous system (imbalance in autonomic system).

THE DIATHESIS-STRESS MODEL

For decades, scientists have debated the relative contribution of inheritance and environment (nature and nurture) to personality and intelligence. While the debate is far from over, one thing seems clear. We do not have to choose between two competing processes. Instead, heredity and environment are complementary processes that interact to influence biological structures and functions. The **diathesis-stress model** integrates hereditary and environmental forces in just this way.

This theory suggests there is an interplay between predisposing and **precipitating factors.** The person's genetic map contributes predisposing factors, as discussed in the preceding section. A lower threshold for stress or an organic weakness makes the person vulnerable to illness. Whether that weakness ever shows up or not depends on the amount of stress, the precipitating force, the person experiences. In a somewhat sheltered and *stressless* environment, even a very vulnerable person might never show signs of the strain. Conversely, a person under severe, continuous strain might respond poorly even though genetic predispositions are strong. Parsons also suggests that evolutionary change continues to work in selecting for behaviors that enable organisms to adapt to stressful environments (Parsons, 1988).

VARIETIES OF PSYCHOLOGICAL STRESS THEORIES

Major psychological theories include the psychodynamic, learning, cognitive, and general systems models. There are several cognitive models, but Richard Lazarus and his associates proposed the most influencial model (Lazarus & Launier, 1978). One extension of the cognitive approach is the **conservation-of-resources** model proposed by Steven Hobfoll (1989). Finally, Carver and Scheier (1981, 1982) and Gary Schwartz (1982, 1983) constructed general systems models, generally called control theories.

The Psychodynamic Model

Sigmund Freud's theory is undoubtedly the accepted standard among psychodynamic models. Freud described two kinds of anxiety in his revised theory. **Signal anxiety** occurs when an objective external danger is present. It corresponds most closely to the stressor-strain (danger-anxiety) relationship. The second, **traumatic anxiety,** was the dominant form of anxiety in Freud's theory. It refers to instinctual, or internally generated, anxiety. Examples include anxiety aroused when coping with repressed sexual drives and aggressive instincts. Anxiety puts a strain on psychic functioning. The resulting symptoms are the "psychopathologies of everyday life," to use Freud's (1966) term. The notion of **conversion** was also important. Conversion is a process that turns a conflicting idea into something harmless. Essentially, the energy from the conflict is converted into a physical symptom.

The Learning Theory View

As an explanation of stress, learning theory generally uses either the **classical conditioning** model, the operant model, or a combination of the two. Russian Nobel laureate Ivan Pavlov pioneered development of the classical conditioning model. The American behaviorist B. F. Skinner developed the **operant conditioning** model.

To illustrate classical conditioning, consider the famous (or infamous) experiment conducted by the father of behavioral psychology, John Watson. Watson (1920) showed 11-month-old Albert a pet rat. Initially, Albert displayed no fear of the animal. Later, Watson arranged that Albert saw the rat immediately followed by a loud noise. Predictably, Albert responded with fear to the loud sound. After just seven repetitions, Albert was afraid of the rat even when no loud sound was present. Fear was also present with a variety of other objects similar to the rat—a rabbit, a sealskin coat, and a Santa's mask (Watson & Rayner, 1920). Figure 1-3 illustrates this conditioning process.

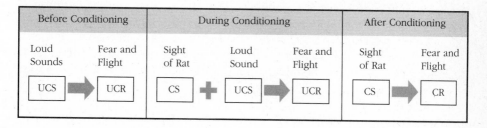

FIGURE 1-3
Classically conditioned fear illustrated with the case of Albert

In classical conditioning, loud noise is one of a general class of stimuli called **unconditional stimuli** (UCS).[6] These are biologically powerful unlearned signals related to survival needs of the organism. When an unconditional stimulus occurs, it evokes an unlearned reflex, or **unconditional response** (UCR). The rat was one of another class of signals called **conditional stimuli** (CS). Before any experience, conditional stimuli may be regarded as novel or neutral stimuli. To have any power, they first must be associated with powerful unconditional stimuli. When a conditional stimulus brings about the response previously produced only by the UCS, it is now a learned reflex or **conditional response** (CR).

Two aspects of the conditioning process are important for stress theory. First, emotional responses, such as fear and anxiety, are complex and include (1) behavioral, (2) psychological, and (3) physiological components. Escape and/or avoidance behaviors keep a person as far away as possible from stressful stimuli. Subjectively, the person experiences a state of internal tension when confronting a feared object or event. The body becomes physiologically aroused, as reflected by increased blood pressure, heart rate, and body temperature. When conditioning occurs, as in Albert's case, all three components are conditioned to the CS (the rat). Later, even very low levels of the stimulus (a picture of a rat) can result in subjective tension and physiological arousal, although the person may not show it outwardly.

Second, anxiety may become anticipatory after the original conditioning has occurred. Anxiety can be aroused just by talking or thinking about the feared stimulus, even when there is no immediate pressure to confront it. Imagine someone afraid of snakes. A friend reports watching an interesting documentary on reptiles. With the mention of snakes, the person may visibly tense, shudder, and redirect the conversation to another topic. If the person cannot control the anxiety while confronting a frightening situation, the anxiety has the potential to be disabling, keeping the individual from enjoying normal pleasures.

Operant theory proposes that behavior changes because it produces either good or bad outcomes. When a behavior produces pleasant outcomes, or rewards, the behavior increases. When a behavior produces unpleasant outcomes, or punishment, the behavior decreases. Explanations of stress from an operant perspective place most emphasis on the acquisition of avoidance behavior and the discriminative control of symptomatic behavior.

Avoidance behavior is an operant response that serves to reduce learned fear or anxiety. For Albert, associating the rat with the loud noise conditioned a fear response to the rat. Fear is an unpleasant emotion that increases internal tension. People generally try to reduce or remove unpleasant tension. Because running away from the rat reduces tension, running away is strengthened. If the rat appears again, the most likely response is flight. In general, any stressful

---

[6]I am departing from the American convention of using "conditioned" in the four basic terms. This was an unfortunate error made in translating from Pavlov's Russian texts into English. It is more accurate to say "conditional," and the meaning is clear: "conditional" means "dependent upon," and "unconditional" means "not dependent upon." Thus, the UCS does not depend on anything for its power while the CS depends on prior associations with the UCS for power.

situation that produces high or unmanageable levels of anxiety is likely to motivate some form of escape or avoidance.

THE COGNITIVE TRANSACTIONAL MODEL OF STRESS

People perceive and label events, store information about their experiences, and retrieve and use that information in different ways. How this influences new encounters is important to the arousal of stress and to the coping strategies employed to deal with stress. Cognitive researchers attempt to understand stress mechanisms in terms of the way in which the brain processes information through its many pathways and way stations.

Cognitive theorists assume that humans are active, reasoning, and deciding beings. They also assume that people construct **schemata,** or mental blueprints. Schemata[7] represent things learned about the world, how it works, and how to relate to it. Certain schemata may be almost universal, such as the schema for gravity. Others always show a high degree of personal uniqueness, such as a schema for teacher/student relationships.

Several cognitive transactional theories have appeared over the years. The most prominent is the model developed by Richard S. Lazarus (Lazarus & Launier, 1978). This theory is outlined here but developed more fully in Chapter 3. As explained by Lazarus, the theory has roots in several scientific soils. These include the cognitive sciences, personality theory, attitude research, social research, health research, and behavioral medicine. Lazarus assumes that stress and health have reciprocal influences. That is, stress can have a powerful impact on health, and conversely, health can change the person's resistance or coping ability.

The central point of the transactional model is that stress is "neither an environmental stimulus, a characteristic of the person, nor a response but a relationship between demands and the power to deal with them without unreasonable or destructive costs" (Coyne & Holroyd, 1982, p. 108). It is apparent that a *relational* analysis is the key to this theory. There are some important implications to be drawn from this.

First, the same environmental event may be interpreted as stressful by one person but not stressful by someone else. This suggests that most external stimuli cannot be defined in any absolute sense as stressful. Instead, it is a personal cognitive appraisal that makes the event stressful or not stressful. Second, the same person may interpret an event as stressful on one occasion but not on another. This may be due to changes in physical condition or changes in psychological states. The person might be physically relaxed and rested on one occasion but tense and tired on another. Emotional and motivational states differ across time, which can also affect the appraisal process.

---

[7]*Schemata* is plural, while *schema* is singular.

CRITIQUE OF TRANSACTIONAL
THEORY AND AN ALTERNATIVE

Although the cognitive-transactional theory continues to evolve and mature, it has encountered numerous criticisms. Stevan Hobfoll (1989) argued that the model is "tautological, overly complex, and not given to rejection" (p. 515). He says that it is tautological because demand and coping capacity are not defined separately. Whether an event is demanding or not depends on coping capacity, and whether coping capacity is adequate is dependent on demand. This situation results, according to Hobfoll, from the excessive emphasis on perception. Because of this, demand and coping can only be inferred after the fact. Refuting the theory is difficult also because both positive and negative instances of coping can be taken as consistent with the model.

In place of the transactional model, Hobfoll argued for a conservation of resources model of stress. According to Hobfoll, people possess resources they value and wish to protect or conserve. These include object resources (a home or business), condition resources (seniority, power, marriage), personal characteristics (self-efficacy and self-esteem), and energies (time, money, and knowledge). Psychological stress occurs when there is a real or perceived net loss of resources or when there is lack of gain after investment of resources.

In this theory, loss plays a central role. Many changes can occur in one's life—changing jobs, buying a new house, ending an intimate personal relationship. These transitions are not stressful in and of themselves. They only become stressful when they entail loss—the change in job means loss of status, power, and income; the mortgage is unmanageable and threatens economic ruin; lost love threatens loss of self-esteem.

According to Hobfoll, people use various means to offset loss. The most direct method is through replacement. A person may leave the company to find a job that preserves status and income. The luxury house can be replaced by one with a manageable mortgage. The jilted person finds a new love.

Another way to offset loss is to reappraise the situation and shift attention. People might focus on what they can gain from job change—reduced responsibility, less pressure, more time with the family. The lost love may be devalued, and blessings may be counted for the end of a relationship that could only bring continued unhappiness.

Although Hobfoll criticized weaknesses of the transactional model, he used similar cognitive concepts. What is the difference, then? Hobfoll argued that existing theories use fuzzy concepts with no normative standard for testing. In addition, some theories emphasize outcomes, while others emphasize process. He believes there must be concrete markers in process. In addition, outcome must be related to process without suffering from either circularity or shifting definitions. Hobfoll tried to suggest one quantifiable marker—loss—that may make stress theories more testable. Still, there does not appear to be a significant difference in the precision, or quantifiability, of loss as opposed to Lazarus's concept of harm (R. S. Lazarus, personal communication, August 13, 1991). While it is important to keep in mind potential weaknesses in a theory, we cannot and should not quickly abandon a strong and well-researched theory on the basis of speculation alone.

VARIETIES OF SOCIAL STRESS THEORIES

Several **social stress theories** focus on integration of the individual into society and tensions that are part of any society. These are **conflict theories.** A major source of tension is that society has to engage in some degree of coercion to get members to comply with social norms. One conflict theorist believes that a crucial problem is affording members of society more life chances or opportunities for growth (Dahrendorf, 1979). Stress occurs when people cannot obtain work, homes, education or technical retraining, or participate in the political process. Conflict theories also look at the stability of social relationships, the distribution of economic goods and services in society (Dooley & Catalano, 1984), and the distribution of interpersonal power and personal control. These conflict variables are related to stress in fairly obvious ways. Theoretically, stress is the inevitable outcome of less stable social relationships, poverty and lack of access to necessary social services, and low power and personal control.

Evolutionary theory views social change and tension as the inevitable result of social development. People must accept the fact of social change and accommodate to it instead of fighting against it. Environmental-ecological theory explains stress in terms of conditions such as crowding, pollution, health hazards from industrialization, and environmental accidents. Finally, **life-change theory** explains stress by reference to life changes that require major adaptations by the person. Death of a spouse, bankruptcy, loss of a job, or life-threatening illness fit the definition of major events that require substantial personal adjustment.

THE HOLISTIC HEALTH MODEL

Holistic theory has many faces. It is a movement with political and economic overtones. It is a pseudoreligion of lifestyle and self-sufficiency practiced with evangelistic zeal by a group of true believers (Alster, 1989). It is a humanistic philosophy with antiscientific sentiments. Finally, it is a reaction to biological reductionism and medical specialization in Western medicine.

In the health arena, holistic theory suggests that it has a new paradigm of health care to offer (Capra, 1982). The intensity with which its values are expressed conveys the impression of a counterculture with anti–medical establishment themes. This is most evident when it suggests that Western medicine is dehumanizing and devalues the role of mental processes in health and healing. Still, holistic health presents itself as a synthesizing movement trying to regain a sense of humane medical treatment and respect for the whole person (Sobel, 1979). Treatment of the whole person is a valued medical tradition that has existed without interruption since ancient times, most visibly in Eastern medical tradition.

According to Burstein and Loucks (1982), there are three trademarks of the holistic health movement. These are "(1) a recognition of human complexity and diversity, (2) an emphasis on the importance of mental events and personal value systems, and (3) a recognition of the desirability of responsibility for oneself" (p. 179). Girdano and Everly (1979) stated that *holistic* is "the concept underlying an approach to controlling stress and tension that deals with the complete lifestyle of the individual, incorporating intervention at several levels—physical, psychological, and social—simultaneously" (p. 20).

While there is research to support the holistic model, it does not generate research itself. Further, it does not have the formal properties of a scientific theory. Alster (1989) is blunt when she suggests that holistic health is a movement without a theoretical framework. She concludes also that the movement has not defined its basic terms and relies on slogans for its support.

CONTROL THEORY: A SYSTEMS MODEL OF STRESS

Each of the preceding theories tried to explain stress and health by focusing on a limited though promising set of variables. Selye focused on the physiological response system but left out social and psychological detail. Learning theory used narrow conditioning constructs with little concern for physiological processes and slight attention to social systems. Cognitive theory emphasized the information processing system, a system that must deal with data from the external social environment as well as from the internal biopsychological environment. Still, cognitive theory gives little detail on physical parameters of stress and health, and it does not explicitly entertain social constructs. Social theory focused almost exclusively on large-scale factors such as poverty, crowding, and rate of social change. Each view has its unique strengths but also its inherent weaknesses.

An alternative to these theories is systems theory. Systems theory is an outgrowth of the attempt to understand self-regulating systems. The origins of systems theory usually are traced to Norbert Wiener's (1961) classic work on **cybernetics.** Cybernetic concepts usually depend on feedback mechanisms and goal-seeking behavior in more or less self-contained units. General systems theory (GST) considers complex, dynamic interactions in multivariate systems, where systems may be hierarchically enmeshed with other systems (von Bertalanffy, 1968). Cybernetic theory, then, is a subset of general systems theory (Schwartz, 1982).

Cybernetics, also called "control theory," suggests that self-regulating organisms compare their current state to some reference to maintain a match. An often-used example is the thermostat. An organism obtains information about current conditions (room temperature) through sensory input (thermometer). If the comparator detects a discrepancy between the current state (68°) and the reference (70°), the organism engages in some act to reduce the discrepancy (switches the furnace on). This will continue until new information provided to the comparator shows a match with the reference standard. The loop is

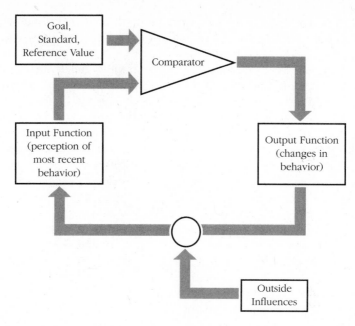

FIGURE 1-4
A simple systems model for feedback of a disturbance from the environment
SOURCE: Carver & Scheier (1982).

called a *negative feedback loop* because it attempts to negate the difference between current and reference conditions. An elementary feedback loop is shown in Figure 1-4.

Probably the most widely known cybernetic system is homeostatic control. With reference to stress, external stressors are disturbances that carry information to the system. When a disturbance produces a discrepancy (extreme tension) from the reference (ideal or moderate tension), the system will engage in self-regulating behavior to restore the ideal state. These are coping actions to reduce or eliminate the source of stress. A more subtle negative feedback loop is found in the regulatory mechanisms of the immune system (Dantzer & Kelley, 1989).

Feedback processes are reactive. Human organisms also engage in feed forward, or proactive self-regulation (Ford, 1990). That is, they act to make good things happen as well as to prevent bad things from happening. This is especially important in reducing existing stress or preventing potential stressors. It is also important in maintaining positive health and preventing ill-health.

Charles Carver and Michael Scheier (1981, 1982) applied control theory to health psychology, a discipline concerned with the ways in which behavior can influence health for better or for worse. Carver and Scheier view the person as a self-contained health-care system that engages in behavior to reduce discrepancies in feedback loops. They suggested that good health is a high-order reference value used to regulate behavior. Good health, though, is related to many different body systems, each with their own low-order reference values. Symptoms are low-order bits of information that tell us something is wrong in a body system.

For example, we monitor a variety of body signals, such as weight, temperature, and blood pressure. If weight becomes undesirably high, we diet and/or exercise to reduce weight. We know that a high temperature may be symptomatic of a cold or flu attack. When this happens, we take appropriate countersteps, such as taking aspirin, fluids, and bed rest. We seek professional help when body signals are weak, such as blood pressure and hypertension, the silent illness. Then we take prescribed medications to reduce symptoms. All these behaviors are control processes that seek to match a current state (presence of body symptoms) with a reference value (normality in the body system) and ultimately with the value of good health.

Gary Schwartz (1982, 1983) and Julius Seeman (1989) argue for a general systems approach in the discipline of behavior medicine. Schwartz's model is called the "biopsychosocial model," even though it has its roots in general systems theory.[8] This is a multicausal and multieffect model of health and illness. It proposes that medical diagnosis should consider the matrix of biological, psychological, and social factors represented in the patient's history and current condition. Further, it suggests that treatment must consider the treatment's interaction with other treatments as well as with the psychosocial system of the patient.

To accomplish this, the biopsychosocial model uses a Patient Evaluation Grid (PEG), as shown in Figure 1-5. From this grid, we can see various ways that stress may influence the course of health, illness, and treatment. The biological axis uses factors such as predispositions, body changes (which may be stress-influenced), and current symptoms. The personal axis considers many cognitive, attitudinal, personality, and adaptive characteristics. The environmental axis contains numerous support systems, life changes, and family and job networks, as well as expectations related to social roles.

Whether we consider any given stress response to have a health consequence or not, this matrix points out that stress is embedded in a multivariate system. Stress also has the potential for multiple effects in systems that range from the function of the body, to the function of psychological processes, to the harmony of home and job. It remains to be seen whether this model will be able to generate data to support it, or whether it will function more as a metatheory, which integrates the results of smaller but more testable theories.

MAKING SENSE OF THE CONFUSION

After reading this assortment of stress and health theories, the reader may feel more confused than enlightened. What is one to think when science can't make up its mind? As a first step, we can borrow the classic parable from Eastern

---

[8]Schwartz appropriately credits Engel (1977) with the first application of GST to medicine.

Dimensions	Contexts		
	Current (current states)	Recent (recent events and changes)	Background (culture, traits, constitution)
Biological	Symptoms Physical examination Vital signs Status of related organs Medications Disease	Age Recent bodily changes Injuries, operations Disease Drugs	Heredity Early nutrition Constitution Predisposition Early disease
Personal	Chief complaint Mental status Expectations about illness and treatment	Recent illness, occurrence of symptoms Personality change Mood, thinking, behavior Adaptation, defense	Developmental factors Early experience Personality type Attitude to illness
Environmental	Immediate physical and interpersonal environment Supportive figure, next of kin Effect of help-seeking	Recent physical and interpersonal environment Life changes Family, work, others Contact with ill persons Contact with doctor or hospital	Early physical environment Cultural and family environment Early relations Cultural sick role expectation

FIGURE 1-5

A patient evaluation grid (PEG) showing the matrix of biological, psychological, and social factors that contribute to illness
SOURCE: Leigh and Reiser (1980).

literature of the dermis probe. Three blind men felt an elephant and each gave their impressions. Each had a different image of reality derived from examining the small area they could reach. If they could combine their solitary sources of information, they might end up with a more complete picture of the elephant.

The science of stress is somewhat like the dermis probe. Many different disciplines are engaged in stress research, each with a slightly different perspective. These different contributions, then, reflect contact with different domains of stress. No one theory has provided a complete picture. Still, each provides important pieces of information that help round out the picture.

As a second step, we should consider the issue of compatibility and compensation. To borrow an analogy from marital relations, strong relations usually come from being compatible. Couples may be strong because they have similar (redundant) competencies and values, or they may be strong because one partner's strengths compensates for the other's weaknesses. The cognitive model of stress and the biological model of stress are compatible in a nonredundant sense. They may turn out to be good partners because each compensates for the other's oversights. Current work shows subtle connections between the cognitive system and body responses that supports this view.

Finally, where does the systems view fit in this scheme? There is nothing inherently incompatible or competitive between the biological model, the cognitive model, and the systems model. The biological subsystem has a job to do in keeping a physical balance, but it interacts with the cognitive system. The cognitive system is the primary self-referent control system that monitors signals and processes information from the biological subsystem and from family, job, and social systems. It works to preserve a psychological balance. Finally, the family system is enmeshed in the larger social system. Each has its job to do in regulating functions within their respective spheres. Each tries to maintain a steady state or balance within its domain. Instead of viewing these theories as competitive, then, we should view them as complementary and compensatory. In this book, I refer to the cognitive system as the self-referent control system that integrates information and orchestrates responses between external social systems and internal physiological systems.

SUMMARY

This chapter has provided working definitions for basic terms used throughout the book. The external source or cause of stress was defined as the *stressor.* The internal tension, be it psychological tension (such as anxiety) or a physical defense reaction, was defined as *stress* or *strain.*

Several theories commonly encountered in stress and health research were reviewed. This review has been selective and brief rather than exhaustive and intensive. It is intended to provide a context and reference point for materials to be presented in subsequent chapters.

KEY TERMS

alarm reaction
anxiety
approach-approach
  conflict
approach-avoidance
  conflict
avoidance-avoidance
  conflict
classical conditioning
conditional response
conditional stimulus
conflict
conflict theory
conservation of
  resources
conversion
cybernetics

diathesis-stress model
distress
eustress
exhaustion
frustration
General Adaptation
  Syndrome
hassles
health
health behavior
holistic theory
homeostasis
illness behavior
life-change theory
operant conditioning
physiological
  toughness

precipitating factors
predisposing factors
pressure
resistance
schemata
secondary gain
social stress theory
signal anxiety
strain
stress
stressors
temperament
traumatic anxiety
unconditional
  response
unconditional stimuli
Yerkes-Dodson Law

REFERENCES

Alster, K. B. (1989). *The holistic health movement.* Tuscaloosa: The University of Alabama Press.

American Psychiatric Association. (1987). *Diagnostic and statistical manual of mental disorders* (3rd ed., rev.). Washington, DC: Author.

Baum, A. (1990). Stress, intrusive imagery, and chronic stress. *Health Psychology, 9,* 653–675.

Berkowitz, L. (1990). On the formation and regulation of anger and aggression: A cognitive-neoassociationistic analysis. *American Psychologist, 45,* 494–503.

Brady, J. V., Porter, R. W., Conrad, D. G., & Mason, J. W. (1958). Avoidance behavior and the development of gastroduodenal ulcers. *Journal of the Experimental Analysis of Behavior, 1,* 69–72.

Budzynski, T. H., & Peffer, K. E. (1980). Biofeedback training. In I. L. Kutash, L. B. Schlesinger, & Associates (Eds.), *Handbook on stress and anxiety* (pp. 413–427). San Francisco: Jossey-Bass.

Burstein, A. G., & Loucks, S. (1982). The psychologist as health care clinician. In T. Millon, C. Green, & R. Meagher (Eds.), *Handbook of clinical health psychology* (pp. 175–189). New York: Plenum.

Cannon, W. B. (1932). *The wisdom of the body.* New York: Norton.

Capra, F. (1982). *The turning point.* New York: Simon & Schuster.

Carver, C. S., & Scheier, M. R. (1981). *Attention and self–regulation: A control–theory approach to human behavior.* New York: Springer-Verlag.

Carver, C. S., & Scheier, M. F. (1982). Control theory: A useful conceptual framework for personality–social, clinical, and health psychology. *Psychological Bulletin, 92,* 111–135.

Coyne, J. C., & Holroyd, K. (1982). Stress, coping, and illness: A transactional perspective. In T. Millon, C. Green, & R. Meagher, *Handbook of clinical health psychology* (pp. 103–127). New York: Plenum.

Dahrendorf, R. (1979). *Lebenschancen.* Frankfurt G. M.: Suhrkamp. Cited in H. Strasser & S. Randall, (1981), *An introduction to theories of social change.* London: Routledge & Kegan Paul.

Dantzer, R., & Kelley, K. W. (1989). Stress and immunity: An integrated view of relationships between the brain and the immune system. *Life Sciences, 44,* 1995–2008.

Dienstbier, R. A. (1989). Arousal and physiological toughness: Implications for mental and physical health. *Psychological Review, 96,* 84–100.

Dooley, D., & Catalano, R. (1984). The epidemiology of economic stress. *American Journal of Community Psychology, 12,* 387–409.

Engel, G. L. (1977). The need for a new medical model: A challenge for biomedicine. *Science, 196,* 129–136.

Fisher, S. (1988). Life stress, control strategies and the risk of disease: A psychobiological model. In S. Fisher & J. Reason (Eds.), *Handbook of Life Stress, Cognition and Health* (pp. 561–602). New York: Wiley.

Ford, D. H. (1990). Positive health and living systems frameworks. *American Psychologist, 45,* 980–981.

Freud, S. (1966). *The psychopathology of everyday life* (A. Tyson, Trans.). New York: Norton.

Fuller, J. L., & Thompson, W. R. (1978). *Foundations of behavior genetics.* St. Louis, MO: C.V. Mosby.

Girdano, D. A., & Everly, G. S. (1979). *Controlling stress and tension: A holistic approach.* Englewood Cliffs, NJ: Prentice-Hall.

Hamilton, V. (1979). "Personality" and stress. In V. Hamilton & D. M. Warburton (Eds.), *Human stress and cognition: An information processing approach* (pp. 67–114). New York: Wiley.

Hanson, P. G. (1986). *The joy of stress.* Fairway, KS: Andrews, McMeel & Parker.

Hinkle, L. E. (1974). The concept of "stress" in the biological and social sciences. *International Journal of Psychiatry in Medicine, 5,* 335–357.

Hobfoll, S. (1989). Conservation of resources: A new attempt at conceptualizing stress. *American Psychologist, 44,* 513–524.

Institute of Medicine (United States). (1979). *Healthy people: The Surgeon General's report on health promotion and disease prevention.* (Government Document No. HE20.2:H34/5). Rockville, MD: U.S. Government Printing Office.

Kanner, A. D., Coyne, J. C., Schaefer, C., & Lazarus, R. S. (1981). Comparison of two modes of stress measurement: Daily hassles and uplifts versus major life events. *Journal of Behavioral Medicine, 4,* 1–39.

Kasl, S. V., & Cobb, S. (1966). Health behavior, illness behavior, and sick-role behavior: II. Sick-role behavior. *Archives of Environmental Health, 12,* 531–541.

Kutash, I. L., Schlesinger, L. B., & Associates (Eds.). (1980). *Handbook on stress and anxiety.* San Francisco: Jossey-Bass.

Lazarus, R. S., & Launier, R. (1978). Stress-related transactions between person and environment. In L. A. Pervin & M. Lewis (Eds.), *Perspectives in interactional psychology* (pp. 287–327). New York: Plenum.

Lewin, K. (1948). *Resolving social conflicts.* New York: Harper & Row.

Matheny, K. B., Aycock, D. W., Pugh, J. L., Curlette, W. L., & Silva-Cannella, K. A. (1986). Stress coping: A qualitative and quantitative synthesis with implications for treatment. *Counseling Psychologist, 14,* 499–549.

Mechanic, D. (1966). Response factors in illness: The study of illness behavior. *Social Psychiatry, 1,* 11–20.

Miller, N. E. (1944). Experimental studies in conflict. In J. McV. Hunt (Ed.), *Personality and the behavior disorders* (Vol. 1, pp. 431–465). New York: Ronald Press.

Nakano, K. (1989). Intervening variables of stress, hassles, and health. *Japanese Psychological Research, 31,* 143–148.

Parsons, P. A. (1988). Behavior, stress, and variability. *Behavior Genetics, 18,* 293–308.

Parsons, T. (1951). *The social system.* New York: Free Press.

Sawrey, W. L., & Weiss, J. D. (1956). An experimental method of producing gastric ulcers. *Journal of Comparative and Physiological Psychiatry, 49,* 269.

Schwartz, G. E. (1982). Testing the biopsychosocial model: The ultimate challenge facing behavioral medicine? *Journal of Consulting and Clinical Psychology, 50,* 1040–1053.

Schwartz, G. E. (1983). Disregulation theory and disease: Applications to the repression/cerebral disconnection/cardiovascular disorder hypothesis. *International Review of Applied Psychology, 32,* 95–118.

Seeman, J. (1989). Toward a model of positive health. *American Psychologist, 44,* 1099–1109.

Selye, Hans. (1956). *The stress of life.* New York: McGraw-Hill.

Selye, H. (1974). *Stress without distress.* Philadelphia: Lippincott.

Selye, H. (1979). The stress concept and some of its implications. In V. Hamilton & D. M. Warburton (Eds.), *Human stress and cognition: An information processing approach* (pp. 11–32). New York: Wiley.

Selye, H. (1980). The stress concept today. In I. L. Kutash, L. B. Schlesinger, & Associates (Eds.), *Handbook on stress and anxiety* (pp. 127–143). San Francisco: Jossey-Bass.

Sobel, D. S. (1979). *Ways of health: Holistic approaches to ancient and contemporary medicine.* New York: Harcourt Brace Jovanovich.

von Bertalanffy, L. (1968). General system theory—A critical review. In W. Buckley (Ed.), *Modern Systems Research for the Behavioral Scientist* (pp. 11–30). Chicago: Aldine.

Watson, J. B., & Rayner, R. (1920). Conditioned emotional reactions. *Journal of Experimental Psychology, 3,* 1–14.

Webster's New Twentieth Century Dictionary, unabridged (2nd ed.). (1979). New York: Simon & Schuster.

Weiss, J. M. (1968). Effects of coping responses on stress. *Journal of Comparative Physiological Psychology, 65,* 251–266.

Weiss, J. M. (1971). Effects of coping behavior in different warning signal conditions on stress pathology in rats. *Journal of Comparative Physiological Psychology, 77,* 1–13.

Wiener, N. (1961). *Cybernetics* (2nd ed.). Cambridge, MA: MIT Press.

Wilson, B. R. A. (1989). Cardiovascular risk reduction. *International Psychologist, 29,* 49–54.

Yerkes, R. M., & Dodson, J. D. (1908). The relation of strength of stimulus to rapidity of habit formation. *Journal of Comparative and Neurological Psychology, 18,* 459–482.

CHAPTER 2

Stress Research:
Logic, Design, and Process

IT IS DIFFICULT TO IMAGINE . . . , A SMALL SPECK OF CREATION TRULY BELIEVING IT
IS CAPABLE OF COMPREHENDING THE WHOLE.
MURRAY GELL-MANN

This discussion of theory and method provides an overview of the logic and techniques used to investigate stress-health connections. Space limitations dictate brevity. As such, I will discuss only those designs essential to understanding studies featured throughout the book. The interested reader will find beginning-level discussions of research design in Christensen (1988) or in Bordens and Abbott (1988). Kasl and Cooper (1987) or Karoly (1985) discuss more technical and specialized methods in stress and health research.

BUILDING THEORIES:
THE METHODS BEHIND THE STORIES

Building useful scientific theories is not a recreational sport. It cannot be done in the comfort of an easy chair. Intuition and hope for a blinding flash of light are of little use. Building theories is, instead, an arduous process marked by single-minded determination, infinite patience, and sometimes the gift of serendipitous discovery.

Theory construction requires understanding the logic of scientific discovery and mastery of several investigative techniques. These techniques have been added and refined as science matured. Also, to build a theory, scientists must be able to make sense of numerous facts and figures. Then they must link these facts and figures in a statement that gives form and substance to the data.

MODES OF THINKING IN SCIENCE

We should not assume that science approaches theory building with uniformity. Our theories of health and illness show great diversity. Gary Schwartz discussed four ways of thinking about nature:[1] formistic, mechanistic, contextual, and organistic (Schwartz, 1982). **Formistic thinking** is categorical, either-or

---

[1]Schwartz credits these to Pepper's (1942) notion of world hypotheses.

thinking. It does not admit middle categories or a series of categories. In this way of thinking, you are either sick or well; you are either Type A or Type B; you are either alcoholic or nonalcoholic. There is no middle ground. Before causal connections can be established, science must first categorize the events it will study. In this sense, formistic thinking is a necessary prelude to more systematic scientific enquiry. Formistic thinking, though, can only lead to overly simplistic, if not primitive, models of environment-behavior relations.

As Schwartz notes, formistic thinking is essential to mechanistic thinking. **Mechanistic thinking** assumes that cause-effect chains are singly determined. That is, one cause is linked to one effect. To the mechanistic mind, a specific germ causes a certain disease. A specific stressor will have one, and only one, effect. A lifestyle choice will produce one fixed outcome. The notion of multiple causes contributing to an effect is foreign to this way of thinking. Similarly, the idea that several different outcomes could emerge from a single cause is incompatible with mechanistic thinking.

Contextual thinking takes the view that any effect depends on context. Contextual thinking is relational and multicausal. In addition, the context of the observer may provide alternate though equally plausible explanations of an event. Stress may be good or bad depending on how you view it. Your point of view depends on personal context, a distinctive blend of dispositions, reinforcement history, and values that make you unique. Disease may be caused by a set of interconnected factors that include decisions to engage in high-risk behaviors that lead to exposure or lowered resistance. Disease also may be related to attitudes toward preventive behavior and compliance with medical regimens.

Finally, **organistic thinking** is systems thinking. An organism's healthy functioning results from the interplay of numerous components both within the organism and between the organism and its environmental context. The interactions are complex, resulting in interactive multicausal, multieffect models. Contextual thinking and organistic thinking are clearly compatible and provide, according to numerous authors, the framework within which satisfactory models of stress and health interactions can be developed.

THE LOGIC OF SCIENTIFIC METHOD

Scientific method is a serial process that seeks to establish cause-effect relationships. The cause is the **independent variable** (IV), and the effect (or outcome) is the **dependent variable** (DV). In the social-behavioral sciences, the independent variable is usually an environmental stimulus, and the dependent variable is some behavior. For example, it is widely assumed that chronic stress causes a decline in health. Stress is the independent variable, and decline in health is the dependent variable.

However, in stress and health research, the variables selected as cause and effect can differ markedly. Stated in other terms, what is cause and what is effect depends on where we decide to cut into the chain of events. This is illustrated in Figure 2-1.

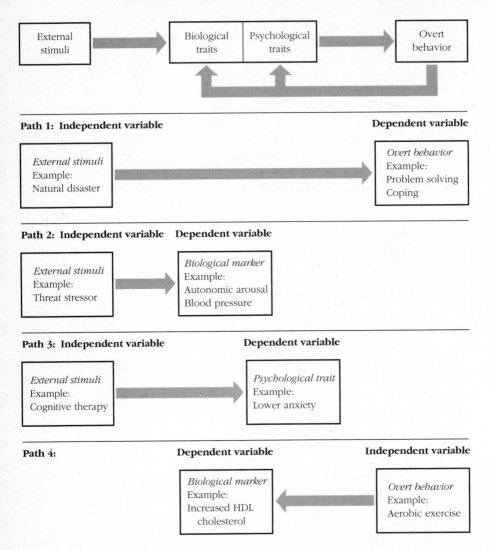

FIGURE 2-1
Possible stimulus-response sequences that structure stress and health research

For this discussion, it is helpful to think of the organism as a complex system influenced by information from external events as well as by feedback from its own behavior. Stimuli may be external physical, or psychosocial, events. They may just as easily be internal biological, or psychological. Outcomes may be internal biological, internal psychological, or overt behavioral. Adding further to the complexity, the person's behavior may be regarded as a stimulus that alters the person's internal biological and psychological states. Here are some examples of these different causal paths.

Independent Variables

A social psychologist might study variations in the type of social support system (intimate-extended versus impersonal-limited) people have and how that protects against the effects of stress. Environmental psychologists might compare reactions to different physical stressors (natural disasters versus technological disasters). Clinical health-care personnel might be concerned about how different therapies (relaxation versus cognitive restructuring) alter subjective reports of stress. In each case, the independent variable is some aspect of the external environment.

Alternatively, we might focus on systematic internal differences in the host organism. For example, we might categorize people in regard to autonomic reactivity (hyperreactive versus hyporeactive) and examine how this influences stress reactions. We could test for differences in levels of trait anxiety and categorize people from high to low on this personality variable. Then we could assess differences in stress reactions related to this trait. In each example, an internal trait is assessed and then categorized as the independent variable. In the first case, we selected a biological characteristic; in the second, a psychological trait.

Finally, we might take differences in behavior patterns as the stimulus event. For example, we might classify people in terms of frequency and intensity of exercise. We could then look at several different dependent measures, such as changes in cardiovascular systems, alterations in physical fitness, or differences in subjective reports of stress.

Dependent Variables

Dependent variables are also defined primarily by their point in the chain of events. Janice Kiecolt-Glaser's group wanted to know if immune competence changes following relaxation training compared to social support or no contact (Kiecolt-Glaser et al., 1985). Their dependent variable was change in natural killer cell activity. Other researchers are concerned about the origins of the Type A personality. Does it result from genetic factors, or does it result from familial patterns of discipline? Here, Type A is measured as an outcome variable. In another context, it might be a stimulus variable similar to trait anxiety in our earlier example. Finally, we might be concerned that coronary risk relates to a mood state, such as chronic intense hostility. In this case, the dependent variable is a cardiovascular measure, such as blood pressure or serum cholesterol, and the independent variable is an internal psychological mood.

A variety of dependent measures focus on internal biological changes. This reflects the notion that biomedical measures somehow are more real than are psychosocial or behavioral measures. Robert Kaplan (1990) made a compelling argument for behavior as the central outcome of health research. He noted that numerous interventions result in clinical improvement, such as reducing blood pressure, but quality-of-life indicators are unchanged. Further, Kaplan cited the highly touted study showing that aspirin reduced deaths from myocardial in-farction. The rest of the story was not publicized; that is, total coronary deaths did not decrease. Aspirin only changed the distribution of deaths among the categories. As Kaplan noted, though, families are rarely as much concerned with how their loved one died as they are that death occurred.

Testing Causal Connections: Educated Guesses

Scientific strategy refers to testing the truth value of a **hypothesis** by directly manipulating the causal variables presumed to influence behavior. A hypothesis is a tentative answer to a research question, a prediction of what behavior we expect under specified conditions.

We will illustrate the process with a prototypic stress-health experiment. Suppose a research group wants to know if relaxation training will reduce migraine headaches. First they inspect the methods and results of previous research in order to become familiar with migraine and its treatment. Based on this review, they state a plausible hypothesis: Relaxation training (IV) will be ef-fective in reducing both the frequency (DV_1) and severity (DV_2) of migraine attacks.

The team then obtains a volunteer group of migraine sufferers. They review medical records (with permission, of course) to ensure that each subject fits the definition of migraine. If they included nonmigraine-pain patients (for example, chronic lower back–pain patients), it would confuse interpretation of results.

Next, the investigators randomly assign subjects to one of two groups, the experimental group or the control group. **Random assignment** is a key feature of scientific research. It permits the assumption that no differences exist be-tween the groups except that introduced by the independent variable. Unfor-tunately, random assignment is not always possible. People cannot be randomly assigned to disease categories, such as coronary heart disease. They cannot be assigned randomly to behavioral or personality profiles, such as the Type A behavior pattern (Friedman & Booth-Kewley, 1987). In this case, the investigator might use a **quasi-experimental design** (Cook & Campbell, 1979).

The **experimental group** receives training in relaxation, while the **con-trol group** receives no training. This difference between the two groups con-stitutes manipulation of the independent variable. In reality, there are very few times when the control group receives nothing. More often than not, the con-trol group receives an **attention placebo.** An attention placebo may be given by having a series of nonspecific informational meetings. Time spent in these meetings would roughly equal the contact time the experimental group receives but would not include relaxation training.

Over time, subjects provide data on the frequency and intensity of their headaches. These measures are the dependent variables. **Baseline,** or pretreat-ment, data will tell the experimenters where the behavior was before treatment and whether the experimental and control groups were equivalent at the outset. After treatment, the data will allow the investigator to either refute or confirm the hypothesis that relaxation changed frequency and intensity of headaches. If the groups were not equivalent in headache measures at the beginning, the outcome of the study could not be assigned reliably to the relaxation treatment. Similarly, if the treatment and control groups were still equal in headaches at the end of the experiment, whether the headaches had been reduced or not, the investigators could not have confidence that relaxation provided an effective treatment.

We should take steps to protect against the chance that subjects know or have guessed the research hypothesis. This could bias the results (Rosenthal, 1966). To prevent this, a special group of collaborators may collect and tabulate the data. These collaborators are special because they do not know the purpose of the experiment, nor do they know to which group the subjects belong. In technical terms, this is a **double-blind control.** If the collaborators are blind to group membership but know the hypothesis of the experiment, it is a **single-blind control.** A recent meta-analysis of modeling procedures to prepare children for surgical operations revealed the importance of this control. That is, treatment effects all but disappeared in experiments using adequate blind procedures but remained quite strong (almost three times the effect size) in experiments not using blind control procedures (Saile, Burgmeier, & Schmidt, 1988).

Good experiments strive for **internal validity.** This is the degree of confidence we have that the outcome can be attributed reliably to the experimental treatment. If other factors change at the same time with the treatment, then other explanations are just as plausible as the hypothesis. We call these uncontrolled variables **extraneous variables.** They confound or confuse interpretation of the results by literally mingling several possible explanations.

Using Subjects for Research: Ethical Dilemmas

An important criterion for conducting responsible research is that subjects must receive information about the basic procedures and any personal risks involved due to their participation. Subjects then sign an **informed consent** form to show they understand the procedures and risks.

Ethical issues in research can be very complicated. When deception is involved, the investigator must be certain that such deception is necessary to test the hypothesis. If deception is used, subjects must receive a **debriefing** to explain what the deception was and to remedy any ill effects that might result. A serious dilemma (exemplified in our prototype experiment) occurs when one group receives a treatment that may be helpful while the treatment is withheld from the control group. This dilemma is usually resolved by offering treatment to the control group after the experimental data have been collected.

Investigators must know local, state, federal, and professional guidelines that pertain to the use of human and animal subjects in research (American Psychological Association, 1982). Any public or private agency that uses federal monies must form an **Institutional Research Board** (IRB) to review projects and ensure that investigators comply with ethical guidelines. It is beyond the scope of this work to delve into issues of this nature. Suffice it to say that federal and discipline-specific guidelines developed over the years guide research ethics while also protecting subjects' safety.

Making Sense of the Numbers

When the project is complete, investigators must try to make sense of the numbers. To reduce the chance that personal bias will influence interpretation, scientists use several statistical tools. In this hypothetical project, the team would compute the average number of headaches and the mean intensity ratings for the experimental and control groups. If the relaxation group showed a sizable decrease in headaches or greatly reduced pain, the hypothesis is confirmed. The problem is to know what constitutes a sizable decrease or change in severity of pain. It is possible that decreases reflect nothing more than uncontrolled chance factors.

The tools scientists use are **inferential statistics.** These enable us to state with mathematical precision how confident we can be that the results were due to chance or that they resulted from the experimental treatment. To be safe, the team sets a confidence level (or level of significance) before the project begins. The **confidence level** defines a statistically significant result by reference to a probability so rare that the results could not have occurred by chance. Conventionally, scientists use confidence levels around $p = .05$ or $p = .01$. A confidence level of .05 states that the results could occur by chance no more than 5 times in 100. A confidence level of .01 states that the results could occur by chance no more than 1 time in 100. Chance factors usually refer to a combination of sampling error, measurement error, or experimental error. If the decrease in frequency or severity of headaches is reliable by statistical test, then the investigators say the hypothesis is true.

Operational Definitions and Repeatability

Scientists take steps to ensure that the procedures used to test hypotheses are explicit and repeatable. They must make certain that special constructs and terms are stated clearly and precisely. Some terms are concrete and have well-defined referents, such as *heart rate.* Other terms are more abstract or theoretical, such as *stress* or *ego* (Clark & Paivio, 1989). When ambiguity exists because a term has several connotations (for example *pain, anxiety, or headache*), then scientists use an **operational definition,** a statement about the procedures the researcher used to establish levels of an independent variable or to measure a dependent variable.

Pain might be defined qualitatively as a particular type of pain—lower back as opposed to headache pain. Then it could be quantified as a score on a standardized pain scale. *Anxiety* might be defined by reference to a score on the

State-Trait Anxiety Scale (Spielberger, Gorsuch, & Lushene, 1970). *Headache* might be defined by reference to medical diagnosis. *Stress* has many operational referents. It is defined as life-events stress, or daily hassles, or a laboratory cold-pressor test, or a medical stress test—running on a treadmill for a specified time. In each case, whether you agree with the definition or not, it is clear what the investigator meant. Also, it is possible for others to repeat the experiment. This is important because science seeks **consensual validation,** which means others obtain the same results.

I selected the preceding terms to illustrate a perennial problem in stress research: many terms used in stress research have a wide range of meanings. A research project may appear elegant in design. But if its central constructs are fuzzy, interpreting results will be an exercise in futility.

Finally, the end of data analysis does not necessarily mean the end of re-searchers' responsibility for their subjects. If the results show that relaxation was effective, the team would provide relaxation training to the control group. This shows again that various ethical problems confront investigators involved in this type of research (O'Leary & Borkovec, 1978).

This statement represents the bare essentials in the logic of experimental design. We now turn to specific research strategies used by investigators in stress and health research. Table 2-1 summarizes the more common strategies. It may be helpful to refer to this table as you read about each design.

CASE STUDIES: THE INTENSIVE ANALYSIS OF ONE

The case study has a long, venerable history in clinical circles. Originally it signified an intensive examination of a single client. Any and all facets of the client's medical, psychological, familial, educational, and social background could provide information crucial to treatment. The **case-study method** also proved useful in opening new areas of inquiry, such as behavior modification research. This led to formal methods for **single-subject designs** and the ex-perimental analysis of behavior, a technique that will be described further in this section. The major limitation of the case-study method is that it cannot directly test hypotheses.

A recent unique example of the case study comes from the work of Nor-man Cousins. It is unique in that the subject and observer were the same per-son. Cousins first gained national recognition as editor of the *Saturday Review.* Later he held a senior lecturer position at the UCLA School of Medicine. When Cousins suffered from a serious collagen disease, he found traditional medical treatment unsatisfactory and left the hospital against medical advice. He docu-mented these experiences in *Anatomy of an Illness* (1979).

Cousins generated a great amount of interest because of what he did after leaving the hospital. He checked into a hotel where he spent several hours a day watching classic comedy movies. He reported that ten minutes of laughter had an anesthetic effect, enabling him to sleep for two hours without the aid of other medications. He also observed a drop in sedimentation rate, an indicator

TABLE 2-1
Comparison of Key Features of Research Designs

Type of design	Degree of control	Method of analysis	Design strengths	Design weaknesses
Case-study method	No control over any variables, whether experimental or extraneous	Subjective (clinical) interpretation Possible comparison to normative data when using standard psychometric exams	Extensive data about the individual May be of heuristic value when it leads to testable hypothesis May be the only way to document rare cases/disorders	Subject to bias of the observer Cannot test causal hypotheses Cannot be repeated Limited generality
Reversal designs	Direct control over experimental or treatment variables Limited or no control over extraneous variables	Graphical—comparison of treatment period to baseline May include some statistical analysis with multiple groups or baselines	Weak causal connections may be inferred Study is repeatable Especially useful in early development of clinical treatments	Usually carried out with very small n Limited generality Cannot eliminate many sources of contamination
Field studies	No direct control over most variables Statistical control over demographic variables	Statistical—yields descriptive values such as means and normative data Comparisons between subgroups with inferences about differences	Potential to obtain quantitative data on many variables from many subjects Establish norms and/or trends May be of heuristic value	Cannot test causal hypotheses May be subject to reporting biases such as selective memory, failures in memory, or expectancies about the nature of the study

			May provide data on social/ecological phenomena that cannot be studied in the laboratory / Can be repeated with most survey studies	Not repeatable with disaster events
Correlational studies	Statistical control over demographic variables	Statistical—results in correlation coefficient and estimate of variance	Identify relations between any number of variables / Identify potentially interesting causal variables for controlled study	Cannot determine causal connections / Significance of the coefficient does not reveal the amount of variance explained
Pre-post designs	Direct control over experimental or treatment variables / Added levels of control depend on type of control group(s) used	Statistical—comparison of target behavior after treatment to pretreatment levels / Comparison to control groups to eliminate competing explanations for change	Stronger inferences of causal link as controls become better / More generality than reversal designs (this depends on sampling and n / Repeatable	Limited causal inferences with no control group or weak controls / Potential ethical questions with untreated controls
Experimental designs	Direct control over hypothesized causal variables / Potential to control most important extraneous variables	Statistical—both descriptive and inferential / Comparison between groups	Most powerful design to establish causal links / Multicausal links / Interactions can be established with extended (factorial) designs	Criticized for using artificial tasks / Can be difficult to interpret with large number of variables / Cannot manipulate some variables for ethical reasons

(continued)

TABLE 2-1
Comparison of Key Features of Research Designs (*continued*)

Type of design	Degree of control	Method of analysis	Design strengths	Design weaknesses
			Repeatable Generality good but related to sampling and task demands	Ethical issues with untreated controls
Epidemiological studies	Varies with specific type of design but potentially very good control Many variables must be controlled by selection rather than by direct manipulation	Statistical—both descriptive and inferential Comparisons between treatment conditions Comparisons between groups exposed to different risk factors	Usually conducted in natural environment Useful for issues of disease etiology and lifestyle disease links Repeatable Generality good	Difficult to obtain good control over many variables Costly in terms of time and effort Outcomes are often still subject to more than one interpretation Ethical issues with untreated controls
Meta-analysis	Only decisional control over how to select and combine studies	Statistical—aggregate effect size Comparison of effect sizes in subsets of studies	Resolves issues from conflicting results Resolves disputes due to disparate methodologies Resolves disputes between competing theoretical models Repeatable	Must work with existing data no matter how clean or dirty the data are Potential bias of using only published studies

of the severity of the inflammation, during laughter. In a short while, he felt he was significantly improved, and he resumed normal activities. Cousins credited this to the healing power of laughter. Cousins also attributed recovery from a heart attack to the "blessed cheerfulness" of his wife (Druss & Douglas, 1988). Numerous studies followed up on Cousins's hypothesis, testing whether laughter is indeed the best medicine. Interest also exists in whether humor is an effective strategy for coping with stress (Martin & Lefcourt, 1983).

FIELD STUDIES:
CONSTRUCTING PLAUSIBLE EXPLANATIONS

Think a moment about how you might try to find answers to these questions. What are the mental and physical health outcomes for victims of a natural catastrophe, such as the San Francisco earthquake of 1989? Can we provide any information to patients, waiting for painful medical procedures, that will minimize their anguish and promote recovery? Are air traffic controllers at increased risk of nervous breakdowns and physical health problems? Does high caffeine consumption increase coronary risk? What is the relationship between physical fitness and coronary risk?

Each of these questions is important and deserves to be answered. Each situation presents a problem, though, in where and how to observe whatever stress–health connection may be present. We cannot create or control an earthquake. Surgery goes on in hospitals, not in research labs. Air traffic controllers may face very different work conditions depending on city size and density of airport traffic. Those conditions cannot be recreated in a laboratory. Caffeine consumption and physical fitness are behaviors whose effects on coronary may not show up for years. These situations, then, require research strategies that differ from the laboratory experiment.

For these questions, the investigator probably would choose from the family of designs called **field studies.** This group includes **survey research, correlational designs, ex post facto designs,** and **field experiments.**

SURVEY RESEARCH: SAMPLING AT LARGE

Survey research is a widely used procedure that seeks to discover typical attitudes or behaviors in large representative samples. Surveys require extensive time for face-to-face interviews or require respondents to fill out lengthy questionnaires. The most elaborate survey research is the U.S. census that occurs every ten years. Other visible examples are Gallup polls and Roper polls, which tap attitudes on social and political issues. They assess changes in behavioral tendencies, such as religious affiliation, sexual mores and conduct, and health behaviors. A recent Gallup poll showed that approximately 59% of the adult population engaged in daily exercise, over twice the number in 1961 (Gallup, 1984).

In 1985, a National Health Interview Survey asked people to respond to a stress questionnaire (Silverman, Eichler, & Williams, 1987). The survey tapped intensity of stress experienced in the previous two weeks, the effect of stress on health, and coping behaviors such as seeking help from family, friends, or professionals. The sample was a nationwide group of civilian citizens 18 years of age or older. The survey reported results in percentages and used a weighted procedure to estimate number of people reporting stress and coping behaviors.

The results showed that roughly 41%, or 34 million people, reported experiencing a lot of stress in the preceding two weeks. Women were more likely than men to report stress (23% versus 18%). One interesting outcome was that respondents with higher levels of education and income reported more stress compared to people with less education and lower income. About 17% of the sample considered seeking help for stress, but only 69% of those considering help actually sought help. Finally, among those who reported the greatest amount of stress, many also reported that they rarely ate breakfast, slept six or fewer hours per night, and were less physically active.

Surveys help indicate trends in attitudes and behaviors. On the other hand, surveys suffer from several limitations. Because survey data is self-report, we must be concerned with the credibility of that report. Most surveys expend little effort to verify data. Surveys often ask people to report blood pressure or other biomedical statistics without cross-checks. The investigator also must hope that respondents interpret questions in a consistent way. Silverman and his colleagues did not make any effort to operationalize stress. The respondents could interpret stress in their own way and respond accordingly. Surveys also may suffer a reactivity effect. That is, respondents may change as a result of being subjects. They may have no opinion before the interview but may form an opinion on the spot to satisfy the social demand characteristics of the interview. Finally, surveys do not allow the investigator to manipulate causal variables or to control for confounding variables. Although statistical controls can be used after data collection, surveys do not permit us to assess causal connections.

CORRELATIONAL DESIGNS: WHAT IS THE RELATIONSHIP?

Correlational research is not experimental in the strict sense of the term. Nonetheless, this type of research can be very useful in tracking down variables that are potentially relevant for more extensive experimental investigations. Correlation is a statistical procedure that assesses the relationship between two or more variables. More precisely, *the correlation coefficient is a quantitative index of the extent to which individuals occupy the same relative position on two scales.* Correlation coefficients, expressed as r, range from +1.00, a perfect positive association; through 0.00, showing no association; to -1.00, a perfect inverse association. A strong negative relationship is just as informative as a strong positive relationship.

A study by Sorbi and Tellegen (1988) illustrates the correlational approach in stress research. Survey studies suggested that stress events frequently precede the onset of migraine headaches. Since no one had tested the strength of this relationship previously, Sorbi and Tellegen decided to do so. Only essential details will be described here because the authors used extensive controls beyond the scope of this work. They treated stress as cause and migraine as effect. In correlational research, stress would be called the **predictor variable** and migraine would be the **criterion variable.**

A group of 29 migraine patients responded weekly to an event-specific coping list. This list contained a stress scale based on the notion that everyday life events are stressful. Stress events could be objectively categorized into threat and challenge. Patients used a diary to record migraine attacks hourly. Sorbi and Tellegen found that threat events preceded migraine, but challenge events did not. The reported correlation was $r = +0.50$. This was significant beyond the .01 level, a result that would be expected to occur by chance less than 1 time in 100.

Several caveats apply to correlational research. First, correlation does not imply causation. Associations may be produced by the operation of another hidden variable, or the association may be simply a matter of coincidence. On the other hand, *there can be no causation unless there is also correlation.* Correlational research can be very useful, then, in identifying patterns of association that may be subjected to closer scrutiny with an experimental method.

Second, even when the observed correlation is high, the explained variance (technically r^2) is smaller. Explained variance, a technical term, can be understood without going into the statistics behind the term. Assume for the moment that a tendency exists for stress to cause migraine headaches. How much of the variability in migraine attacks can be reliably attributed to stress? Certainly we would not expect stress to be solely responsible for migraine. It is reasonable to assume that biomedical factors could also explain some of the variability in migraine attacks. The correlation observed in the Sorbi and Tellegen study suggests that stress explains no more than 25% ($r^2 = .50^2 = .25$) of the variability in migraine headaches. About 75% of the variability is unexplained by this relationship and must be due to the operation of other factors, such as biomedical variables.

EX POST FACTO STUDIES: LOOKING BACK

One special type of field study is the ex post facto design. This design is unique in field research because the investigator must select variables to study after the event has already happened. Natural and technological disasters call for an ex post facto study. Suicide, abuse, and rape also are cases where an ex post facto design is needed. Obviously, there is no way to exercise control over variables leading up to these events.

As an example of this research approach, Shirley Murphy (1984) went into the Mount Saint Helens (Washington) region following a natural catastrophe. She collected data on a variety of physical and emotional symptoms. Catastrophe research might use **archival data** from social and governmental agencies. Researchers may also inspect medical records. Door-to-door surveys with preset questions can provide clues to alterations in physical and mental health status. More extensive face-to-face interviews may then probe deeper into victims' experiences. A descriptive analysis that summarizes the traumas reported by the group may then be provided. With careful planning and execution, it is possible to test hypotheses about likely changes following such an event. It would still be impossible to test hypotheses directly about what precipitated an event such as suicide or abuse.

Scientists still regard the laboratory experiment as the pinnacle of research procedure. Nonetheless, one can learn much from designs implemented in the natural environment or with small groups of clients in a clinical setting. These designs share great *heuristic* value. That is, they generate hypotheses that in turn may be tested in the more optimal conditions of the laboratory.

CLINICAL RESEARCH: PRE-POST INTERVENTION DESIGNS

Clinical research usually works with clients who seek help for distressing or painful symptoms. Migraine sufferers seek help to reduce the pain and cope better with stress. Victims of trauma, such as rape or abuse or war, seek help for *post-traumatic stress syndrome*—that is, help to control fear and reduce physical symptoms that often accompany the trauma.

Clinical researchers try to find the best treatment to use with a specific type of client who presents a distinct set of symptoms. The time when simple comparisons of two or three treatments would suffice is becoming increasingly rare. More often than not, we also need to understand the origins, the **etiology,** of the disorder. In addition, we are rarely satisfied with the knowledge that a treatment works. We also want to know *how* it works. Often, this means we want to identify the effective agent of change in the treatment. For example, several investigators wondered about the active ingredients in biofeedback and relaxation for the treatment of headache pain. They concluded that the success of these treatments had nothing to do with reduced muscle tension or autonomic arousal. Instead, it seemed that a cognitive process, positive change in self-efficacy (a feeling that "I can make things happen"), was the common core.

It should come as no surprise, then, that clinical reseach may appear to be as much theoretical as applied. It is probably better to think of clinical research as a give-and-take between lab, clinic, and field settings. Hypotheses generated in the field or the clinic may eventually be tested in the controlled setting of a laboratory. On the other hand, insights gained from laboratory studies may become the rationale for practical interventions.

Single-Subject Research: Baseline Reversal Design

The simplest clinical study is the single-subject design. While many variations are possible, the most general is the **baseline reversal,** or *AB* design. In a

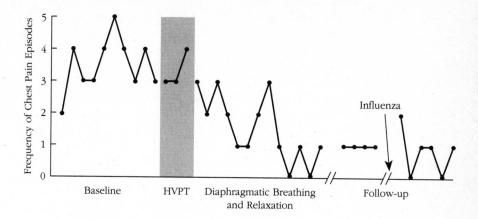

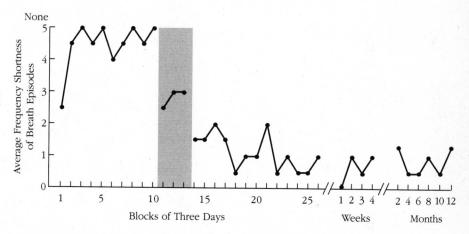

FIGURE 2-2
Frequency of chest pain episodes and average frequency of shortness of breath episodes
for patient G. A. for baseline, treatment, and follow-up
SOURCE: Hegel et al. (1989).

baseline-reversal design, the clinician obtains baseline data for a time before
beginning therapy. This tells the therapist how frequent or intense the behavior
is at the outset. Then the clinician selects a therapy that, hypothetically, should
improve the symptoms. The treatment phase is roughly the same length of time
as the baseline phase. Finally, the clinician compares the treatment data to baseline
data. If the symptoms are gone or reduced, there is reason to believe this treatment will be successful for this symptom in the future. For example, Mark Hegel
and his colleagues worked with three women who displayed hyperventilation
syndrome (Hegel et al., 1989). They taught each patient to use controlled dia-
phragmatic breathing plus the relaxation response. As Figure 2-2 shows for one
patient, chest pain and shortness of breath episodes declined systematically after
introducing this treatment. The treatment gains were still evident 12 months
later. Results were similar for the other two patients.

To be sure that the treatment, and not some coincidental outside factor, produced the improvement, baseline conditions may be restored. If the symptoms reappear, we have even more confidence that the treatment was the effective agent. This is an *ABA* design. Finally, the design may be extended to reinstate the effects of the treatment, an *ABAB* design. Leaving the client under baseline conditions would be unethical, especially when the treatment has proven effective. These designs are helpful, but they lack control and generality is limited when conducted with a single subject. It should be noted, however, that nothing prevents using multiple subjects in a baseline-reversal design. When this occurs, the design is usually called a **pre-post design.**

Pre-Post Designs:
The Aspirin of Therapy Research

In a pre-post design, a group of clients with common symptoms responds (pretesting) to a standard scale (or set of scales). This shows us how severe the symptoms are before treatment. Then all clients receive treatment for a set time. In a posttest, clients respond to the same scale (usually an equivalent form of the same scale). We compare scores on the pretest to scores on the posttest to find out whether the treatment was effective or not.

This design seems elegantly simple on the surface, but it is also subject to control problems. It is possible that factors external to the intervention really produced the change. For example, clients may obtain informal therapy from family, friends, or ministers. These informal therapies may have been as responsible for the change as the formal therapy was. Clients with acute stress reactions may improve because the stressor retreats as quickly as it entered. In the absence of a control group, we cannot tell.

Pre-post design with untreated control To solve this problem, we may use an untreated control group having the same clinical symptoms as the treatment group. One way of managing this is the **wait-list control,** diagrammed in Table 2-2. Volunteers may be solicited through local advertising. After the pretest, we randomly assign roughly half the volunteers to a wait list. To do this, we must construct a convincing cover story. We might say that the clinic can provide treatment to only a few people at a time. As soon as space is available, they will receive treatment.

TABLE 2-2
Pre-Post Design with Wait-List Control Group

Nonfactorial design with wait-list (untreated) controls			
Group assignment	*First step*	*Second step*	*Third step*
Treatment group	Pretest (T1)	Give treatment	Posttest (T2)
Wait-list control	Pretest (T1)	Waiting period	Posttest (T2)

When the treatment group completes therapy, we treat the wait-list group. Before beginning treatment, though, they again fill out the scales that were used in pretesting. The logic is straightforward. If the treatment group improved while the wait-list group did not, then the treatment must be responsible, not external factors. This design is superior to both the baseline-reversal and the pre-post design, but it still has flaws. For example, we know that if clients simply believe in a therapy, there is greater chance for cure. This is the **placebo effect.** To solve this problem, we use an attention-placebo control group.

Pre-post design with attention placebo control   A study at the Sloan-Kettering Cancer Center led by Sharon Manne illustrates this approach[2] (Manne et al., 1990). Manne and her associates were concerned about the extreme distress experienced by children undergoing invasive, painful chemotherapy. Children often must be physically restrained for venipuncture procedures. Manne cited evidence that these children receive as many as 300 venipunctures in the course of treatment. The procedure usually becomes more aversive as the veins become less accessible.

Manne's team designed a behavioral-cognitive treatment program with four components. First, children could divert attention by using a party whistle during venipuncture. Second, paced breathing substituted for undesirable behaviors such as struggle and refusal to sit still. Third, children could earn cartoon or celebrity stickers as positive reinforcement for cooperation. Finally, parents received instructions to encourage use of the party whistle and paced breathing.

Of the 23 children who participated, 13 were in the treatment group and 10 in the attention-placebo group. All subjects provided baseline data during a scheduled venipuncture procedure and three data sets following intervention. Parents in the attention-placebo group received instructions to use whatever procedures had been successful in previous sessions. For both treatment and control dyads, psychologists were present during venipuncture sessions. One flaw existed in the design: they could not use blind control. The treatment team, including medical personnel, knew whether the dyads belonged to the treatment group or the attention group.

Mann's team rated each child's distress over three trials. The results of the experiment were clear. The behavioral-cognitive treatment significantly reduced the amount of observed child distress. Children in the treatment group required less physical restraint after intervention than before and significantly less than the control group. The control group also improved, but not as much. This illustrates the role of attention that would be obscured by an untreated control design. (See Figure 2-3.) Parents also rated their child's pain as much lower following intervention. The intervention was successful with both young children (3 years old) and older children (9 years old) and with both boys and girls. However, treatment children did not report lower subjective pain. This suggests that

---

[2]The procedures and analysis are simplified to highlight the main design features and outcomes. Also, Manne and her associates used sophisticated statistical analyses that are beyond the scope of this text.

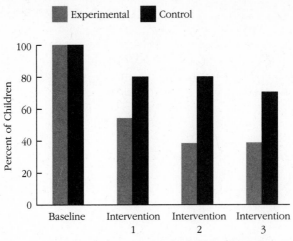

FIGURE 2-3
Mean frequency of use of restraint across baseline and three intervention trials (percentage of children)
SOURCE: Manne et al. (1990).

behavioral control under distress and subjective experience of distress are not necessarily linked.

Factorial Designs: Combining Independent Variables

The previous designs manipulated only one independent variable.[3] They are easy to interpret but of doubtful generality. Events in the real world are rarely if ever determined by just one factor. **Factorial designs** combine two or more independent variables in a single experiment. We gain significant information with this strategy. Each independent variable can be tested as though a single-variable experiment is under way. At the same time, *interactions* can be tested. Interactions reflect the way multiple factors combine to produce outcomes not predicted by the operation of variables studied in isolation. No single-variable experiment, no matter how well designed, can ever provide information about interactions. Neither can we link a group of single-variable experiments to obtain information about interactions. The only way to study interactions is to combine the influence of suspect variables in one experiment.

---

[3]This is similar to the single-cause, single-effect mechanistic thinking discussed earlier. However, we should not jump to the conclusion that investigators are locked in to mechanistic thinking because they choose to restrict their observations to the effect of one variable. Often they are aware of the complex net of causal variables, but they choose to isolate one at a time to better understand each variable's effect before making observations with several variables in play at once.

A study conducted by Kenneth Allred and Timothy Smith (1989) illustrates the factorial design. Allred and Smith were following a line of inquiry begun by Suzanne Kobasa on the hardy personality. Numerous studies suggested that people who display a hardy personality are resistant to stress-induced illness. Investigators usually attributed this to an adaptive cognitive style and reduced physiological arousal but without directly testing their speculations. Allred and Smith decided to test the notion directly.

To do this, Allred and Smith used two independent variables, personality hardiness and threat as a stressor. First, Allred and Smith used the Abridged Hardiness Scale and the Revised Hardiness Scale. They divided their male subjects into high- and low-hardiness groups by taking the combined median split of the two scales.[4] This shows one way to obtain discrete levels of an independent variable—through assessment. When using this method, the investigator must consider the reliability and the validity of the scales used to assign to groups. **Reliability** means the scale provides the same outcome each time it is used. If a scale does not measure consistently, the experimental procedure is flawed by error. **Validity** means the scale measures what it is supposed to measure. Using a scale that measures dominance is of no use when the personality construct to be measured is hardiness.

Second, Allred and Smith randomly assigned subjects to receive either a high evaluative threat condition or a low-threat condition. Subjects in the high-threat condition believed they would take a test that could predict academic and vocational success. Subjects in the low-threat condition believed they would provide physiological measures while doing a cognitive task where the answers were unimportant. Each independent variable had two levels, resulting in a typical 2 × 2 factorial design. This design is shown in Table 2-3. The dependent variables were systolic and diastolic blood pressure as well as a self-statement inventory to assess positive and negative thoughts.

Analysis of the data showed that hardy subjects had only marginally lower arousal when they were waiting for the task to begin. Hardy subjects had higher systolic blood pressure, perhaps because of more active coping efforts. High-hardy subjects in the high-threat condition also had more positive thoughts than did low-hardy subjects in the same condition. The results supported the hardy cognitive style but raised questions about the presumed physiological links between hardiness and health status.

EPIDEMIOLOGY: THE SCIENCE OF EPIDEMICS

Epidemiology, the science of epidemics, seeks to understand the distribution and etiology of disease (Lilienfeld & Lilienfeld, 1980). The historical origins of this science are ancient and venerable, but the modern era may be traced to the work of John Snow around 1850. Snow, a founding member of the London

---

[4] A median split divides the group into two equal halves. If the subject scored in the same half on each median split, they stayed in the study. Otherwise, they were dropped from the study.

TABLE 2-3
Schematic Representation of the 2 × 2 Factorial Design Allred and Smith
Used and the Expected Outcome for the Dependent Variables

	High threat	Low threat
High hardiness	Low arousal Positive thoughts	No change compared to low hardy
Low hardiness	High arousal Negative thoughts	No change compared to high hardy

SOURCE: Allred & Smith (1989).

Epidemiological Society, noted that death rates were 8 to 9 times higher in a London district south of the Thames. Snow discovered that one particular company supplied water to this region and that this was the only company to draw its water from a highly polluted area of the Thames. Snow inferred from this that cholera comes from "poison" transmitted by polluted water.

Epidemiologists use many dependent measures not typically encountered in psychosocial research. The most common are **mortality, morbidity, incidence, prevalence,** and **relative risk.** Mortality is a period death rate per population base. For example, the annual death rate from cardiovascular disease is approximately 326 cases per 100,000 people. Morbidity measures the presence of disabling symptoms in a population. Heart patients may experience severe fatigue, require corrective surgery, or suffer nonfatal strokes.

The rate at which new cases of a disease appear in a given period is incidence. Prevalence is the number of cases of a disease that exist at a given time. Thus, prevalence is total cases, whether old or new. The rapid change in AIDS during the mid-1980s illustrates these two measures. Early in 1986, the total number of cases—prevalence—was about 18,907. At that time, new cases began to appear at an alarming rate—incidence. In this case, the incidence statistic was much more important than the prevalence statistic. Finally, relative risk (RR) is the measure of association between a marker trait and the disease. It is expressed as a ratio:

$$RR = \frac{\text{Incidence of disease in exposed group}}{\text{Incidence of disease in nonexposed group}}$$

Grobbee and his colleagues used this measure in their report on caffeine and cardiovascular disease in men (Grobbee et al., 1990). Men who drank four or more cups of coffee per day (whether caffeinated or decaffeinated) had a relative risk of 1.04. In concrete numbers, 589 non–coffee drinkers suffered some cardiovascular disorder compared to 613 men who drank four or more cups of coffee per day (613 ÷ 589 = 1.04). This difference was so small that it could be explained by sampling differences or measurement error. One interesting result was that men who drank decaffeinated coffee had a relative risk of 1.67 (572 nonexposed compared to 1002 exposed); this was statistically significant. The authors conclude that nothing exists to support the notion that coffee consumption increases risk of coronary heart disease or stroke.

The logic of epidemiology follows the usual scientific progression from description to explanation to prediction and control (Kleinbaum, Kupper, & Morgenstern, 1982). In general, epidemiology first tries to describe a population's health status. It counts current cases of illness (prevalence) or measures the rate at which new cases of an illness appear in a given period (incidence). Using these measures, comparisons can be made between subgroups of the population, as Snow did for people living below the Thames as opposed to those living above. Differences between subgroups may lead to useful, testable hypotheses (for example, pollution of the water caused the illness).

The second step is to explain the etiology, or origins, of a disease. Etiology constructs a coherent picture of the factors that contribute to an illness. Numerous markers may be identified, including demographic characteristics (sex, age, ethnic group), biological and genetic factors, environmental variables, socioeconomic variables, and personal health habits and lifestyle (such as coffee consumption). The emphasis is on groups at risk. No attempt is made to predict illness in individuals (Cockerham, 1982).

Epidemiology may test models developed in stage two by trying to predict prevalence and distribution of diseases. If predictions are accurate, there is increased confidence that the etiological model is correct. Finally, they may use the knowledge gained in prior studies to control diseases. This could include preventive steps, eradication, prolongation of life, or improving the health status of afflicted persons.

There are many variations to epidemiological studies, more than we can discuss here. I will use a common procedure, the **clinical trial,** to illustrate. A clinical trial is a field experiment to verify that a therapeutic agent is effective. The study presented also illustrates the prospective approach, which is discussed later in this chapter.

Recent research in medical nutrition suggested that beta carotene may act as a dietary anticarcinogen. Animal models suggested that carotenoids slow down development of tumors but do not reduce the number of tumors (Krinsky, 1989). Case-control studies showed that increased consumption of fruits and vegetables with high beta carotene reduced the risk for cancer. Case-control studies do not allow us to eliminate competing explanations because we cannot control for many other variables.

Greenberg's group reported the results of a large-scale, randomized, double-blind clinical trial in people with a prior history of nonmelanoma skin cancer (Greenberg et al., 1990). For this study, Greenberg's research group randomly assigned 1805 patients to one of two groups. (Random assignment to groups is a key feature of clinical trials.) The treatment (exposed) group (913 patients) received 50 mg of beta carotene daily. The placebo (nonexposed) group (892 patients) received capsules identical in appearance to the carotene capsules.

The team monitored compliance with the therapy through regularly scheduled questionnaires. If subjects did not take the pills, or compliance between the groups differed substantially, no firm conclusions could be made. Greenberg's group anticipated another potential problem: that the nonexposed group might obtain black-market supplies of beta carotene. To check on compliance, subjects provided blood samples, which were tested for beta carotene level. This is called a **manipulation check.** Patients in the exposed group had an eightfold increase in beta carotene, whereas patients in the placebo group showed no change from prestudy levels.

Patients received routine medical examinations at yearly intervals over a five-year study period. There were two dependent measures: time to the occurrence of new skin cancer, and number of new skin cancers. The results clearly conflicted with earlier case-control studies: beta carotene did not protect the exposed group against recurrence of skin cancer. The exposed group had an average of .29 new cancers per study year, while the placebo group had an average of .25 new cancers. The rates also did not differ at checkpoints during the five-year study time. The authors point out that their study used subjects with a particular type of cancer. From this sample, then, it would be unwise to conclude that beta carotene offers no protection for any cancers.

This study demonstrates a **prospective design.** It followed subjects through the natural history of a disorder. In contrast, a **retrospective design** attempts to reconstruct probable causes by looking back on a disorder after it has already occurred.

Epidemiology built its reputation by discovering the causes of disease such as scurvy, smallpox, syphilis, and cholera. Now, a new tool, **psychosocial epidemiology,** shows promise as a way to discover relationships between psychosocial variables and health status. The current focus on components of the Type A behavior pattern and coronary risk exemplifies this approach. Although psychosocial epidemiology bears a different name, its logic and method is similar to classical epidemiology as just described. Numerous epidemiological studies, both classical and psychosocial, will be reported later in this book.

META-ANALYSIS: ANALYZING THE ANALYSES

Meta-analysis is the "new kid on the block" when it comes to analyzing experiments. Richard Light, a Harvard statistician, and David Pillemer, a Wellesley College psychologist, developed the technique in the early 1970s (Light & Pillemer, 1984). It was Gene Glass (1976), however, who coined the term. Meta-analysis is observational, not experimental. It generates new data, but only through use of old data, not through manipulation of causal variables. It is a statistical technique that sums up the results of studies concerned with similar hypotheses. In its short life, meta-analysis has had some impressive results. For example, it changed prevailing medical beliefs about the effectiveness of aspirin as a preventive treatment for recurrence of heart attack.

Historically, science has progressed by contributing a volume of studies that probe the breadth and depth of an issue. In the process, a group of studies might seem to converge to a common solution only to be upset by another group of studies showing discrepant results. Wading through the mass of data to figure out the basis for the discrepancies was a formidable task. Nonetheless, when a critical mass accumulated, some undaunted soul would pore through the results and try to snatch order from the jaws of chaos. The written record of this effort was a **qualitative literature review** (or a narrative review). Entire journals are devoted to such reviews (*Psychological Bulletin* and *Psychological Review*).

Qualitative reviews suffer from the bias of expert opinion. No matter how expert the reviewer is, a qualitative review still involves subjective judgment. Further, qualitative reviews lack methodological rigor, and they place undue emphasis on the level of significance of studies under review (Johnson, 1989).

By contrast, meta-analysis provides an objective tool for conducting a **quantitative literature review.** Presumably, the results of a meta-analysis can be placed in the public domain for scrutiny, whereas expert opinion cannot. Also, the process is subject to replication and should lead to the same outcomes and interpretations.

In brief, meta-analysis accounts for the magnitude of effect, which is defined as the absolute size of the difference between experimental and control conditions. It is not based solely on statistical significance. By pooling the results of many studies, the effect of certain stimulus variables can be seen more clearly. In several situations, meta-analysis led to conclusions far different from those obtained from a narrative review.

As an example of this approach, we will discuss a study by Ephrem Fernandez and Dennis Turk (1989). Their research programs revolved around issues of pain management. Health care personnel recognize that pain is a subjective event with multicausal origins. Even in the absence of biomedical evidence for a physical source of pain, people report distressing levels of pain. Enough research now has accumulated to suggest that psychosocial factors contribute to people's perception of pain (Turk, Meichenbaum, & Genest, 1983). Based on this knowledge, Dennis Turk and others are testing the efficacy of behavioral and cognitive therapies to reduce pain.

Fernandez and Turk (1989) used a pool of 46 articles with a composite sample of 2000 subjects. They showed that previous qualitative and quasi-statistical studies led to confusion about the potency of cognitive coping strategies. Earlier reviews suggested that acknowledging pain was the most effective method of altering pain perception, and neutral imagery was the least effective. *Meta-analysis showed the opposite results.* On one matter, though, all the analyses agreed: cognitive strategies produce substantive improvement over untreated or placebo controls.

Although meta-analysis has had remarkable success, it is not a panacea; it has its pitfalls and critics. The investigator must make many decisions about which studies to include and exclude, how to group studies where definitions vary, how to treat missing data, and so on. Stanford statistician Ingram Olkin, an early leader in developing meta-analysis, said that "doing a meta-analysis is easy. Doing one well is hard" (cited in Mann, 1990, p. 477). Friedman and Booth-Kewley (1987), in their meta-analysis of the disease-prone personality, find fault with the excessive speculation that has often resulted from meta-analyses. They point out that the most valuable product of meta-analysis should be more refined empirical work to resolve discrepancies. Finally, some are concerned that meta-analysis distances us even further from the client whose well-being is the primary concern of much of the research.

SUMMARY

In this chapter, we have discussed several methodologies for probing stress-health connections. Table 2-1 compares key features of the research designs presented. We began by looking at case studies and field studies. Case studies look in great depth at a single individual but do not establish cause-effect relations. Field studies observe many behaviors that occur in natural settings. However, most do not control for extraneous variables and thus cannot provide information about cause and effect. Yet they have more ecological validity than laboratory experiments and are of heuristic value. That is, they generate new ideas or hypotheses that may be tested through more controlled laboratory methods.

At the most primitive level, clinical experiments use single-subject designs and compare baseline data to data following treatment. Extensions of this basic design include the single-group pre-post design, the pre-post design with an untreated control group, and the pre-post design with an attention-placebo control group. Each design improves on preceding designs by increasing control that eliminates alternate explanations for the success of the treatment. Factorial designs are the first step to multicausal hypotheses. They combine two or more independent variables and allow us to test how these variables interact to produce outcomes not predicted from studying the variables in isolation.

Epidemiological research assesses the distribution of diseases in a population. It also seeks to discover the etiology, or causes, of disease. When changes in mortality (deaths) and morbidity (disabling symptoms) occur at different rates in subgroups of a population, important clues may appear to guide further research. One of the most common research designs in epidemiology is the clinical trial. This method randomly assigns subjects to different therapies and then tests the success of each therapy for a certain disease. Psychosocial epidemiology is now extending these methods to study relations between psychosocial factors and health status.

Meta-analysis is a newcomer to the quantitative analysis of data. It works on data from already completed studies. The technique analyzes effect size, the size of the difference between the experimental and the control group. This enables investigators to evaluate the consistency of findings, assess the importance of either demographic or situational variables used by previous investigators, and resolve contradictions between existing studies.

KEY TERMS

archival data
attention placebo
  group
baseline measures
baseline reversal
  design
case-study method

clinical trial
confidence level
consensual validation
contextual thinking
control, double-blind
control, single-blind
control group

correlational research
  design
criterion variable
debriefing
dependent variable
epidemiology
etiology

experimental group
ex post facto study
extraneous variables
factorial designs
field experiment
field study
formistic thinking
hypothesis
incidence
independent variable
inferential statistics
informed consent
Institutional Research
  Board
internal validity

manipulation check
mechanistic thinking
meta-analysis
morbidity
mortality
operational
  definitions
organistic thinking
placebo effect
predictor variable
pre-post design
prevalence
prospective design
psychosocial
  epidemiology

qualitative literature
  review
quantitative literature
  review
quasi-experimental
  design
random assignment
relative risk
reliability
retrospective design
single-subject design
survey research
validity
wait-list control

REFERENCES

Allred, K., & Smith, T. W. (1989). The hardy personality: Cognitive and physiological responses to evaluative threat. *Journal of Personality and Social Psychology, 56,* 257–266.

American Psychological Association. (1982). *Ethical principles in the conduct of research with human participants.* Washington, DC: Author.

Bordens, K. S., & Abbott, B. B. (1988). *Research design and methods.* Mountain View, CA: Mayfield.

Christensen, L. B. (1988). *Experimental methodology* (4th ed.). Boston: Allyn & Bacon.

Clark, J. M., & Paivio, A. (1989). Observational and theoretical terms in psychology: A cognitive perspective on scientific language. *American Psychologist, 44,* 500–512.

Cockerham, W. C. (1982). *Medical sociology* (2nd ed.). Englewood Cliffs, NJ: Prentice-Hall.

Cook, T. D., & Campbell, D. T. (1979). *Quasi-experimentation: Design and analysis issues for field settings.* Chicago: Rand McNally.

Cousins, N. (1979). *Anatomy of an illness.* New York: Norton.

Druss, R. G., & Douglas, C. J. (1988). Adaptive responses to illness and disability: Healthy denial. *General Hospital Psychiatry, 10,* 163–168.

Fernandez, E., & Turk, D. C. (1989). The utility of cognitive coping strategies for altering pain perception: A meta-analysis. *Pain, 38,* 123–135.

Friedman, H. S., & Booth-Kewley, S. (1987). The "disease-prone personality": A meta-analytic view of the construct. *American Psychologist, 42,* 539–555.

Gallup, G., Jr. (1984). *The Gallup poll: Public opinion 1984.* Wilmington, DE: Scholarly Resources.

Glass, G. V. (1976). Primary, secondary, and meta-analysis of research. *Educational Researchers, 5,* 3–8.

Greenberg, E. R., et al. (1990). A clinical trial of beta carotene to prevent basal-cell and squamous-cell cancers of the skin. *The New England Journal of Medicine, 323,* 789–795.

Grobbee, D. E., Rimm, E. B., Giovannucci, E., Colditz, G., Stampfer, M., & Willett, W. (1990). Coffee, caffeine, and cardiovascular disease in men. *The New England Journal of Medicine, 323,* 1026–1032.

Hegel, M. T., Abel, G. G., Etscheidt, M., Cohen-Cole, S., & Wilmer, C. I. (1989). Behavioral treatment of angina-like chest pain in patients with hyperventilation syndrome. *Journal of Behavior Therapy and Experimental Psychiatry, 20,* 31–39.

Johnson, B. T. (1989). *DSTAT: Software for the meta-analytic review of research literatures.* Hillsdale, NJ: Lawrence Erlbaum Associates.

Kaplan, R. M. (1990). Behavior as the central outcome in health care. *American Psychologist, 45,* 1211–1220.

Karoly, P. (1985). *Measurement strategies in health psychology.* New York: Wiley.

Kasl, S. V., & Cooper, C. L. (1987). *Stress and health: Issues in research methodology.* New York: Wiley.

Kiecolt-Glaser, J. K., Glaser, R., Williger, D., Stout, J., Messick, G., Sheppard, S., et al. (1985). Psychosocial enhancement of immunocompetence in a geriatric population. *Health Psychology, 4,* 25–41.

Kleinbaum, D. G., Kupper, L. L., & Morgenstern, H. (1982). *Epidemiologic research: Principles and quantitative methods.* New York: Van Nostrand Reinhold.

Krinsky, N. I. (1989). Carotenoids and cancer in animal models. *The Journal of Nutrition, 119,* 123–126.

Light, R. J., & Pillemer, D. B. (1984). *Summing up: The science of reviewing research.* Cambridge, MA: Harvard University Press.

Lilienfeld, A. M., & Lilienfeld, D. E. (1980). *Foundations of epidemiology* (2nd. ed.). New York: Oxford University Press.

Mann, C. (1990). Meta-analysis in the breech. *Science, 249,* 476–480.

Manne, S. L., Redd, W. H., Jacobsen, P. B., Gorfinkle, K., Schorr, O., & Rapkin, B. (1990). Behavioral intervention to reduce child and parent distress during venipuncture. *Journal of Consulting and Clinical Psychology, 58,* 565–572.

Martin, R. A., & Lefcourt, H. M. (1983). Sense of humor as a moderator of the relation between stressors and moods. *Journal of Personality and Social Psychology, 45,* 1313–1324.

Murphy, S. A. (1984). Stress levels and health status of victims of a natural disaster. *Research in Nursing and Health, 7,* 205–215.

O'Leary, K. D., & Borkovec, T. D. (1978). Conceptual, methodological, and ethical problems of placebo groups in psychotherapy research. *American Psychologist, 33,* 821–830.

Pepper, S. C. (1942). *World hypotheses.* Berkeley: University of California Press.

Rosenthal, R. (1966). *Experimenter effects in behavioral research.* New York: Appleton-Century-Crofts.

Saile, H., Burgmeier, R., & Schmidt, L. R. (1988). A meta-analysis of studies on psychological preparation of children facing medical procedures. *Psychology and Health, 2,* 107–132.

Schwartz, G. E. (1982). Testing the biopsychosocial model: The ultimate challenge facing behavioral medicine? *Journal of Consulting and Clinical Psychology, 50,* 1040–1053.

Silverman, M. M., Eichler, A., & Williams, G. D. (1987). Self-reported stress: Findings from the 1985 National Health Interview Survey. *Public Health Reports, 102,* 47–53.

Sorbi, M., & Tellegen, B. (1988). Stress-coping in migraine. *Social Science and Medicine, 26,* 351–358.

Spielberger, C., Gorsuch, R., & Lushene, N. (1970). *Manual for the State-Trait Anxiety Inventory.* Palo Alto, CA: Consulting Psychologists Press.

Turk, D. C., Meichenbaum, D., & Genest, M. (1983). *Pain and behavioral medicine: A cognitive behavioral perspective.* New York: Guilford Press.

PART TWO
BIOPSYCHOLOGICAL FOUNDATIONS OF STRESS

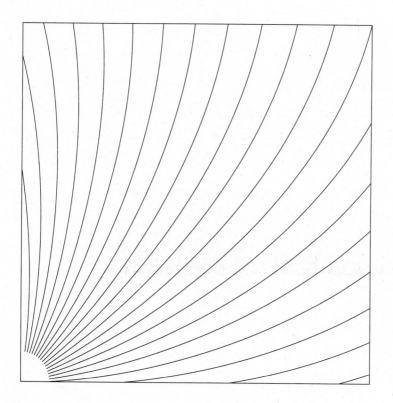

CHAPTER 3

The Cognitive Stress System: Attitudes, Beliefs, and Expectations

IF PLEASURES ARE GREATEST IN ANTICIPATION, JUST REMEMBER THAT THIS IS ALSO
TRUE OF TROUBLE.
EBERT HUBBARD

Your clinic appointment ends with arrangements made for admission to the hospital. "We have to run some tests," the doctor says. You reply, "Tests? What tests? What do I have? Tell me what's going on. I need to know."

Your supervisor stops by to summon you to a meeting with management in one hour. "We have to discuss the production record of your group" is the only clue. Your response is to the point. "What's wrong with our work?" "I can't say anything more until the meeting. See you then," your supervisor replies.

Your teenager calls to say, "I don't know how to tell you this, but, ah, I just wrecked the car." "You did what? Were you hurt? Was anyone with you? How did it happen? Where are you now?"

These very different events share a common problem: each is ripe for many different interpretations. You may welcome the hospital diagnostics for the prospect of rest, discovery, and the end of uncertainty. On the other hand, you may dread the tests because of what might be found or because you expect the procedures to be uncomfortable, if not painful. The production record may be good or bad; the supervisor's comments do not provide any clues.

The youngster who has to relay the unwelcome news to his parents also faces a variety of uncertainties. He cannot be sure how his parents will react, and he might lose future use of the family car. Also, the parents can only imagine what their car might look like. At one extreme is the image of a scratched car; at the other, the image of a demolished car.

LABELS, GUESSES, AND GAPS

The most common cognitive response to uncertainty is **labeling,** assigning meaning to the event. Hospital tests mean a serious health problem. A meeting with management spells trouble, reprimands, probably a diminished chance for promotion, and so forth. Labeling will occur very early in cognitive processing, even prior to one's having all the relevant information. The process is private and goes unnoticed for the most part. Still, it plays a vital role in transactions with the people we meet daily. It sets the stage for a distress reaction or a positive encounter (Brewin, 1988).

A second process occurs simultaneously. That is, people tend to fill gaps in available information with *guesses,* or inferences about the unknown. "What's wrong with our work?" not only labels the supervisor's summons as a threat, it shows that the person has already guessed the likely script for the meeting. The inference is that the news is bad, that management will chew out the group for poor production.

The true purpose of the meeting might be much different, though. Management may want to use the group for a special project that needs the group's production ability. Instead of reprimanding, management intends to honor. The pessimistic guess about what is going on nudges the process to the negative side of stress. Our knowledge of the **literal brain**[1] suggests that physical arousal will occur. Blood pressure may increase, and adrenaline may flood the system. Metabolic rate quickens, and sweating could occur. Based on extensive studies of **pessimistic explanatory styles,** Chris Peterson and Martin Seligman (1984, 1987) came to believe that this pessimistic style is a major problem in transactions that lead to depression, stress, and illness.

Most events hold some uncertainty because only a small amount of information is available at any given time. We actively seek data to fill these gaps. Information seeking can be an important coping strategy, but obtaining information is also time dependent. The doctor does not know what to expect or what will be found. It may be several days before test results are available. The supervisor could disclose nothing until the meeting. That gives you at least an hour to worry and fret. The teenager can verbally relay only bits and pieces of the total picture. Meanwhile, the mind works overtime drawing its own pictures of what happened or what will happen. These three processes—assigning meaning, filling in gaps, and seeking information—continue in cycles. Only when the mind has achieved a satisfactory evaluation and integration will it cease its struggle to give meaning.

ANTICIPATIONS: HOPE AND DESPAIR

Herbert Lefcourt (1976) related one of the most dramatic examples of the powerful effect of labeling. A woman had been mute and socially withdrawn for nearly ten years. She was in a psychiatric hospital, confined to a ward known to patients as the "chronic hopeless" ward. Then hospital management decided to redecorate. To simplify the work, hospital staff moved these patients to a new location with a special meaning. Patients recognized the new ward as the exit ward—the last step before going home. Shortly after being moved, the mute woman started talking and seemed very happy with her new social life. Workers soon finished redecorating the chronic hopeless ward, and the residents had to move back. In Lefcourt's (1976) words, "Within a week after she had been

[1]See pages 60 and 118 for more details on the literal brain.

returned to the "hopeless" unit, the patient . . . collapsed and died. The subsequent autopsy revealed no pathology of note, and it was whimsically suggested at the time that the patient had died of despair" (p. 10).

COGNITIVE SCIENCE: PROBING THE MYSTERIES OF MIND

Observations of voodoo deaths and placebos provide strong supporting evidence that thoughts, labels, and expectations powerfully influence stress reactions and health processes. A great many slings and arrows of modern living might never be suffered were it not for the way we think about our daily transactions.

Stress is not so much a physical property of a situation as it is a transaction between person and environment (Lazarus & Launier, 1978). It is more a product of our cognitive processes, the way in which we think about and evaluate the situation. In much the same way, how we cope and how effective our coping is depends largely on how we think about our resources, how we select coping strategies, and what coping skills we have nurtured.

Labels, thinking, and expectations are the province of the mind. They fall within the domain of **cognitive science.** This new science of the mind is concerned with all the ways in which humans know, think, reason, and decide. Considered private and inaccessible for decades, the mysteries contained in the hidden recesses of the mind are now the subject of intense discussion and investigation. These mysteries are opening up gradually to the probing eyes of cognitive scientists in laboratories around the world. The discoveries of these scientists may hold the key to understanding why one person's distress is another's challenge.

Cognitive scientists first tried to construct general theories about the basic processes in cognition. Now, they also think about the cognitive processes involved in stress and health. In addition, cognitive therapists have begun to develop ways to help people alter self-defeating thoughts and build a sense of control. This chapter concerns cognitive processes such as **perception, attention, appraisal,** and **information seeking.** Later in this chapter, we will discuss a highly regarded model of cognitive processing. Finally, we look at research on pessimistic explanatory styles and health beliefs as they influence health status.

A MODEL OF MIND: INFORMATION PROCESSING

Cognition is defined as all the ways of knowing, thinking, reasoning, and deciding. It includes attention, perception, memory, problem solving, and creativity. In short, cognition is everything we have come to associate with intelligence. To describe how the mind works, cognitive scientists borrowed a computer model from the fields of language and communication. This is the

information processing model.[2] It states that the person's transactions with the environment can be likened to an elaborate computer data-processing task. For any task, there are at least three stages: input, throughput, and output. A feedback system also is present to correct errors and to modify output based on internal decision rules.

Our sensory systems serve as input channels. After sensory input comes throughput processes such as memory, reasoning, planning, and problem solving. These mental functions require some internal organization and rules for managing the flow of information. For computers, an outside programmer must write the program and provide the rules. We write our own programs using organizational schemes and rules assembled through experience. Speaking is an output process, as is behaving.

Cognitive scientists hope to discover what goes on at each stage. They also try to find connections between brain structures and cognitive processes. They look for feedback circuits that allow for error correction and flexible processing.

SCHEMATA AND PERSONAL CONSTRUCTS

As experiences accumulate, some ideas about how the world operates become functional parts of long-term memory. We group these ideas in mind files that contain as much information about a certain event or class of events as we have. In addition, we organize the information within a file in a meaningful, coherent way. This allows us to predict with some accuracy what the outcome of personal action should be. We cannot say with certainty how this is done, but two theories propose similar solutions. First is George Kelly's (1955) **personal construct** theory, a model that evolved from personality research. Second is the **schema theory** from the developmental research of Jean Piaget.[3]

Both personal constructs and schemata are subjective constructions of reality. Both can influence perceptions and reactions. According to Kelly, constructs are not part of reality. Instead, we impose constructs on reality to give it meaning. Constructs are predictive guesses that are tested in reality: The world is just or unjust. Bosses, spouses, and acquaintances are bad or good, happy or sad, friendly or hostile, warm or aloof, charitable or uncaring. Any construct that refers to others also can refer to self. Some constructs become rigid and impermeable to new information, and other constructs remain flexible and permit a wide range of new information.

A key idea in Kelly's (1955) thinking is that people become mentally channeled by the way they anticipate events. Anticipations are similar to putting blinders on a horse—they restrict the view to a very narrow range of the track. Different interpretations simply do not exist because they are outside the restricted channel set by expectations.

---

[2]Currently, a new model, the neural network model, is challenging the information processing model. Still, the work relevant to stress and health is rooted in the information processing model.
[3]For a comprehensive, readable introduction to Piaget's theory, see Ginsburg and Opper (1979).

A clinical anecdote talks of a couple who came close to divorcing because the husband thought the wife was unfaithful. She had begun to engage in mysterious, secretive behavior. As it turned out, she had concocted an elaborate ruse to surprise her husband with a special gift. His construct of reality allowed him to see only one interpretation—that she was having an affair with someone else.

In Piaget's theory, the mind alters sensory input so it will fit with a previously developed schema. This is called **assimilation.** As new information becomes available, the schema becomes more elaborate. This is **accommodation** to meet external demands. We have schemata for cars: what they are like, how they operate, and how we can operate them. Our schema for bosses probably carries a much different meaning from our schema for colleagues or for lovers. Our schema for mothers differs from our schema for fathers. A schema for situations, also called a *script,* contains the rules for situationally appropriate behavior (Schank & Abelson, 1977). Self-concept is an important personal schema. Negative self-schemata may increase vulnerability to depression in the presence of stressful life events (Hammen, Marks, Mayol, & deMayo, 1985). On the other hand, anticipatory schemata of success or failure can influence the way people approach a situation (Bandura, 1989). In this way, schemata act as the primary *meaning systems* in cognition.

PERCEPTION: STRESS IS IN THE EYE OF THE BEHOLDER

If schemata are the central organizing files of the mind, perception is the selective and organizing gateway to the mind. Ulric Neisser (1976), dean of cognitive scientists, stated that perception is the most fundamental cognitive act. This is appropriate in the case of stress and health as well. One review of work stress noted that employee perceptions of stressful situations influenced employee health and well-being (Beehr & Newman, 1978).

Perception is defined as the interpretation and organization of information provided to the brain by the senses. *Interpretation* suggests that we attach meaning and make value judgments about the information. One basic judgment is whether the event is pleasant and valuable or unpleasant, if not painful. *Organization* implies that we make links to experiences stored in long-term memory. We classify new information; that is, we put it in the same memory bin with similar information. This adds to our store of experiences. In the future, this stored experience will add color also to the perceptual process.

Even from the first breath of life, these positive and negative evaluations are not random. Research in behavioral genetics showed that inherited emotional sets and the cumulative effect of experience influence **perceptual biases** (Buss & Plomin, 1975; Thomas, Chess, & Birch, 1970). These emotional sets lead some people to see things negatively and to react accordingly. Other people seem to view most events, even catastrophic events, as positive (Hamilton, 1979).

Misperceptions and Stress

One basic problem is that perception is not perfectly veridical. In other words, mental representations are not always congruent with external reality. Perception falls prey to numerous distortions or subtle alterations in the message. Two of the best known and most severe forms of **perceptual distortions** are delusions and hallucinations. A **delusion** is a mistaken belief, such as "I am Jesus" or "Everyone is out to get me." **Hallucinations** are tricks the brain plays on some people. These people firmly believe they have seen or heard something that does not really exist.

What about something less extreme, like an imagined threat or the thought that a doctor's examination could be negative? An interesting research project sheds some light on this issue. John (1967) designed an experiment to answer basic questions about how the brain responds to a real physical object. The crucial point in the experiment came when John stopped presenting the geometric forms that subjects saw earlier. At this time, he simply asked the subjects to *imagine* the forms were on the blank screen in front of them. The results were unexpected—there were no differences in the recorded brain waves from the real forms and the imagined forms! In other words, the brain could not distinguish between the perception of the object and its own thought of the object. This led Kenneth Pelletier (1977) to call the brain the *literal brain*.

Such observations help explain how people can become upset when they recall an emotionally distressing event. It also explains why people may panic when merely thinking about surgery or an upcoming major exam. The thought is as real to the mind as the actual event, and the effect on the body is just the same.

Perceptual Vigilance and Attention

The perceptual system appears to have some elaborate processes built in to ensure continued alertness or attention to changes in the environment. As defined by cognitive scientists, **attention** is the process by which we choose what stimuli are important and where to focus our mental energy. "Choosing" may be involuntary, impulsive, and automatic; or voluntary, deliberate, and selective.

A car crash in front of the house, a firecracker placed under your chair by a mischievous friend, or the cry of "fire!" in a theater will almost always lead to automatic attending. Features of physical stimuli that demand our attention include size, intensity, and motion. In addition, surprise, novelty, and complexity shift the process in the direction of involuntary attention.

A process called **selective attention** protects against overload; helps focus on relevant information, thus improving efficiency; and blocks out unimportant stimuli. Selective attention combined with voluntary sustained attention is **perceptual vigilance.** This requires extreme concentration and deliberate control over competing irrelevant information. Vigilance is vital to certain jobs, such as air traffic control and medical practice. Several serious accidents and near-misses have occurred because of the intense pressure on air traffic controllers, especially in high-density airports such as Boston, New York, and Chicago. In hospitals, medical staff often monitor patient life signs over long periods. Anesthesiologists must be alert every instant to signs of change in vital functions during prolonged surgery.

Sustained attention can produce a variety of problems. For example, vigilance suffers greatly even over short intervals. Within a few hours, an air traffic controller may begin to lose the high level of concentration required for peak accuracy. In addition, the level of arousal required to sustain vigilance appears to take a toll physically and psychologically. Controllers working in congested airports have a much higher rate of physical illness (compared to overall population morbidity), such as high blood pressure and gastric difficulties. They also report more migraines and subjective stress.

Another vigilance problem occurs when patients receive disturbing news of a serious disease or treatment that will affect their future. Some people prefer the path of least resistance, using denial to protect themselves. Some become aroused and vigilant and actively seek any information they can find about their disease and prognosis. They seem to prefer being active and participating in their treatment to sitting back passively. Others become vigilant to the extreme. Janis (1982) called this state **hypervigilance,** when people are on guard constantly as though they must detect the smallest signal to keep on top of the disease. In the long run, hypervigilance usually interferes with decision making. It results in chronic physical and emotional arousal, which may then hinder healing processes.

Perceptual Defense: Hear No Evil, See No Evil?

When attention serves to protect us from sensitive or undesirable information, we call it **perceptual defense.** The idea of perceptual defense dates back to the work of Leo Postman in 1948. Postman's group observed that people responded more slowly to "bad" or obscene words than to neutral or good words (Postman, Bruner, & McGinnies, 1948).

Recent research showed how perceptual defense might work when people confront stressful information. In one study, researchers asked their subjects to view a very unpleasant film (Suedfeld, Erdelyi, & Corcoran, 1975). Results showed that subjects allocated more time to process negative information than to process positive information. In addition, subjects turned away to avoid prolonged threatening exposure. The implication is clear: Whether they used mental or physical resources to avoid threat, the subjects were out of perceptual circulation for a while. During this time, then, they could not attend to new information.

Evidence of this type supports the notion of a perceptual defense process. It also points to a danger not previously suspected, the likelihood of missing new and important information. This process may account for gaps that occur in memory regarding anxiety-filled transactions. As an example, think about a hit-and-run accident. You might be transfixed by horror just long enough to miss identifying information that could enable police to locate and prosecute the offender.

PERCEPTION, DEPRIVATION, AND OVERLOAD

A large body of research built up over nearly 50 years shows that stimulation levels influence stress. We all have our preferred levels of stimulation and try to avoid the extremes of **deprivation** and **overload.** In the preferred middle ground, the emphasis is on novelty and quality. Sameness and sheer quantity are less desirable. Excessive stimulation aggravates existing stress or is a source of stress itself.

Stimulus Deprivation: Boredom and Stress

Bexton's study of stimulus deprivation at McGill University is almost legendary (Bexton, Heron, & Scott, 1954). Volunteers received $20 per day to lie in bed and sleep. To most students, this seemed like an easy buck. They could quit when they wanted to, and until that time, their basic needs were satisfied. There was only one catch. They had to lie in a cubicle with hands and arms padded and with translucent goggles on their eyes. The subjects could not even hear external sounds because of a masking noise presented through a speaker system.

Bexton's group did not predict what happened. Most of the volunteers quit in the first 24 to 36 hours, and no one went beyond 72 hours. The volunteers slept for the first few hours and enjoyed the relaxation. Soon, though, most of them experienced boredom, restlessness, and increasing anxiety. They tried to generate stimulation by singing, whistling, and talking to themselves. Nonetheless, they experienced a gradual deterioration of intellectual efficiency, followed by unsettling, if not terrifying, experiences. That is, many began to have hallucinations. Some hallucinations were mild, but they seemed to increase in bizarreness and intensity with time. Most were simple geometric forms, but some were more grotesque. One subject saw eyeglasses that turned into deformed, long-legged people walking on the horizon of a small world. To most of the students, the experience was emotionally disturbing and unpleasant. It was too much time with too little input.

How can we explain this result? One possible explanation has to do with the reticular formation, a structure that lies in the brain stem. The reticular formation is the brain's arousal center. It keeps activity going even in the absence of external stimulation. Contact with the outside world, though, is necessary for reality testing. Without it, the brain improvises. It generates its own activity and makes up its own images. As these internal forms stray farther and farther from the norm, they take on the appearance of hallucinations. To use a metaphor, there are no quality controls to ensure that the internal production matches the external blueprint.

This suggests that we need a minimum level of input to keep the cognitive system operating smoothly. It also shows that reduction of input below a minimum level produces stress. Reports from people who function in stimulus-deprived environments such as underwater exploration, polar expeditions, radar operation, and long-distance truck driving confirm these conclusions. Formal research on this issue has helped people prepare to work in such conditions.

Stimulus Overload: Too Much Equals Chaos

Too much stimulation may translate to psychological overload. The expression "this place is a zoo" implies that too much is going on at a pace too fast for the individual's preferred stimulation level. The simple solution, of course, is to get away, be alone, reduce the rate of stimulation even for a short time. When feasible, this coping strategy may be all that is necessary. When this strategy is not feasible, other measures may be called for, such as family problem solving (Chapter 6), more effective management of space and reduction of noise (Chapter 9), and cognitive coping strategies (Chapter 10 and 12).

MEMORY: I DON'T REMEMBER IT THAT WAY

How often have you heard statements such as these? "I don't remember it happening that way." "No, you were the one who said. . . ." "Your memory is going. It was nothing like that." These comments reflect a fundamental vagary of human existence, the fragility of human memory. Perhaps it would be fairer to say "the vulnerability of human memory." This is not to dispute research over the past century that suggests human memory is both powerful and permanent. It is only to note that memory is also subject to numerous forces that selectively discard, suppress, or creatively reconstruct memory to fit personal motives and needs.

Two important memory processes are redintegration and reconstruction. **Redintegration** means reuniting or restoring to a new condition. We recall a set of related bits of information as a unit when we recall one item. For example, during a trial, an attorney prompts a witness to recall some detail from a murder. At that moment, a flood of data related to the prompted recollection may arise. For the most part, redintegration is valuable. However, there is just one problem: Some of the facts recalled never happened. They are inferences or guesses about what must have occurred. Redintegration fills in gaps through a logical fabrication to make complete what is otherwise incomplete. In the heat of battle, it is all the more difficult to distinguish fact from fiction because the recollection makes sense.

In **reconstruction,** we shape memory to fit expectations, beliefs, knowledge, or schemata. A classic study shows how we do this. Before World War I, an English psychologist by the name of Frederic Bartlett (1932) presented subjects with a story called "The War of the Ghosts." The story was part of the oral tradition of Indians who lived on the west coast of Canada a century ago.

It reflected the Indian schemata of world order but obviously had little to do with English schemata. Bartlett asked subjects to recall the story anywhere from several hours to several years later. All the records showed evidence of distortions in recall. Subjects omitted details and changed facts. New bits of information appeared that had nothing to do with the original story. This outcome is really not startling in itself, but the systematic changes that occurred revealed much about memory.

First, each successive recall of the story produced a shorter story, a process called *leveling*. In addition, some details became more prominent, a process called *sharpening*. Subjects changed the story to make it more consistent with English culture. "Hunting seals" became "fishing" and "canoe" became "boat." Elements of the story that were unintelligible without knowledge of the Indian culture were simply discarded or completely changed. This shows that memory can change selectively to fit personal schemata. Errors that lead to interpersonal conflict (marital disputes, for example) may result from inferential, redintegrative, and reconstructive processes.

APPRAISAL PROCESSES IN STRESS

Probably the most influential cognitive model of stress comes from the work of Richard Lazarus and his group (Lazarus & Launier, 1978). We discussed the basic tenets of this model in Chapter 1. Lazarus defined stress as a mismatch between demands and coping resources. Two cognitive processes, appraisal and coping, are important to the person/environment transaction. *Appraisal* means literally to set a value on or judge the quality of something. **Coping** means to engage in behavioral and cognitive efforts to deal with environmental and internal demands and with conflicts between the two (Coyne & Holroyd, 1982).

Lazarus suggested three appraisals that provide meaning and influence the coping process. These are primary appraisal, secondary appraisal, and reappraisal. **Primary appraisal** gives the initial evaluation about the type of situation. Lazarus (1991) said that primary appraisal "concerns the stakes one has in the outcome of an encounter" (p. 827). Secondary appraisal judges the match between coping skills and situational demands. Primary appraisal answers the question "Am I in trouble or not?" **Secondary appraisal** answers the question "What can I do about it?" **Reappraisal** is based on feedback from transactions that occur after the first two appraisals. This may lead to a change in primary appraisal, which may in turn influence the perception of the skills available to deal with it.

There are three types of primary appraisal. Some events are simply **irrelevant** to the person. They contain no threat and require no response. A loud, unnerving shout on the street may be recognized immediately as a driver who is irate with another driver for taking a coveted parking space. The shout can be discarded as irrelevant to your well-being as long as you are not the other driver. Other events are **benign-positive.** They are desirable or, at worst, neutral. They make no serious demands on personal skills.

Events evaluated as **stressful** vary in at least two ways. First, they vary in the nature of the threat to the person. Second, they vary in the nature of

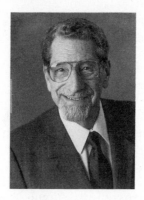

Richard Lazarus, proponent of the cognitive-transactional view of stress
SOURCE: Courtesy of Richard Lazarus.

the demand placed on personal coping resources and skills. Stress begins when we perceive (primary appraisal) that a situation presents some physical or psychological harm, either real or imagined, for which we have no effective response (secondary appraisal). Stress may end because we alter the meaning of the event so that threat is no longer present. Stress may also end because we use a coping method that removes or neutralizes the threat.

Lazarus proposed three stressful appraisals. The first type of stressful appraisal is **harm-loss.** Events of this nature usually involve real or anticipated loss of something that has great personal significance, such as the death of or separation from a spouse or a child. Loss of a job, prestige, or money is another example. Damage to self-esteem is a psychological loss. The sudden loss of a friend or lover is both loss of support and an ego loss. Wills and Langner (1980) noted "there is no self-esteem threat more powerful than rejection by an intimate partner" (p. 163). Diagnosis of a long-term or terminal illness, mastectomy for breast cancer, and loss of eyesight or hearing are physical harm-losses.

Appraisal of **threat** occurs when a situation demands more coping capacity than is available. The emotional tone of the evaluation is negative. **Challenge** refers to a situation we evaluate as demanding and potentially risky, but the emotional tone is one of excitement and anticipation. In addition, we believe the demands can be met whatever they are. The distinction between threat and challenge is still somewhat muddy and not resolved to everyone's satisfaction (Coyne & Lazarus, 1980), but an example might help to clarify. A novice climber climbs small mountains but becomes incapacitated by fear if asked to climb a sheer rock face. For the novice, this extreme demand is a threat. An experienced climber, on the other hand, not only relishes the thought of tackling the dangerous climb but feels honored to be involved.

FACTORS CONTRIBUTING TO STRESSFUL APPRAISALS

What determines whether we appraise an event as stressful or not stressful? At least three factors are critical. These are **emotionality** associated with the event,

uncertainty, because we lack the information needed to evaluate the situation or because we cannot cope with ambiguity, and **evaluation of meaning.**

Emotionality

The connection between emotions and cognitions has been a controversial issue for decades. One camp adopts the view that emotions are primary and influence the form and focus of cognitions. Another camp takes the view that cognitions are primary and give rise to emotions. Consistent with a transactional view, Lazarus suggested that cognitions and emotions are linked in an ongoing flow of negotiations related to environmental stimuli (Folkman, Schaefer, & Lazarus, 1979; Lazarus, 1991). Cognitions and emotions are thus interdependent. In this view, emotions can influence adaptive transactions and coping processes in four ways.

First, emotions serve as an early warning signal that something is wrong. These emotional reactions are related to biologically primitive survival themes. As transactions with the environment turn out positively or negatively, our memory system stores emotional impressions in the same bin with details for the event (Anderson, 1990). Later, when the same event (or a similar event) occurs, it is likely that our perception of the event will be colored by the stored emotional tone.

Second, emotions interrupt ongoing behavior. In this sense, emotional evaluations are attention-getters. They redirect our focus to something that is more important because of the danger or threat involved. If the situation is powerful enough to "demand" our attention, we are likely to evaluate the event as stressful.

Third, emotions can interrupt cognitive tasks in process and start tasks that are necessary to meet new demands. This is why concentration on practical affairs can be difficult after a highly emotional incident. For example, the death of a loved one may disrupt or intrude on thought processes for months or years. An extreme example is when the bereaved person becomes so obsessed with thoughts of the deceased that he or she cannot carry on day-to-day activities.

Finally, emotions can be motivators. Some emotions are pleasant; we will engage in a variety of behaviors to maintain those emotions or put ourselves in situations where there is hope that they will be recreated. Marvin Zuckerman (1971) believes that this is even true of the intense emotions aroused in activities such as mountain climbing, skydiving, hang gliding, or bunge cord jumping. Zuckerman called those who seek out these intense thrills **sensation seekers.** Once they have experienced the intense high provided by their chosen sport, they feel compelled to repeat it to reinstate the high. On the other hand, some emotions are unpleasant; we will do whatever we can to get rid of them. Stress usually results from unpleasant emotional events. In either case, pleasant or unpleasant, emotions can increase behaviors that will control, preserve, eliminate, or reduce internal tension.

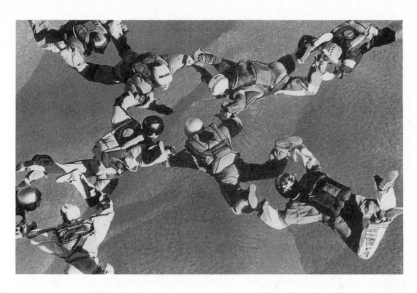

High flyers: While falling at a comfortable 120 mph, skydivers maneuver into formation thousands of feet above the ground. The sport parachutists will break off from the formation and open their parachutes more than 2000 feet above ground.
SOURCE: AP/Wide World Photos.

Uncertainty, Predictability, and Stress

The second factor contributing to a stress appraisal is uncertainty. We may experience uncertainty in several ways. First, an event may be unpredictable, such as a bombing raid or a tornado. Second, an event may require more knowledge than we have available. We can call this a quantitative deficit. Third, an event may be more complex than our schemata can accommodate. We can call this a qualitative deficit.

Mishel (1984) studied a group of 100 patients in a Veterans Administration hospital. He found that scheduled medical events alone did not produce stressful appraisals. It was lack of clarity and lack of information about the medical procedures that accounted for the patients' report of stress. Thus, a strong relationship existed between uncertainty and stress.

The Lazarus group thinks uncertainty is confusion over meaning (Folkman, Schaefer, & Lazarus, 1979). They suggested that we do not have readily available schemata to interpret each and every situation. This makes the event unpredictable, and the person does not know what behavior is appropriate. Given this **unpredictability,** a feeling of helplessness or futility may overwhelm and lead to a stress reaction.

We know from numerous studies that unpredictability is both psychologically and physically debilitating. When we have no way of predicting an event, we experience chronic arousal. Both subjective tension and bodily strain occurs. Chronic physical arousal results in ulcers in laboratory animals (Brady, Porter, Conrad, & Mason, 1958; Weiss, 1968, 1971).

An event preceded by a signal is predictable. Rosenhan and Seligman (1989) noted that when a signal precedes an aversive event (for example, an impending SCUD attack in Tel Aviv), a person will be terrified during the signal but can relax when the signal is off. Also, if the person can do something when the signal occurs to offset the impending doom (for example, get to a shelter), then the person will not experience the same ill effects as when he or she can do nothing.

Two personal traits govern whether uncertainty will result in a stress reaction or not. The first is **tolerance for ambiguity.** The second concerns information-seeking skills. We say an event is ambiguous when it is susceptible to different interpretations, when it is vague or obscure. Tolerance means the ability to withstand or endure.

When uncertainty occurs, we can search for new data that will remove the uncertainty. Several investigators conclude that information seeking is one of the most important coping strategies a person can develop. When we search for relevant information, it is assumed that we can tolerate ambiguity until we obtain the necessary information. Uncertainty seems to result in stress only if we do not have the ability to prevail while we check out possible meanings. If we do persevere, new facts may enable us to transform an unpredictable event into a predictable event.

In addition, successful coping depends on our ability to predict what will happen and on our ability to engage in controlling behaviors. A prerequisite to the ability to control is belief in the ability to control. One study obtained an interesting result in this regard. Jerry Suls and Brian Mullen (1981) wanted to know if perceptions of control and desirability of life events would have any effect on subsequent health in a college sample. They found that undesirability of life change by itself did not produce change in later illness. Lack of control over life change also did not produce change in illness. If undesirable and uncontrollable events occurred together, though, or unwelcome events of uncertain control occurred, there was a significant impact on illness in the following month. The results suggest that information may be important to the extent that it both reduces uncertainty and increases the perception of personal control.

Meichenbaum and Jaremko (1983) proposed that we should engage in **perspective taking** when unalterable stress occurs. This coping strategy involves remembering that most problems are time limited, that other areas of life still provide many rewards, and that bad outcomes can still be bearable.

Evaluation of Meaning

The final factor influencing stress appraisal is evaluation of meaning. We have shown several ways that appraisals contribute to meaning. Primary perceptual processes combined with self-schemata and event-schemata contribute to meaning. As an event unfolds, new information may lead to a change in our perception of the event; this change calls up a new schema or event script. Then we may change the meaning of the event from stress to irrelevant or benign-positive.

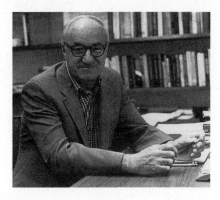

Albert Bandura, author of self-efficacy theory
SOURCE: Courtesy of News and Publications Service, Stanford University. Photo by Chuck Painter.

SECONDARY APPRAISAL, SELF-EFFICACY, AND MASTERY

As defined earlier, secondary appraisal is concerned with whether we have the skills needed to meet the demands of the situation. Albert Bandura (1977, 1989) proposed a related notion, **self-efficacy.** Self-efficacy is the perception of capability, the belief that we possess the personal skills and performance abilities that will enable us to act correctly and successfully in given situations. It is a self-schema about personal competency and mastery.

Bandura's theory distinguishes between efficacy expectations and outcome expectations. Each time we engage in a behavior, it has some good or bad consequence. These consequences are rewards for appropriate acts or punishments for inappropriate acts. As we mature, we develop **outcome expectations.** That is, we learn to anticipate which behaviors are most likely to lead to which outcomes. An **efficacy expectation** is the belief that we can successfully perform the behavior that will produce the outcome. In Bandura's (1977) words, "expectations of personal mastery affect both initiation and persistence of coping behavior. The strength of people's convictions in their own effectiveness is likely to affect whether they will even try to cope with given situations" (p. 193).

Belief that one's skills are poor (low self-efficacy) would lead to the secondary appraisal that an event is unmanageable and thus stressful. Belief in one's ability to deal with anything that comes along is more likely to lead to the appraisal that the event is irrelevant or benign. Numerous studies show that self-efficacy increases with coping success (Bandura, Reese, & Adams, 1982).

Stress Reappraisals

According to the transactional model, every stress situation is a series of negotiations that continues until we control the stress through coping efforts or until the stressor ends spontaneously. Feedback related to coping actions and from people who are involved provide information on both our coping success and the meaning of the event itself. As feedback goes on, we reevaluate the situation, possibly adjusting both coping strategies and meanings in the process.

There are at least three ways in which we deal with stressful events during reappraisal. These are rationalizing, changing the meaning of the event, and reducing the significance of the event. In rationalizing, we attach a personally desirable meaning to an event, although an unbiased analysis would show that the meaning is not appropriate. Consider, for example, someone who has just been fired. After the first shock, he or she might suggest that dismissal is the long-awaited sign to go into private business. Everyone else, though, would consider the chances of this person's becoming a successful business entrepreneur nonexistent.

As noted earlier, changing the meaning of an event may be warranted if new information provides some basis for it. For example, a manager receives word of reassignment to an office in a different region of the country. At first, the manager feels hurt, rejected, and shuffled aside. Later, discussions with management clarifies responsibility, projects, pay, and locale. It becomes obvious that the new arrangement will mean a freer hand, more creative opportunities, a larger work force, and a more relaxed lifestyle for the family in a less overwhelming city. This new data may lead to a significant change in the meaning of the new assignment. In fact, the manager may reinterpret the new post with positive meanings of challenge and opportunity instead of threat and loss.

Another process that occurs in reappraisal is reduction of the meaning of the event. Imagine a union negotiating a new contract where initial talks hint at a sizable pay increase. Planning begins for new investments, perhaps even luxury purchases that have been postponed a long time. Then union and management reach settlement on the contract, but the anticipated large pay raise is little more than a token increase. Initially, employees feel frustrated. They may direct anger toward both union and management. Soon the planned investments and purchases are gradually and quietly reduced in significance. "Well, we really didn't need that anyway." "We got along without it all this time, we can make it a while longer." This type of cognitive process seems to operate most frequently in cases where outcomes are essentially out of personal control.

ATTRIBUTIONS, BELIEFS, AND HEALTH

A major concern in cognitive models of stress is the extent to which attributions and beliefs contribute to high-risk behaviors. Two theories deal with these cognitive processes. First, Christopher Peterson and Martin Seligman (1984) developed a theory of pessimistic explanatory style to explain how cognitions influence health. Second, Irwin Rosenstock (1966) and his associates proposed the **Health Belief Model** to describe how perceptions of vulnerability and beliefs about illness influence health behavior. We will discuss briefly the major tenets of these two models.

TABLE 3-1
Possible Causal Attributions by a Person Driving a Car That Caused a Fatal Auto Accident

	Internal		External	
	Stable	*Unstable*	*Stable*	*Unstable*
Global	I've never been good with mechanical things.	I can't do anything right when I'm tired.	There are too many jerks on the road today.	The signs (zodiac) were not good for today.
Specific	I'm just a very poor driver.	I'm not a good driver when I'm tired.	That corner causes a lot of accidents.	A truck blocked my view.

Pessimistic Attributional Style

The notion of pessimistic explanatory style is an outgrowth of Martin Seligman's work on learned helplessness. Seligman defined learned helplessness as a cognitive-motivational deficit that results from inconsistent but inescapable punishment. Most organisms learn very quickly to escape from aversive stimulation. If punishment occurs on an unpredictable schedule with no hope for escape, the organism will quit trying to escape. Then, even if escape is possible, the organism will fail to escape; it has learned to be helpless. Learned helplessness has been used as a major explanatory construct for depression, and it may be related to deficits displayed by individuals with histories of abuse (Rosenhan & Seligman, 1989).

Seligman's group observed significant differences in people's responses to uncontrollable events. They modified the learned helplessness model in an effort to better account for these differences (Abramson, Seligman, & Teasdale, 1978). This resulted in a general theory of explanatory style that has been applied to numerous outcomes, including failure, depression, illness, and even presidential behavior (Zullow, Oettingen, Peterson, & Seligman, 1988). Explanatory style is the habitual way we explain bad events. In other words, it is how we attribute cause. This theory suggests that causal attributions vary on three dimensions: internal or external; stable or unstable; and global or specific. Table 3-1 provides an example of these dimensions.

To illustrate these dimensions, consider the plight of a rape victim. She may say, "It's my fault. I shouldn't have been out that late alone." This is an internal attribution. On the other hand, she might conclude that poor lighting and lack of visible police protection were at fault. This is an external attribution. Internal attributions generally lead to more passivity and lowered self-esteem following adversity than do external attributions (Peterson, Seligman, & Vaillant, 1988).

Second, she might believe the conditions that led to her attack are permanent. This is a stable attribution. If she thought the conditions were temporary, this would be an unstable attribution. A stable attribution would probably lead to a chronic feeling of vulnerability, whereas an unstable attribution might lead to a quicker resumption of normal lifestyle.

Finally, the victim might have a pervasive feeling of vulnerability, a feeling that she might not be safe at any time or any place (Janoff-Bulman, 1988). This is a global attribution. On the other hand, she might recognize that the factors contributing to this incident were limited, a specific attribution. A pessimistic explanatory style exists when we consistently use internal, stable, and global explanations for adverse events. The outcomes of this explanatory style are thought to be passivity, poor achievement, and signs of depression.

One study tried to evaluate the connection between attributional style and personal hardiness (Hull, van Treuren, & Propsom, 1988). Personal hardiness, a trait that will be discussed in Chapter 4, is thought to result in resilience to stress and positive health. The authors of the study provided strong evidence that attributional style plays a mediating role in the hardy personality. Specifically, hardy persons tend to give internal, stable, and global attributions for positive events, and external, unstable, and specific attributions for negative events. Persons low in hardiness are the opposite, giving internal, stable, and global explanations for negative events. As noted, this generally results in poor outcomes.

A longitudinal study examined the connection between pessimistic explanatory style and physical health (Peterson, Seligman, & Vaillant, 1988). Chris Peterson's team used a sample of male Harvard University graduates from the classes of 1942 to 1944. These people agreed to participate in a long-term project on adult development. They provided extensive data on both psychological and physical health, including factual medical records to verify health status. Also, in 1946 they responded to an open-ended questionnaire.

Peterson's group used a technique called CAVE (Content Analysis of Verbatim Explanations) to analyze statements the subjects made. These statements provided scores that allowed the team to classify subjects on the basis of pessimistic versus optimistic styles. Peterson's group wanted to test the hypothesis that men who used internal, stable, and global explanations for bad events would show worse health outcomes than men who used external, unstable, and specific explanations. The results supported the hypothesis. The strongest relationship between pessimistic explanations and health status occurred 20 years later when most of the men were about 45 years old. Results were also significant at 50, 55, and 60 years of age, but the correlations were smaller than those observed at 45.

Although the theory of explanatory style is appealing, it has its critics. Brewin (1988) noted, for example, that the theory is strong when dealing with accidents and illness. On the other hand, the presumed link to depression following stressful events is far from clear. Carver (1989) also pointed to flaws in the theory and scaling techniques used. He noted that the model is a multicomponent model (three attributions, presumably with different contributions), yet most research has not bothered to test the specific contribution of the individual components. In this case, he argued, we might see premature closure similar to what occurred with the Type A behavior pattern.

The Health Belief Model

Irwin Rosenstock (1966) developed the Health Belief Model (HBM) from field theory and value expectancy theory. Early surveys of health beliefs provided descriptive support without testing the model's predictive power (Kirscht, Haefner, Kegeles, & Rosenstock, 1966). Since then, many investigators have elaborated and tested the model with different populations (Calnan & Moss, 1984), in varied settings, and with various health/illness behaviors (Cockerham, 1982). The model probably is most applicable to higher socioeconomic groups with above-average education. Notably absent, though, is research on children's beliefs about health, although this lack may be short-lived (Peterson & Harbeck, 1988). The model continues to enjoy popularity, perhaps because it assumes that beliefs are subject to modification. Thus, educational or clinical interventions may be expected to bring changes that could have a positive impact on health status.

Figure 3-1 shows the basic components of the Health Belief Model. The model is multicausal in one sense. It proposes that health behavior results from the joint influence of psychosocial factors, including demographic and social cues aimed at changing risk behaviors. At the core of the cognitive system is a set of personal beliefs about illness. These beliefs mediate the perception of threat and thus affect the likelihood of taking action against illness.

First, the model assumes that people hold beliefs about the *seriousness of disease*. This is a motivating factor that makes health issues important. Someone who believes that death from lung cancer is a likely outcome of smoking probably will be motivated to quit. Support for this part of the model is not as strong as for the rest of the model. Still, David McClelland (1989) has argued that motivational factors have a more important connection to health status than first believed.

Further, each person has a **perception of vulnerability** or susceptibility to disease. This is a personal estimate of the chance of contracting a disease. Some people worry constantly about getting sick. Others think of themselves as the "Rock of Gibraltar," immune to illness. This usually leads to reduced efforts to avoid risks. Even if a smoker believes that lung cancer could occur, they might believe it will never happen to them.

Finally, each person has a set of beliefs about the *benefits of taking action* to prevent or combat disease. These include perceptions of costs and barriers to action. People might feel that the risk of lung cancer warrants quitting and that they are personally at risk. Still, they might not be willing to endure the side effects that accompany withdrawal from smoking. They might calculate that quitting will lead to a weight increase, which they regard as negative. They might also fear loss of companionship with smoking friends. These would be barriers to quitting.

Rosenstock, Strecher, and Becker (1988) provided a revised explanatory model that incorporates Bandura's (1977) self-efficacy concept. They noted that the early Health Belief Model ignored efficacy expectations because the researchers focused on acute medical distress and simple preventive actions such

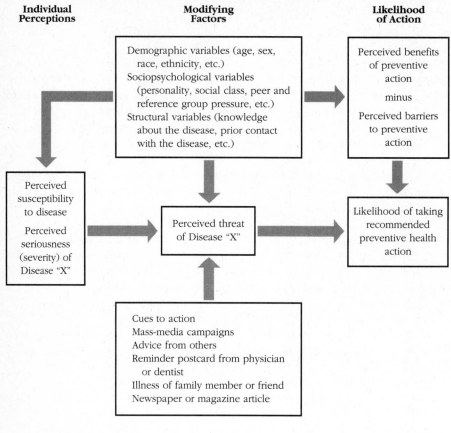

FIGURE 3-1
The Health Belief Model
SOURCE: Becker (1974).

as inoculations or dental care. Chronic illness, however, did not fit as well with the Health Belief Model. Long-term health behaviors such as diet and exercise also were not as well predicted by the model. Complying with strict medical regimens or making significant long-term lifestyle changes requires belief in personal competency (self-efficacy) to undertake the change.

At the same time, Rosenstock and his colleagues warned against uncritical acceptance of self-efficacy theory as a "patent medicine" cure. They noted that self-efficacy theory often incorrectly assumes that a client has adequate incentives to change, feels threatened by environmental events, believes outcomes can be influenced by behavior, and does not face barriers to taking actions. These assumptions are contradicted by data collected with the Health Belief Model.

SUMMARY

In principle, the cognitive system encompasses everything that has to do with mental activity from the simplest to the most complex. This discussion was necessarily selective instead of exhaustive and focused on those parts of the cognitive system that are influential in stress and health. These include primary perception, attention, and memory. A central theme of this discussion is that cognitive schemata serve to organize information from our myriad transactions with our environment. These schemata in turn enable us to assign meaning during new transactions.

We reviewed the transactional model of stress and the evidence that supports the theory. The core of the theory is that stress is a relation between the person and the context. Appraisal processes evaluate the presence of threat or challenge as well as the resources available to meet the demands. When the person has adequate resources to meet the demand, there is no stress.

Finally, we reviewed important theoretical models that look at relations between specific cognitive processes and health behaviors or health outcomes. When people habitually attribute bad outcomes to internal, stable, and global causes, they display a pessimistic explanatory style. This cognitive set predicts poor health outcomes.

The Health Belief Model assumes that perceptions of seriousness of disease combine with perceptions of vulnerability and cost benefits to influence health behaviors. The authors of this model revised it recently to incorporate the notion of self-efficacy to better explain long-term coping behaviors.

KEY TERMS

accommodation
appraisal
assimilation
attention
challenge appraisal
cognition
cognitive science
coping, transactional
    model
delusion
efficacy expectation
emotionality and
    appraisal
evaluation of meaning
hallucinations

harm-loss appraisal
Health Belief Model
hypervigilance
information process-
    ing model
information seeking
labeling
literal brain
outcome expectation
perception
perception of
    vulnerability
perceptual biases
perceptual defense
perceptual distortions

perceptual vigilance
personal constructs
perspective taking
pessimistic ex-
    planatory style
primary appraisal
    benign-positive
    irrelevant
    stressful
reappraisal
reconstruction
redintegration
schema theory
secondary appraisal
selective attention

self-efficacy	threat appraisal	uncertainty
sensation seeker	tolerance for	unpredictability
stimulus deprivation	ambiguity	
stimulus overload		

REFERENCES

Abramson, L. Y., Seligman, M. E. P., & Teasdale, J. D. (1978). Learned helplessness in humans: Critique and reformulations. *Journal of Abnormal Psychology, 87,* 49–74.

Anderson, J. R. (1990). *Cognitive psychology and its implications* (3rd. ed.). New York: W. H. Freeman.

Bandura, A. (1977). Self-efficacy: Toward a unifying theory of behavioral change. *Psychological Review, 84,* 191–215.

Bandura, A. (1989). Human agency in social cognitive theory. *American Psychologist, 44,* 1175–1184.

Bandura, A., Reese, L., & Adams, N. E. (1982). Microanalysis of action and fear arousal as a function of differential levels of perceived self-efficacy. *Journal of Personality and Social Psychology, 43,* 5–21.

Bartlett, F. C. (1932). *Remembering: A study in experimental and social psychology.* London: Cambridge University Press.

Becker, M. (Ed.). 1974. *The Health Belief Model and personal health behavior* (p. 334). San Francisco: Society for Public Health Education, Inc.

Beehr, T. A., & Newman, J. E. (1978). Job stress, employee health, and organizational effectiveness: A facet analysis, model, and literature review. *Personnel Psychology, 31,* 655–699.

Bexton, W. H., Heron, W., & Scott, T. H. (1954). Effects of decreased variation in the sensory environment. *Canadian Journal of Psychology, 8,* 70–76.

Brady, J. V., Porter, R. W., Conrad, D. G., & Mason, J. W. (1958). Avoidance behavior and the development of gastroduodenal ulcers. *Journal of the Experimental Analysis of Behavior, 1,* 69–72.

Brewin, C. R. (1988). Explanation and adaptation in adversity. In S. Fisher & J. Reason (Eds.), *Handbook of life stress, cognition and health* (pp. 423–439). New York: Wiley.

Buss, A. H., & Plomin, R. (1975). *A temperament theory of personality development.* New York: Wiley.

Calnan, M. W., & Moss, S. (1984). The Health Belief Model and compliance with education given at a class in breast self-examination. *Journal of Health and Social Behavior, 25,* 198–210.

Carver, C. S. (1989). How should multifaceted personality constructs be tested? Issues illustrated by self-monitoring, attributional style, and hardiness. *Journal of Personality and Social Psychology, 56,* 577–585.

Cockerham, W. C. (1982). *Medical sociology* (2nd ed.). Englewood Cliffs, NJ: Prentice-Hall.

Coyne, J. C., & Holroyd, K. (1982). Stress, coping, and illness: A transactional perspective. In T. Millon, C. Green, & R. Meagher, *Handbook of clinical health psychology* (pp. 103–127). New York: Plenum.

Coyne, J. C., & Lazarus, R. S. (1980). Cognitive style, stress perception, and coping. In I. L. Kutash, L. B. Schlesinger, & Associates (Eds.), *Handbook on stress and anxiety* (pp. 144–158). San Francisco: Jossey-Bass.

Folkman, S., Schaefer, C., & Lazarus, R. S. (1979). Cognitive processes as mediators of stress and coping. In V. Hamilton & D. M. Warburton (Eds.), *Human stress and cognition: An information processing approach* (pp. 265–298). New York: Wiley.

Ginsburg, H., & Opper, S. (1979). *Piaget's theory of intellectual development* (2nd ed.). Englewood Cliffs, NJ: Prentice-Hall.

Hamilton, V. (1979). "Personality" and stress. In V. Hamilton & D. M. Warburton (Eds.), *Human stress and cognition: An information processing approach* (pp. 67–114). New York: Wiley.

Hammen, C., Marks, T., Mayol, A., & deMayo, R. (1985). Depressive self-schemas, life stress, and vulnerability to depression. *Journal of Abnormal Psychology, 94,* 308–319.

Hull, J. G., van Treuren, R. R., & Propsom, P. M. (1988). Attributional style and the components of hardiness. *Personality and Social Psychology Bulletin, 14,* 505–513.

Janis, I. L. (1982). *Stress, attitudes, and decisions.* New York: Praeger.

Janoff-Bulman, R. (1988). Victims of violence. In S. Fisher & J. Reason (Eds.), *Handbook of Life Stress, Cognition and Health* (pp. 101–113). New York: Wiley.

John, E. R. (1967). *Mechanisms of memory.* New York: Academic Press.

Kelly, G. A. (1955). *The psychology of personal constructs* (Vols. 1 and 2). New York: Norton.

Kirscht, J. P., Haefner, D. P., Kegeles, S. S., & Rosenstock, I. M. (1966). A national study of health beliefs. *Journal of Health and Human Behavior, 7,* 248–254.

Lazarus, R. S. (1991). Progress on a cognitive-motivational-relational theory of emotion. *American Psychologist, 46,* 819–834.

Lazarus, R. S., & Launier, R. (1978). Stress-related transactions between person and environment. In L. A. Pervin & M. Lewis (Eds.), *Perspectives in interactional psychology* (pp. 287–327). New York: Plenum.

Lefcourt, H. M. (1976). *Locus of control: Current trends in theory and research.* Hillsdale, NJ: Lawrence Erlbaum Associates.

McClelland, D. C. (1989). Motivational factors in health and disease. *American Psychologist, 44,* 675–683.

Meichenbaum, D., & Jaremko, M. E. (1983). *Stress reduction and prevention.* New York: Plenum.

Mishel, M. H. (1984). Perceived uncertainty and stress in illness. *Research in Nursing and Health, 7,* 163–171.

Neisser, U. (1976). *Cognition and reality: Principles and implications of cognitive psychology.* New York: W. H. Freeman.

Pelletier, K. (1977). *Mind as healer, mind as slayer: A holistic approach to preventing stress disorders.* New York: Delacorte/Delta.

Peterson, C., & Seligman, M. E. P. (1984). Causal explanations as a risk factor for depression: Theory and evidence. *Psychological Review, 91,* 347–374.

Peterson, C., & Seligman, M. E. P. (1987). Explanatory style and illness. *Journal of Personality, 55,* 237–265.

Peterson, C., Seligman, M. E. P., & Vaillant, G. E. (1988). Pessimistic explanatory style is a risk factor for physical illness: A thirty-five-year longitudinal study. *Journal of Personality and Social Psychology, 55,* 23–27.

Peterson, L., & Harbeck, C. (1988). *The pediatric psychologist.* Champaign, IL: Research Press.

Postman, L., Bruner, J. S., & McGinnies, E. (1948). Personal values as selective factors in perception. *Journal of Abnormal Psychology, 43,* 142–154.

Rosenhan, D. L., & Seligman, M. E. P. (1989). *Abnormal psychology* (2nd ed.). New York: Norton.

Rosenstock, I. M. (1966). Why people use health services. *Milbank Memorial Fund Quarterly, 44,* 94–124.

Rosenstock, I. M., Strecher, V. J., & Becker, M. H. (1988). Social learning theory and the Health Belief Model. *Health Education Quarterly, 15,* 175–183.

Schank, R. C., & Abelson, R. (1977). *Scripts, plans, goals, and understanding.* Hillsdale, NJ: Erlbaum.

Suedfeld, P., Erdelyi, M. H., & Corcoran, C. R. (1975). Rejection of input in the processing of an emotional film. *Bulletin of the Psychonomic Society, 5,* 30–32.

Suls, J., & Mullen, B. (1981). Life events, perceived control and illness: The role of uncertainty. *Journal of Human Stress, 7,* 30–34.

Thomas, A., Chess, S., & Birch, H. (1970). The origin of personality. *Scientific American, 223,* 102–109.

Weiss, J. M. (1968). Effects of coping responses on stress. *Journal of Comparative Physiological Psychology, 65,* 251–266.

Weiss, J. M. (1971). Effects of coping behavior in different warning signal conditions on stress pathology in rats. *Journal of Comparative Physiological Psychology, 77,* 1–13.

Wills, T. A., & Langner, T. S. (1980). Socioeconomic status and stress. In I. L. Kutash, L. B. Schlesinger, & Associates (Eds.), *Handbook on stress and anxiety* (pp. 159–173). San Francisco: Jossey-Bass.

Zuckerman, M. (1971). Dimensions of sensation seeking. *Journal of Consulting and Clinical Psychology, 36,* 35–52.

Zullow, H. M., Oettingen, G., Peterson, C., & Seligman, M. E. P. (1988). Pessimistic explanatory style in the historical record. *American Psychologist, 43,* 673–682.

CHAPTER 4

Personality and Stress: Traits, Types, and Biotypes

BODILY TRAITS ARE NOT MERELY PHYSICAL, NOR MENTAL TRAITS MERELY PSYCHIC.
NATURE KNOWS NOTHING OF THOSE DISTINCTIONS.
C. G. JUNG [PARAPHRASED]

The notion that personality is somehow related to coping and health has almost the status of an idée fixe in Western society. It is so ingrained in Western philosophy, medicine, and psychology that many people probably would believe a link exists even if scientific evidence disputed it. Research has shown that personality does correlate with both the type and intensity of the stress response. It is related to certain types of health problems. In addition, personality may be related to a variety of sick-role behaviors that affect the time course and prognosis for recovery from illness.

Before delving into these issues, however, it is necessary to understand how the term **personality** is used by those who study it most. We all have some idea of what it means to have a pleasant personality. We may also feel quite confident that we know what we are talking about when we describe someone as having a rotten disposition. However, if pressed to define personality precisely and then to measure differences in personality accurately, we would find the job much tougher. That is the problem investigators face in trying to pin down the relationship between personality and stress or health. In the next few pages, we will examine the concept of personality and the major theories of personality that relate to stress and health. Evidence will then be presented linking personality types to a variety of stress reactions and health problems. In some cases, the evidence seems quite strong and indisputable. In other cases, however, the claims are still on shaky ground and should be accepted only with healthy skepticism. Later in this chapter we will discuss positive personality traits that seem to increase resilience to stress.

PERSONA: WHAT LIES BEHIND THE MASK

The concept of personality has changed many times. As originally used by the ancient Greeks, the term *persona* meant a mask such as an actor would wear on stage for theatrical plays of that time. Later, *persona* came to mean the roles individuals played in different aspects of their lives.

More recently, *persona* has come to mean some characteristic or set of characteristics within a person. In figurative terms, personality is the essence of the person behind the mask. It makes the person both real and unique. Personality is also stable and enduring, providing a private reference point in the midst of constant flux and change. Presumably, this durability also allows an outsider to look inside and predict with some accuracy how the person typically behaves.

CLASSIC AND CONTEMPORARY DEFINITIONS OF PERSONALITY

Definitions of personality are relatively easy to come by. But agreement on what personality really refers to is more difficult to find. The most commonly encountered definition of personality was provided by Gordon Allport (1961), who said that personality is "the dynamic organization within the individual of those psychophysical systems that determine his characteristic behavior and thought" (p. 28). Personality so defined is the hub or meeting point for all the biological and psychosocial forces that come to bear on the individual during the course of development.

In spite of disagreement on what personality is, most definitions share common themes such as *uniqueness, organization*, and *style of adapting or coping*. The perceptions, thoughts, feelings, and behaviors of each individual are organized in different patterns. This difference in patterns makes each person in some way different from every other person and determines the characteristic style of responding.

Theodore Millon (1982) is a personality theorist concerned about personality in relationship to stress and health. His view is roughly consistent with the psychodynamic view, which is that personality summarizes the person's style of defending against anxiety, resolving interpersonal stress, and dealing with psychological conflicts. Similarly, Millon views personality as the coping style the individual uses to deal with stressful situations.

VARIETIES OF PERSONALITY THEORY

Different types of personality theories have been popular at one time or another. These include (1) the **psychoanalytic,** (2) the **dispositional,** (3) the phenomenological, and (4) the behavioral-cognitive. The psychoanalytic and dispositional theories have received the most attention, especially in regard to stress-health connections. Phenomenological theory has not been systematically developed to deal with the stress-health issue. Further, although behavioral-cognitive components are included in several models of stress and health, there is not a unified behavioral-cognitive theory of stress and health as such. Because of this, I will summarize only the psychoanalytical and dispositional approaches and discuss the relevance of each to current concerns in stress and health research.

Psychoanalytic Theory in Stress and Health

Psychoanalytic theory, epitomized by the work of Sigmund Freud, describes personality by reference to intrapsychic conflict. The nature of the conflict and the developmental stage during which the conflict first occurred are presumably important in determining the formation of the person's personality.

During the Golden Age of psychoanalysis, many attempts were made to interpret stress responses and health problems in terms of psychoanalytic theory. Most of these attempts were part of the early work in **psychosomatics.** A psychosomatic disorder is one in which a real physical ailment (such as ulcers, asthma, colitis, or cardiac arrhythmia) is caused by or influenced by a psychological process, such as ongoing stress or anxiety.

A prominent psychoanalyst, Franz Alexander (1950), was a leading proponent of this view. He proposed that the asthmatic person is a victim of three correlated events. First, a genetically determined weakness in one organ of the body makes it likely that the organ will break down when stress occurs. This can be likened to a "weak link" theory. Second, a specific psychological conflict weakens the person's defense system if and when stress occurs. Third, some threatening situation arises. Presumably, life stress (the threat) arouses the unresolved conflict (the psychological risk), and the person is not able to defend against it. As a result, the weakest link in the body, in this case the lungs, expresses the stress in asthmatic attacks.

After a lengthy literature review, Kutash and Schlesinger proposed that in allergy patients strong dependency needs are combined with maternal domination or paternal weakness (Kutash, Schlesinger, & Associates, 1980). Others point to a relationship between personality and the person's reaction to asthma (Jones, Kinsman, Dirks, & Dahlem, 1979) as well as to the course of recovery (Kaptein, 1982). However plausible this sounds, little evidence has been found in favor of the psychoanalytic theory of asthma.

Dispositions, Personality Types, and Traits

The second type of theory is the dispositional theory. Dispositional theories generally propose that there are "enduring, stable personality differences which reside within the person" (Liebert & Spiegler, 1982, p. 157). The two most commonly encountered dispositional theories are the typology approach and the trait approach. A **typology** looks for a small number of dispositional clusters that occur with some frequency. A **trait theory** looks for a large number of dispositions that allows description of an individual on each of the dispositions. Presumably, people may have many traits but fit only one type.

Jung's typology   Perhaps the best known typology is the approach proposed by the Swiss psychiatrist Carl Jung. According to Jung, there are only two types of people, the **introvert** and the **extravert**. The introvert is described as socially withdrawn, reflective, not given to displays of emotion, and somewhat closed off from the external world. The extravert is characterized as outgoing, socially active, free in the expression of emotions, and rather open.

Biotypes   In contemporary stress and health research, attempts have been made to relate certain personality traits to particular diseases. As the reasoning goes, genetic mechanisms determine constitution, temperament, and intellect in each person. The interplay of these factors in turn leads to the emergence of a unique personality, which may be as strong and resilient as genetic endowment can provide. Or it may be a personality given to weakness or excess. In the latter case, the nature of the genetics-personality link may produce risks for stress and health-related problems. One personality type might be more prone to coronary attacks, while another personality type might be more prone to ulcers, and so on.

One major difficulty in trying to establish the personality-illness connection is the proverbial chicken-and-egg problem. That is, do health problems change personality, or do personality disorders contribute to health problems? Another problem is that biotype theories tend to convey either the impression that genetics is destiny or a very closely related misperception that personality types are irreversible. Both these notions are unfortunate. Personality, as described earlier, is the hub of all the influences—whether biological, psychological, or social—that weave their way into the fabric of personality from conception. Thus, genetic factors may be pushed or shoved in different directions, to more extreme or less extreme expressions, depending on the forces that come into play after birth. In addition, while the stability of personality is often emphasized, there are indications that changes in personality function can and do occur throughout life.   /

Trait Anxiety and State Anxiety

Charles Spielberger (1966) believes there is a basic difference between **trait anxiety** and **state anxiety**. Trait anxiety tends to be relatively stable across time and place. People who are high in trait anxiety have a much greater tendency to be anxious whatever the situation and relatively more anxious all the time compared to those low in trait anxiety. For the high–trait-anxious person, it takes relatively less external stress to trigger a stress reaction. On the other hand, people who are low in trait anxiety are more relaxed all the time, regardless of the situation. It takes relatively higher levels of stress to trigger an anxiety response in them.

In contrast to trait anxiety, state anxiety is specific to a situation. Job interviews, driving tests, and solo music performances are situations that can produce high anxiety. Students experience a form of state anxiety called **test anxiety**. People in a variety of professions take certifying exams that can make or break a career. A person high in trait anxiety combined with high test anxiety might be overwhelmed or panicked by the test. On the other hand, someone with low trait anxiety might manage with no difficulty as long as test anxiety did not become extreme. State anxiety can vary a great deal within a person.

A person might be low in trait anxiety but experience extreme state anxiety when confronted with a robber. The same person caught in a dangerous winter storm might handle the situation very calmly.

The concept of state–trait anxiety is important to stress research because of the belief that stress reactions, especially chronic stress, may be related to trait anxiety. Trait anxiety has been associated with illness behavior in patients with myocardial infarction, and state anxiety has been related to willingness to admit to the presence of a serious illness (Byrne & Whyte, 1983–1984).

GENERAL MODELS: THE PERSONALITY-HEALTH CONNECTION

Before discussing research on personality and disease, it may be helpful to conceptualize plausible models. As Friedman and Booth-Kewley (1987) point out, "it is silly to postulate a psychological model of disease causation that is physiologically impossible" (p. 541). Four possible models are presented in Figure 4-1. First, it is possible that a given personality profile causes a disease to appear. The Type A–coronary heart disease connection in its most primitive form is an example. This is the typical psychosomatic model that argues for the influence of a psychological variable on a somatic process.

Second, a personality profile may result from a disease process. Depression may be a natural outcome of being diagnosed with cancer. Anger and hostility may mount when the disease is terminal. In this view, disease is caused by a biological agent. The personality pattern occurs after the fact and plays no role at all in the etiology of the disorder. This **somatopsychic** model argues for the influence of the physiological system on psychological process.

Third, personality may be a perceptual filter through which the disease is viewed and a characteristic response to the disease is organized. In this model, the cause of the disease is still viewed as a biological insult, but the course of the disease is tempered by how the person responds to it. Someone with a preexisting tendency to depression may view the diagnosis of cancer more fatalistically than someone with a positive personality profile. This person also may respond more passively, which may exacerbate the health problem and lead to an overall faster deterioration and poorer prognosis for recovery.

Fourth, personality may be a filter, but it may also act through some subtle feedback loop to influence the biological mechanisms that are involved in the disease process itself. In this view, a personality trait may lead to increased autonomic arousal, hormonal flooding, or some combination of both. If maintained over long periods of time, these altered body functions could lead to physiological changes and further biological insult.

CORONARIES, TYPE A, AND HYPERTENSION

Are there coronary-prone, depression-prone, and cancer-prone personalities? Are there special dispositions that predispose a person to drug dependency or

Model 1: Psychosomatic Model

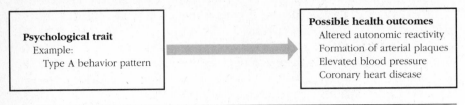

Model 2: Somatopsychic Model

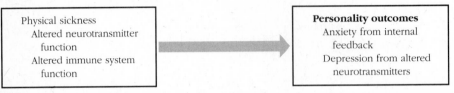

Model 3: Perceptual-Filter Model

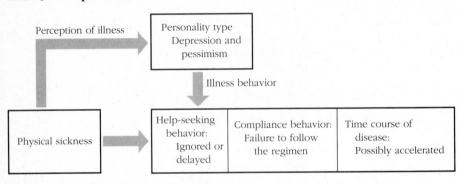

Model 4: Interaction Model

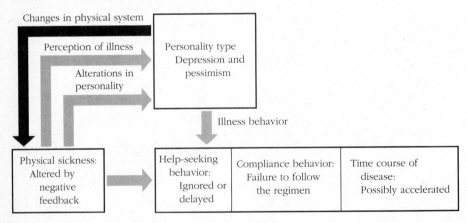

FIGURE 4-1
Possible models of personality/health relations

TABLE 4-1

Comparison of the Most Prominent Theories of Personality-Disease Connections

Biotype	Assumed toxic core	Assumed disease link	Empirical status
Type A behavior pattern	Anger directed in and task-oriented anger with chronic activation	Increased risk for coronary artery disease	Converging data from laboratory and from epidemiological studies provide the most convincing evidence
Cancer-prone personality	Internalized anger and aggression with abnormal release of emotions	Increased risk for cancer	Methodologically and empirically weak Grossarth-Maticek's work, if replicated, may be strongest evidence yet
Smoking and personality	High tension and anxiety	Physical addiction with increased risk for lung cancer and coronary disease	Weak evidence
Alcoholic personality	Genetically set psychological vulnerability Ineffective psychosocial skills Chronic stress	Physical addiction Possible risk for breast cancer	Inconsistent and weak evidence at best
Disease-prone personality	Depression (primary) Anger Anxiety	Any one of several diseases including heart disease, arthritis, asthma, ulcers, and headaches	Based on meta-analysis of 101 studies Inconclusive as yet

to smoking? If so, what special traits make people vulnerable to their own brand of illness or addiction? What hope is there, if any, that the risks can be reduced? If there are no specific biotypes, might there still be a general set of personality traits that disposes people to increased vulnerability? These are some of the questions to be addressed in the next few pages. Table 4-1 summarizes the variety of personality-illness theories that will be discussed throughout the chapter.

The Type A Behavior Pattern

Perhaps the most widely publicized and popularly discussed biotype is the **Type A behavior pattern** (TABP). The idea of a Type A behavior pattern was first described by two doctors, Meyer Friedman and Ray Rosenman (1974). There are

several popular tales of how Friedman and Rosenman came to discover the connection between Type A behavior and **risk of coronary thrombosis** attacks.
According to their own story, however, they were led to the discovery by an
upholsterer who came to their office to repair furniture. He commented that
the doctors must treat a lot of worried people. When they questioned the basis
of his opinion, he pointed out the excessive wear on the leading edges of the
couches and chairs. This was a sign to him that many of the doctors' clients
were literally "on edge." Following this bit of serendipity, Friedman and Rosenman launched the line of research that was to lead to a veritable Type A industry.

The Type A person is described as one who is time driven, impatient, insecure of status, highly competitive and aggressive, generally hostile, and incapable
of relaxing. Time urgency is always prominent in the list of symptoms, but as we
shall see later, it is not the core problem. Type A people seem to run with a faster
internal clock and perceive time differently than do Type B people (Mueser,
Yarnold, & Bryant, 1987). Type A people tend to work rapidly, pushing themselves
to complete things at a rapid pace (Yarnold & Grimm, 1982b), and they set higher
performance standards (Grimm & Yarnold, 1984). Type A people report more
stress symptoms than Type B people do. They are more dominant in interpersonal relationships with Type B people (Yarnold & Grimm, 1982a) and impatient in competitive situations (van Egeren, Fabrega, & Thornton, 1983). They
also smoke more and exercise less (Howard, Cunningham, & Rechnitzer, 1976).

Rosenman and Friedman (1974) refer to this pattern as the *hurry sickness*.
They listed 13 important trademarks for Type A behavior. These criteria have
been translated into a question format in Exercise 4-1. It may be instructive to
answer these questions before going on. In doing so, stick with your first impressions of how you behave most of the time. Try not to edit answers or to
answer based on what you think a Type A person should or should not be. You
will find an approximate scoring method at the end of this chapter.

Type A and Coronary Risk

Is Type A behavior related to increased risk for coronary disease, as Friedman and Rosenman suggested? There are two distinct phases of research that
attempted to answer this question. A large body of literature provided early
evidence that people with the Type A behavior pattern have a much greater risk
for heart attacks than people who do not display the hurry sickness. Recent
research, however, challenges the simple notion but shows that there is a core
of Type A that may be lethal. We will begin by reviewing the structure of early
arguments. Then we will discuss the new theory of Type A and coronary risk.

Biomedical research identified several risk factors that were reliably
associated with risk for coronary disease. These include (1) age, (2) sex, (3) high
cholesterol levels, (4) hypertension, (5) smoking, (6) inactivity, (7) diabetes
mellitus, (8) parental history of heart disease, and (9) obesity (Rosenman et al.,
1970). In the normal population, approximately 1 of every 162 Americans will
suffer a heart attack, although that rate has been dropping for 30 years (Sytkowski,
Kannel, & D'Agostino, 1990). David Glass (1977) suggested that no matter what

EXERCISE 4-1
Criteria Used to Identify Type A Behavior Pattern

1. Do you overemphasize some words in speech and hurry the last words in your sentences?	Yes _____	No _____
2. Do you always move, eat, and walk rapidly?	Yes _____	No _____
3. Are you generally impatient and get irritated when things do not move fast enough for you?	Yes _____	No _____
4. Do you frequently try to do more than one thing at a time?	Yes _____	No _____
5. Do you generally try to move the topic of conversation to your own interests?	Yes _____	No _____
6. Do you feel some sense of guilt when you are relaxing?	Yes _____	No _____
7. Do you frequently fail to take note of new things in your environment?	Yes _____	No _____
8. Are you more concerned with getting than becoming?	Yes _____	No _____
9. Do you constantly try to schedule more activities in less time?	Yes _____	No _____
10. Do you find yourself competing with other people who are also time-driven?	Yes _____	No _____
11. Do you engage in expressive gestures, clenching a fist or pounding the table to emphasize a point, while engaged in conversation?	Yes _____	No _____
12. Do you believe that your fast pace is essential to your success?	Yes _____	No _____
13. Do you score success in life in terms of numbers, numbers of sales, cars, and so on?	Yes _____	No _____

SOURCE: Adapted from Friedman & Rosenman (1974).
See footnote on page 94 for scoring guide.

combination of these risk factors was used, they still failed to detect most new cases of coronary disease. Presumably, the presence of the Type A behavior pattern could predict coronary disease better than could all the other risk factors put together. Rosenman and Friedman (1961) reported a threefold to sevenfold higher rate of diastolic hypertension in Type A women (34.8%) compared to Type B women (4.5%). In the 39–49 age bracket, Type A men were 6.5 times as likely to have a heart attack (Suinn, 1975). This relationship was first established in a classic longitudinal research project, the **Western Collaborative Group Study**, involving 3500 subjects (Rosenman et al., 1964). As we will see later, though, this finding could not be replicated in the Multiple Risk Factor Intervention Trial (MRFIT) (Kuller, Neaton, Caggiula, & Falvo-Gerard, 1980).

    Other studies pointed to the existence of a coronary-prone personality with a core of impatience and overactivity from the Type A pattern (Lloyd & Cawley, 1983). A second cluster included **depression** and high levels of anxiety presumably caused by an overreactive sympathetic system (van Doornen, 1980). Several teams observed this sympathetic reactivity and suggested that Type A people had an increased risk for several stress-related illnesses, not just for coronary (Goldband, 1980; Irvine, Lyle, & Allon, 1982). Lovallo and Pishkin also observed more blood clotting, higher cholesterol levels, and increased triglyceride levels under stress in Type A people (Lovallo & Pishkin, 1980). All of this led some investigators to believe that coronary-disease victims experience no more stressful events than healthy subjects but that they translate emotional upsets into bodily symptoms more frequently.

Attempts to relate Type A behavior to demographic factors have been somewhat confusing. A history of parental coronary disease is not strongly related to Type A behavior (Newlin & Levenson, 1982). Type A behavior tends to increase with socioeconomic status (Shekelle, Schoenberger, & Stamler, 1976). For some time, Type A was thought of as primarily a male pattern. But now it seems that Type A behavior depends more on age, employment, and marital status than on gender. One study found more men than women with Type A behavior, but mostly in the 18- to 25-year age range (Waldron et al., 1977). Women showed higher Type A scores in the better educated, employed 25- to 39-year-old group. In most cases, as the authors of this study surmised, these women were employed and rearing a family as well. This same study compared Whites with African-Americans and found that Whites had higher Type A scores than African-Americans had. Finally, Type A scores tend to decrease with age.

The Changing Face of the Type A Behavior Pattern

It is an understatement to say that current views of the Type A behavior pattern have changed dramatically. The most significant issue is that the alleged relationship between Type A and coronary disease began to evaporate after about 1977. There were also unexpected findings that Type As had lower mortality after a first coronary event than did Type B patients (Dimsdale, 1988). Ragland and Brand's (1988) data are especially surprising because they showed that Type Bs had twice the mortality rate of Type As after a first coronary attack.

The Toxic Core of Type A Behavior

These unexpected reversals posed a challenge that is now being answered. This required that both the theory and the method be subjected to more intense scrutiny. One major effort tried to dissect Type A behavior into its component parts. TABP is usually measured by the Structured Interview (SI) or the Jenkins Activity Survey (JAS) (Jenkins, Zyzanski, & Rosenman, 1965), an objective paper-and-pencil test of Type A behavior. Research on the properties of these scales

---

Approximate scoring for the Type A scale:
If you answered most of the questions "yes," you would be described as a Type A person. If you answered "yes" to over half of them, you might still be regarded as Type A but not an extreme Type A.

show that they tap a complex pattern with several behavior and affect factors, including strong hostility and anger. Wright (1988) and others (Matthews, Glass, Rosenman, & Bortner, 1977) suggested that these measures are largely measures of **Type A anger**.[1] Must all Type A components be present at some threshold level to increase risk for Coronary Heart Disease (CHD), or is some subset of TABP factors more toxic than others? Why is CHD absent in some people who nonetheless demonstrate strong time urgency and hostility? Further, why do some people not classified as Type A still experience CHD (Contrada, 1989)? Could there be a common toxic agent, a component of the TABP, that is highly related to CHD in both the Type A and non–Type A?

Researchers amassed evidence during the 1980s suggesting that the toxic ingredient was hostility/anger (Blumenthal, Barefoot, Burg, & Williams, 1987; Dembroski & Costa, 1987). The Western Electric Study showed that high-hostility men had five times the incidence of CHD (Shekelle, Gale, Ostfeld, & Paul, 1983). A recent meta-analysis of 83 studies points to negative affect as the most important ingredient, although depression also emerged as a strong component (Booth-Kewley & Friedman, 1987)[2].

Based on this emerging evidence, Logan Wright and his colleagues set out to determine more precisely the importance of TABP components (Wright, 1988). First, they identified a cluster of factors that accounted for more of the association between TABP and coronary risk than either global measures or single components. This cluster included *time urgency, chronic activation*, and *multiphasia*. Time urgency has already been described in this chapter. Chronic activation is a tendency to be "wired" on a long-term basis, to stay aroused and keyed up from sunup to sundown, day in and day out. Chronic activation is more than just high energy and fast-paced activities. It is also muscular tension and hormonal flooding. Research suggests that the hormones associated with anger may be metabolized differently depending on whether one can respond with a large-muscle response or the response is bottled up.

Multiphasia is the tendency to engage in multiple activities at the same time, a type of double-timing to crowd more and more into less and less time. Examples might include the person who must read a technical article while exercising on a stationary bike, the business manager who must take work along on vacation, or the student who works on a term paper while attending a recital.

The emergence of this cluster provided support for the argument that a subset of the TABP would provide a better prediction of CHD than would global Type A measures. Still, it lacked the hostility/anger factor that other studies had shown to be important. Wright's group believed that anger might have to be broken down into smaller components. In this view, one can experience anger related to tasks or situations, such as dirty or demeaning jobs that have to be done.

---

[1]A controversy exists over the value of the JAS as a measure of Type A. (Boyd & Begley, 1987). In addition, Scherwitz and his colleagues showed substantial variations in scoring speech characteristics that make it difficult to compare Type As from one study to Type As from another (Scherwitz, Graham, Grandits, & Billings, 1987).

[2]One research group headed by Larry Scherwitz also proposed a self-involvement factor, but this has not generated much support in the literature (Scherwitz et al., 1986).

One can be angry with persons, such as when they stand in the way of personal achievements. In such cases interpersonal relations may be tainted with aggression. One can also be angry with oneself. Whatever type of anger is present, it might be contained and bottled up, or it might be expressed outwardly, thereby ventilating emotional energy.

To test this notion, Wright used a variety of measures to tap anger-in and anger-out. Anger-in proved to be the strongest element predicting risk for CHD. Another factor, anger-out, collapsed to time urgency and chronic activation. This indicates that time urgency and activation reflect task-oriented anger. Yet another factor was the traditional Rosenman and Friedman TABP. In the end, Wright's (1988) program pointed to the multicausal nature of coronary artery disease. Wright's group identified five separate paths to coronary artery disease: inherited risk based on family history, risks that accrue from personal lifestyle choices such as overeating and lack of exercise, anger directed inward, anger directed outward combined with a sense of time urgency and chronic activation, and finally, the traditional Type A pattern identified by Rosenman and Friedman.

Intervening in Type A Behavior

The techniques used to change Type A behavior run the gamut from Rosenman and Friedman's philosophical reeducation to detailed behavior management programs focused on narrowly defined aspects of the Type A pattern (Rosenman & Friedman, 1977). Many individuals identified as Type A have changed dramatically to a more temperate lifestyle. One reason for caution in interpreting these results is that many studies worked with people who had suffered a coronary attack. In many cases, the attack was life threatening. The intrinsic motivation in such a scare may be all that is necessary to get people to change their lifestyle. Thus, how much the treatments contributed to change is not clear. It may be that the motivation to change and information on what to change is more important than the specific means of change.

The Hypertensive Personality

A concept related to the Type A behavior pattern is that of the **hypertensive personality.** Franz Alexander (1939) believed hypertensive patients fight an internal struggle between two strong but incompatible feelings. On one hand, the person feels passive and dependent. On the other hand, the person has strong aggressive and hostile impulses. Because expression of hostility is threatening, the person must fight continuously to keep it under control. Theoretically, this internal conflict should produce long-term autonomic arousal, constriction of blood vessels, and increased blood pressure. Over a period of time, permanent arterial changes occur, and hypertension results.

Alexander's theory was largely speculative and was based on clinical observations of patients as opposed to carefully thought-out, controlled studies. More recently, attempts to identify a specific pattern of traits common to hypertensives yielded inconsistent results (Sparacino et al., 1982). For example, one study looked at the relationship between blood pressure and scores on several widely used personality scales. The research group reported that hypertensives tended to demean themselves while suppressing their feelings. In addition, they were described as neurotic, emotionally immature, guilt-prone, and tense (Pilowsky, Spalding, Shaw, & Korner, 1973). Unfortunately, a number of flaws compromised the usefulness of this information. The study did not use a control group, and the hypertensive sample was small. Most important, the procedure used in the experiment involved a rather stressful catheter implant, which could have in-fluenced the outcome.

After a lengthy review, Iris Goldstein (1981) concluded that there is no sup-port for the notion that hypertensives are psychologically different from nor-mals. Goldstein could find no sound evidence that hypertensives are any more neurotic than people with normal blood pressure. Further, there seems to be little or no support for Alexander's idea that hypertensives are struggling to in-hibit aggression.

THE DEPRESSION-PRONE PERSONALITY

"Depression is the common cold of mental illness" (Rosenhan & Seligman, 1989, p. 307). It afflicts literally hundreds of thousands of people. At any moment, about 1 of every 15 Americans suffers moderate to severe depression. The chances are one in three that sometime in your life you could have a depressive episode severe enough to require clinical treatment. For some, the affliction is barely noticeable, a blue Monday that turns into Tuesday. For others, it is an unhappiness with self and all that life has to offer, an unhappiness that colors all waking perceptions. And for others, depression is the beginning of the end, the bottomless pit of sorrow and despair leading to hospital isolation, attempted suicide, or death.

As this description suggests, depression runs along a continuum of severity. But there is also a body of evidence pointing to distinct types of depression. A genetic mechanism may play a major role in distinguishing less severe de-pression from severe depression. The most severe form, **bipolar depression,** is present in no more than 5% to 10% of cases. It appears to be genetically determined, while most other forms of depression appear to result from daily pressures.

To say that a person is depressed describes the emotional tone, to be sure. But there is much more than that. Depression is a condition so pervasive it changes virtually all the activities normally considered part of daily life. Depres-sion is a disturbance in mood, a prolonged emotional state that colors all men-tal processes. The most significant mood seems to be a feeling of hopelessness coupled with helplessness. The person may lose weight because of loss of pleasure in eating. Sleep disturbances also occur frequently. Some people sleep a great deal when they become depressed, but at odd hours so that normal activities are disrupted. Others may go to sleep readily but wake up early and not be able to get back to sleep. With both eating and sleeping problems, the person tends to feel fatigued and run down all the time. Normal reserves of energy are depleted, and motivation suffers.

Depression also says something about how the person thinks. It is more than just sluggish thinking. The person feels personal worthlessness to one degree or another. He or she may have vague feelings of being guilty of some type of transgression. In the depressed person's mind, this sin accounts for why people don't care. Concentration suffers, so sticking to any kind of task that requires sustained attention becomes difficult, if not impossible. In some serious cases thought disturbances may occur, including suicidal thinking and delusions of persecution or of serious illness, such as cancer.

Several observations make the study of depression relevant to the study of stress and health. First, a number of physical illnesses (including coronary heart disease, asthma, headaches and ulcers) seem to be commonly associated with depression (Friedman & Booth-Kewley, 1987). Risk for illness may increase because depression tends to increase the circulation of adrenaline and cortisol. These in turn may result in suppression of the immune system. Illnesses may also occur because of the cumulative effect of loss of appetite, poor eating habits, lack of exercise, fatigue, and sleep disturbances.

Second, many illnesses are accompanied by depression because of the sheer strain of dealing with the illness. For example, chronic low-back pain usually results in serious depression when the pain has lasted for more two years (Garron & Leavitt, 1983). Depression occurs in this case even when there is no evidence of depressive episodes before the back pain.

Third, depression seems to be one major reaction to personal crises or to failure to cope with a crisis. It also seems to be a common reaction to a number of stressors such as loss of work, loss of savings and investments, and divorce or separation. Finally, depressed people experience more stress in their daily lives, yet they seem to have fewer personal resources and social supports to deal with the stress than do their nondepressive counterparts (Mitchell, Cronkite, & Moos, 1983).

Stress, Depression, and Suicide

Suicide and depression are often linked in folklore. There is good reason to be concerned about the potential for suicide when depression has dragged on for some time. What is often overlooked is that people rarely commit suicide while in a state of depression. This is because both the mental processes required to plan and execute the act and the physical stamina needed to carry out the act are not available. The most dangerous period is when the person is swinging back to a more normal mood state. Unfortunately, this shift tends to make the impact even more devastating for the family.

Suicide is the second leading cause of death for college students. In White adolescent males, suicide increased by 64% from 1970 to 1977. (U.S. Department of Commerce, 1979). In 1987, one in six suicides involved a 15- to 24-year-old male (Subcommittee on Juvenile Justice, 1985). In a study of gifted high school students, Ferguson (1981) discovered that stress and suicidal thoughts tend to go together. That is, the more stress builds up, the more likely the person is to think about suicide and self-destructive behavior. There does not appear to be any difference in this tendency, however, when gifted adolescents are compared to normally intelligent adolescents.

THE CANCER-PRONE PERSONALITY

Cancer is one of the most terrifying diseases of our time. Approximately one in four people will be diagnosed with cancer at some time in their lives, while two in three families will have to deal with the disruption, pain, and suffering caused by cancer. The search for a cure has led in all directions—to medicines, surgery, radiation therapy, vitamins, diet, carrot juice, and apricot pits. Many people, desperately seeking to hang on to life and loved ones, grasp at any straw that seems to offer a hope of understanding and beating the dread disease.

But treatment looks beyond just controlling or curing, to eliminating the threat of cancer. In turn, eliminating cancer depends on identifying more precisely the causes of cancer. This is all the more problematic because cancer is not a single disease but an array of nearly 100 different types. The search for causes has led through many genetic, biochemical, physiological, and environmental studies to a partial understanding of what happens *after* abnormal cell growth is triggered. In some cases, it is even possible to trigger a cancerous growth process in the cell experimentally. But cancer's origins are still largely a mystery.

In recent years, attention has turned to possible connections between psychosocial stressors and cancer (Cunningham, 1985; Levy & Wise, 1987). Some of this work is worthy of consideration and shows promise of filling in additional pieces of the puzzle. But much of it is flawed, some of it probably worthless, and some possibly even dangerous. Barofsky (1981) pointed out that evidence linking stress, psychological conflicts, and personality characteristics to cancer has been extensively reviewed and found methodologically and empirically deficient. The next few paragraphs will present evidence on the **cancer-prone personality** and identify the psychosocial processes that have been reliably linked to cancer.

The personality characteristics most frequently attributed to cancer patients are internalized anger and aggression. Numerous studies reviewed by Morrison and Paffenbarger (1981) showed that cancer patients tend to have higher levels of depression, anxiety, anger, hostility, denial, and repressed emotionality. It should be noted, however, that four of these emotional traits (depression, anxiety, anger, and hostility) are associated with other diseases such as asthma, headaches, ulcers, coronary heart disease, and arthritis (Friedman & Booth-Kewley, 1987). This suggests that the emotional tones may be part of, but not unique to, the cancer-prone personality.

Suggestions abound that these emotional problems are linked to childhood trauma, an unhappy childhood, or family maladjustment. Separation from a parent or death of a parent or sibling has been found in cancer patients' histories more frequently than in those of other patients (Kissen, 1967). One writer even suggested that vulnerability to cancer relates to lack of breast feeding in infancy (Booth, 1969). Family histories of cancer patients reveal more unhappy home lives, domestic strife, and neglect during childhood. This may contribute to the feelings of loneliness, desertion, and denial seen in many cancer patients. Unfortunately, most of the studies that provided evidence for these statements suffered from one or more inadequacies. They lacked control groups, used patients who already knew their diagnosis, and/or analyzed the data improperly.

In spite of improved controls, there is still conflicting information. For example, one team found more repression and less "self-reported" depression relative to a control group (Dattore, Shontz, & Coyne, 1980). Paula Taylor's group used life events, repression-sensitization, and **locus of control** to predict presence of cancer (Taylor, Abrams, & Hewstone, 1988). They found that these variables could explain no more than 8% of the variance. One of the better controlled studies was carried out using women with breast cancer (Greer & Morris, 1975). The pattern of suppressed anger and abnormal release of emotions was verified in this group. They could find no evidence for the personality traits previously attributed to cancer patients.

Even granted that this difference in anger and release of emotions is the crucial difference between cancer-prone and non–cancer-prone people, there is still the issue of how the differences could be physically translated into cancer. Before discussing one model, it should be noted that no one would probably suggest that psychosocial stress could, in and of itself, produce cancer (Levy & Wise, 1987). The assumption is that predisposing factors interacting with host traits trigger the disease with suitable precipitating conditions. One part of the precipitating matrix could be reduced resistance due to psychosocial stress. One general model of this type, proposed by Barofsky (1981), is shown in Figure 4-2.

The hypothesized path from psychological conflict to tumor production may involve any one of several mechanisms. The most frequently suggested path is via elevated adrenocortical production resulting from stress. This produces suppression in the immune surveillance system, which controls the production of Killer-T cells involved in the detection of cancer cells. As a result of this suppression, tumors form with little or no resistance.[3]

As the model shows, diagnosis of cancer and the resulting treatment add to the load of stress. Additional conflict, anger, hostility, denial, and depression generally occur as a result of cancer. The intensity and duration of such conflict may be related to personal coping resources. But even the strongest will go through some period of disruption as they integrate the information about their uncertain future. Many of the early studies are criticized, however, because they

[3]More will be said about this in Chapter 5.

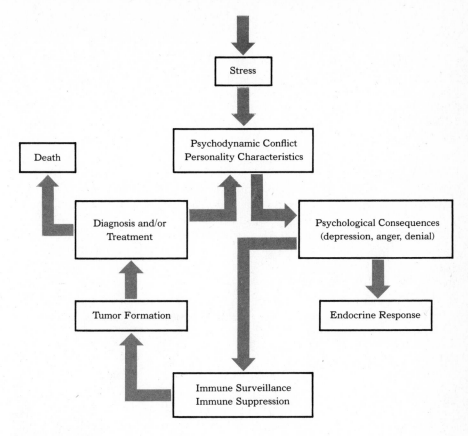

FIGURE 4-2
A theoretical model of how psychosocial stress and personality may influence the production of tumors
SOURCE: Barofsky (1981).

used patients with already-diagnosed cancer. It is impossible under such circumstances to separate the psychological characteristics due to the illness from those that have led to the illness. In other words, it would be impossible to distinguish between the somatopsychic hypothesis and the psychosomatic hypothesis in these conditions.

As already noted, defensive coping reactions can significantly influence the course of a disease process. Katz and his colleagues provided some insight on this issue in their study of a group of women hospitalized for breast biopsy (Katz et al., 1970). At the end of the study, they concluded that being in a stress situation alone does not account for arousal of either the emotions or the physical emergency reactions so often expected from a stressor. Rather, both emotional defenses and physical arousal of the adrenal system appear to depend on how the stress is cognitively perceived, interpreted, and defended against. They found that high rates of adrenal reactivity were associated with apprehension, worry, fear, dejection, discouragement, and despair. On the other hand, low adrenal reactivity was associated with hope, faith in God, fate, and pride in one's ability to handle a life-threatening situation.

An interesting line of research on psychosocial factors in cancer has been carried out in Yugoslavia by Grossarth-Maticek and reported by Hans Eysenck (1987). The major finding of this research was that chronic helplessness was related to an increased incidence of cancer. After reviewing this and other research, Eysenck echoed the prevailing opinion that acute stressors activate cortisol, which in turn suppresses immune function, leading to increased risk for cancer.

A final issue concerns the attitudes and emotions that are curative and that enable one to survive the threat of cancer. It is well known, if quietly admitted, that the best medicine may be to no avail when administered to someone who has already given up the struggle for life. Even if no strong relationship exists between the origins of cancer and some personality type, the evidence suggests that the way in which a person responds to the threat may have a lot to do with surviving the physical insult of cancer. The Katz study is one example of this. Chronic worry, fear, hopelessness, and despair generally hasten the destructive disease process. On the other hand, hope, faith in a supreme power, and personal courage generally operate to marshal the best body defenses available.

PERSONALITY AND SMOKING

Smoking is considered a high-risk, self-defeating behavior that probably serves to reduce tension for many people. It is thus of great significance in considering both health and stress. Because of the potential harm of smoking, an increasing number of programs have been designed to help people quit smoking or to reduce the number of people, especially adolescents, who take up smoking for the first time. The first type of treatment deals with the forces that keep people smoking once they have started. The second type of program deals with the factors that induce people to start.

There are many theories about what maintains smoking. One theory is that smoking is physically or psychologically addictive or both. Another theory suggests that smoking is primarily a tension release for people who are overly anxious. Support for this notion comes from reports that frequency of smoking increases and decreases with the rise and fall of stress. Theories on what motivates people to start smoking point to peer pressure and peer reinforcement, parental modeling, some set of personal traits, or some combination of all of these.

To this point, little research has been done relating personality traits to smoking. In general, the smoker is described as extraverted, somewhat neurotic, and tense. There is a sex difference, however, in that higher anxiety is found in female smokers than in male smokers. It is noteworthy that these findings relate to the factors that cause people to begin smoking, not to what keeps people smoking (Spielberger & Jacobs, 1982).

From the standpoint of stress research, the findings are consistent with an interaction model. They suggest that people with higher levels of tension and anxiety may be more vulnerable to pressures to start smoking. Given stress of the right type and intensity, they are more likely to become trapped in the smoking habit. On the other hand, strong parental models, suitable outlets for tension, guidance for constructive emotional release, and educational programs that enable teenagers to cope with pressure from peers may prevent the habit from starting. Getting people to quit smoking is just as problematic but involves another level of complexity. As indicated in the preceding paragraph, there is no evidence of personality factors related to sticking with the habit. But there is mounting evidence that smoking is a physically addictive process (Russell, 1976). This is a significant barrier to quitting.

THE ALCOHOLIC PERSONALITY

The concerns that prompted research on personality and smoking also prompted a great deal of research on the **alcoholic personality.** Drinking is related to a variety of stress-reduction and escape behaviors that indicate ineffective coping skills. Drinking also tends to increase and decrease relative to the amount of stress experienced. Alcoholics generally have higher risks for illness, more rapid mental and physical deterioration (Porjesz & Begleiter, 1982), and a higher death rate compared to nonalcoholics. Arthur Schatzkin's team found that moderate alcohol consumption increases risk for breast cancer by 50 to 100% (Schatzkin et al., 1987). The personal and social costs of drinking are staggering. The road slaughter that occurs each year because of alcohol-related auto accidents is enough to suggest that society must come to grips with this major killer.

It is now generally accepted that alcoholism has a genetic component that may be expressed in a different basal metabolism or some other physical system (Stabenau & Hesselbrock, 1983). Presumably, this makes the person more vulnerable to the addictive properties of alcohol. In addition, there is a pattern of **positive assortative mating** (alcoholics marrying alcoholics) that increases the risk of alcoholism for offspring (Hall, Hesselbrock, & Stabenau, 1983). Still, many factors intervene in the person's development to determine whether the person actually becomes alcoholic or not.

The diathesis-stress model may be one of the best theoretical models available to describe the overall mix of factors contributing to alcoholism. This model states that predisposing (risk) factors will be expressed only if a precipitating (stress) event of sufficient intensity is encountered. According to Alterman & Tarter (1983), the predisposing factors include a genetically transmitted psychological vulnerability. These factors include conduct disorders in childhood, hyperactivity, and attentional problems. Stress factors include a disordered family and disturbed family interactions, type of peers associated with, ethnic background, and deprived environment.

The emerging portrait of the alcoholic is of a person with chronic distress, externally controlled (Apao & Damon, 1982), combined with weak or ineffective psychosocial skills (Nerviano & Gross, 1983). Difficulty in psychosocial skills usually revolves around feelings of personal inadequacy, higher levels of fear than normal, and problems with concentration. These traits are revealed in conflict with authority, more frequent and intense expressions of hostility, and aggressiveness. This combination of factors may serve to reduce effectiveness on the job and in a variety of interpersonal relationships from casual social to intimate personal relationships. In the end, though, it may be an alcohol-induced myopia, the inability to process information outside a narrow range, that also contributes to the lowered inhibition on impulsive responses that leads to difficulty for the alcoholic (Steele & Josephs, 1990).

When an alcoholic hits the road, some of these characteristics may be intensified. This only serves to increase the likelihood that something bad will happen. Donovan's group proposed a model that integrates personality factors with behavior leading to **"high-risk driving"** (Donovan, Marlatt, & Salzberg, 1983). This model is presented in Figure 4-3.

BIOTYPES OR THE DISEASE-PRONE PERSONALITY: THE FINAL SCORE

This extended analysis should make one thing clear: the issues confronted by those working in this arena are very complex. The problems are of great interest and may have important practical outcomes, even though the results seem at times to be weak, inconsistent, and diffuse. On the surface, it may seem that this gives grist to the medical mill's contention that the lingering acceptance of a personality-disease connection is little more than folklore (Angell, 1985).

Friedman and Booth-Kewley (1987) take the view that the issue may not be resolved by looking at specific biotypes but in looking for a **disease-prone personality.** They conducted a meta-analysis of 101 studies that dealt with five personality variables and five diseases. The personality variables were anxiety, depression, an anger-hostility-aggression complex, an anger-hostility complex, and extraversion. The diseases were asthma, headaches, ulcers, arthritis, and heart disease. Cancer was not included because of the numerous cancers that exist.

The results are instructive. First, Friedman and Booth-Kewley obtained modest support for a personality-disease link. This comes from the fact that each disease is linked to each of the personality factors in a common fashion. In general, a higher level of any of the personality factors (more depression for example) is related to a greater likelihood of the disease. While the relationships are weak, they are statistically reliable. If there is a dominant trait, it is depression. This led the authors to suggest that depression may have been neglected in favor of the anger trait suggested by Type A research.

What is one to conclude from this finding? From this limited sample of personality variables and disease, it is apparent that the notion of biotypes is not supported. The biotypes notion would be supported only if one disease

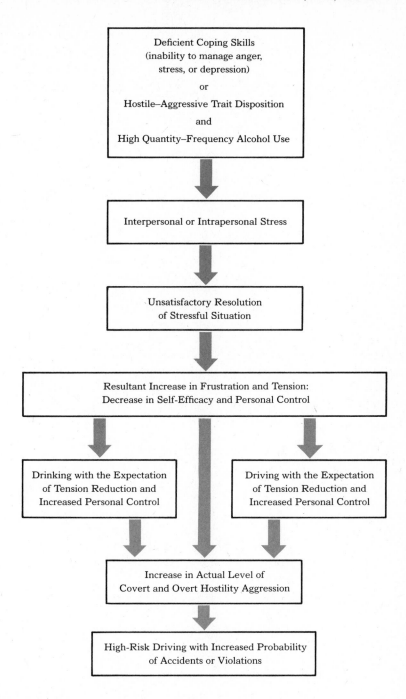

FIGURE 4-3
Hypothetical model of the effects of social-skill deficits, heavy alcohol use, and hostile-aggressive disposition on high-risk driving
SOURCE: Donovan, Marlatt, & Salzberg (1983).

reliably connected to a specific trait while another disease reliably connected to a different trait. On the other hand, the notion of a generic disease-prone personality may be acceptable. Friedman and Booth-Kewley suggest that, like diet, personality may produce imbalances that can predispose one to disease. It is not so much the specific thing you eat, but the lack of balance that presents the problem. The commonality of the traits-diseases relationship also argues against the psychosomatic model (a specific personality causes a specific disease) and against the somatopsychic model (a specific disease causes a specific personality profile).

Finally, the small correlations obtained remind us once again that health status is determined by multiple causes (Wright, 1988). These multiple paths to disease rule out simplistic explanations. The logic of this is based on the small correlations. Small correlations indicate that personality accounts for only small amounts of variability in disease. Numerous other factors must be drawn into the equation to explain the origin and progress of a disease. At the same time, as Friedman and Booth- Kewley note, the mere fact that the explained variance is small should not lead us to think it is inconsequential. The number of lives involved even in a small amount of variance can be of great consequence.

CONTROL, HARDINESS, AND SELF-ESTEEM

Three traits will be discussed here that have been linked to stress and health. These are locus of control, **psychological hardiness,** and **self-esteem.**

Locus of Control, Coping, and Mastery

The concept of locus of control comes from the work of Julian Rotter (1966, 1990). Bonnie Strickland (1989), recent president of the American Psychological Association, recognized its importance and reviewed uses of the construct in current research. Rotter (1990) believes that the thousands of studies stimulated by the construct proves its heuristic value. He suggests further that numerous other control concepts, including self-efficacy, are more or less variations on the locus of control construct.

Locus of control refers to the expectancy that personal actions will be effective to control or master the environment. In Rotter's model, people vary on a continuum between the two extremes of **external** and **internal locus of control.** Lefcourt (1976), a protege of Rotter's, defined external control as the perception that positive or negative events are unrelated to one's own behavior and thus are beyond personal control. External people view most events as dependent on chance or controlled by powers beyond human reach.

The internal person, on the other hand, feels that few events are outside the realm of human influence. Even cataclysmic events may be altered for good through human action. Lefcourt (1976) defined internal control as the perception that positive or negative events are a consequence of personal actions and thus may potentially be under personal control. If the theme song of the external is "Cast Your Fate to the Wind" the theme of the internal is "I Did It My Way."

Internal people as a group seem to have more efficient cognitive systems. They expend a substantial amount of mental energy obtaining information that will enable them to influence events of personal importance. They expend greater efforts to cope with or achieve mastery over their personal, social, and work environments (Phares, 1976). Internal people also show a greater tendency to implement a specific plan of action. As Phares (1976) noted, "Whether one terms it action taking, confronting, or mastery, internals seem to be more disposed toward behavior that will enhance their personal efficacy, even in the sense of rectifying inadequacies" (p. 66). In this way, a sense of mastery may develop that enables them to cope more successfully with stressful events. Phares's research also suggests that locus of control is malleable.

A number of investigations have linked locus of control to coping with stress and dealing with family or personal health problems (Donham, Ludenia, Sands, & Holzer, 1983; Ludenia & Donham, 1983). One review (Averill, 1973) outlined three major types of personal control. These are behavioral control, which involves some direct action; cognitive control, which primarily reflects a personal interpretation of events; and decisional control, which means the person has a choice among several different courses of action. The author stated that

> each type of control is related to stress in a complex fashion, sometimes increasing it, sometimes reducing it, and sometimes having no influence at all . . . the relationship of personal control to stress is primarily a function of the meaning of . . . control . . . for the individual. (Averill, 1973, p. 286)

Locus of control seems to be important in health behavior. One study of tubercular patients showed that internally oriented patients had much more knowledge about their disease than externally oriented patients did. This is noteworthy because the information they obtained was negative. Results such as this are interpreted as consistent with the idea that internals are knowledge seekers. The results may also relate to internals' belief that they can do something positive to influence the outcome of the disease process if they have appropriate information (Lefcourt, 1976).

Health service providers face several difficult problems with their clients. These include the facts that people (1) are not highly motivated to engage in effective preventive health care and (2) do not follow prescribed medical programs very carefully when sick. Abella and Heslin (1984) guessed the problem might be related to locus of control. That is, people who are internally oriented might be motivated to control aspects of their environment related to their own health. On the other hand, externally oriented people might not be so motivated, because personal actions are perceived to be unrelated to either positive or negative outcomes. The outcome of the study suggests that the person who both values health and has an internal locus of control is most likely to engage in preventive health behavior.

Psychological Hardiness

Some people seem especially resilient and unflappable. Stress rolls off with little or no apparent disruption to their actions or feelings. Suzanne Kobasa (1979a, 1979b) provided evidence that personality plays a significant role in helping us resist stress-related illnesses. She says resilient people have psychological hardiness. According to Kobasa, three major traits contribute to hardiness: control, commitment, and challenge. *Control* is defined and measured as locus of control, described in the previous section. *Commitment* is a sense of self and purpose. *Challenge* reflects the degree to which safety, stability, and predictability are important. Those with high hardiness are described as having a well-integrated sense of self and purpose. In addition, they see change as stimulating and as providing them with opportunity for growth.

In one study of 137 male business executives, Kobasa and her colleagues looked at both hardiness and exercise as buffers against illness (Kobasa, Maddi, & Puccetti, 1982). They found that stressful life events increased illness, whereas both hardiness and exercise reduced illness. In this sample, the more stress increased, the more exercise and hardiness proved their worth as buffers. Executives who were rated lowest in hardiness and exercised the least had the highest rate of illness. Conversely, those who were rated high in hardiness and exercised the most had the lowest rate of illness. Kobasa (1982) also observed the positive buffering effect of hardiness in a sample of lawyers.

Since then, many studies have focused on the relationship of hardiness to health behaviors. Hannah (1988) observed that hardiness results in more appropriate health behaviors only when it is also combined with high health concern. Nagy and Nix (1989) showed that hardiness is related to both lower stress and preventive health attitudes. Susan Pollock (1989) showed that hardiness is related, directly or indirectly, to physiological and psychological adaptation in chronically ill adults. The direct route is the influence of hardiness on the perception of illness. Pollock suggested that hardiness directly influences the perception of illness. She also believes that coping efforts and social supports indirectly influence adaptation. Hardy people appear to engage in more active coping and draw on more resources than the less hardy do.

Contrada (1989) showed that hardiness is associated with reduced diastolic blood pressure under conditions of laboratory stress. This relates specifically to the challenge component of hardiness. Contrada also assessed TABP using the traditional SI and JAS and found that the hardiness construct added significantly to the prediction of diastolic blood pressure (DBP) beyond the Type A construct. Those who were strongest Type B and strongest on the hardiness measure had the lowest DBP. Allred and Smith (1989) found that hardy subjects gave more positive self-statements under conditions of threat, but they question the presumed organic link of hardiness and health.

Hannah and Morrissey (1987) found that hardiness develops with age in adolescents. Hardiness or resiliency also may explain the extraordinary adaptation of children and adolescents raised in adverse environments (Neiman, 1988; Richmond & Beardslee, 1988). It buffers against burnout in stressful occupations such as intensive-care nursing (Lambert & Lambert, 1987; Rich & Rich, 1987). In the case of intensive-care nursing, commitment appears to be the main hardiness ingredient.

Since Kobasa proposed the hardiness construct, it has been subjected to close and critical scrutiny. There is evidence that hardiness has many faces. The existential constructs of self-actualization and inner-directedness bear more than just surface similarity (Campbell, Amerikaner, Swank, & Vincent, 1989). Another term frequently used is *resiliency* (Werner, 1984). Gary Leak and Dale Williams (1989) noted that the commitment component of hardiness is similar to Alfred Adler's notion of social interest.

Frederick Rhodewalt and Joan Zone (1989) conducted one of the more interesting studies of hardiness. They compared adult women who were divided into hardy and nonhardy groups. Their results support the contention that hardiness may be more important when it is absent than when it is present. In this view, nonhardy people tend to appraise more events as undesirable and report that negative events require more adjustment. Thus, negative affect combined with more difficulty in coping may be the core of higher stress, more so than hardiness providing special resiliency.

Self-Esteem, Stress, and Coping

The term *self-esteem* is frequently used to refer to a sense of positive self-regard. In the simplest possible terms, it is feeling good about yourself. Self-esteem is sometimes confused with **self-concept**. *Self-concept* is a very broad term that includes all the ways in which people compare themselves to others and evaluate themselves physically, mentally, and socially. Self-esteem thus feeds into self-concept. Recent research suggests that self-esteem is made up of three psychosocial factors and two physical factors (Fleming & Courtney, 1984). The three psychosocial factors are self-regard, social confidence, and school ability. The two physical factors are appearance and ability.

The relationship of self-esteem to coping is complex. It includes feedback from many previous successful or unsuccessful attempts at coping. When people feel good about themselves, they are less likely to respond to or interpret an event as emotionally loaded or stressful. In addition, they cope better when stress does occur. This feeds back positive information that further increases self-esteem.

Many investigators have been trying to determine what specific aspects of self-esteem are more closely related to coping failure and success. When low-esteem people are put in a threat situation, they tend to show both poorer overall coping and lower overall competency. According to Rosen, Terry, and Leventhal (1982) the difficulty with coping in low-esteem people can be traced to two basic negative self-perceptions. First, low-esteem people have higher levels of fear under threat than do high-esteem people. Second, low-esteem people perceive themselves as having inadequate skills to deal with threat. They are less interested in taking preventive steps and seem to have more fatalistic beliefs that they cannot do anything to prevent bad things from happening. They are a step behind at the start because they believe they cannot cope.

SUMMARY

In this chapter, a variety of personality theories have been reviewed that are specifically related to issues of stress and health. Several biotypes have been shown to have at best weak links to health, while others appear more strongly related to vulnerability to stress or specific health problems. The Type A behavior pattern was reviewed at some length. This action-emotion complex appears to have a strong toxic core of hostility that more accurately predicts coronary risk than global Type A measures do. Two general themes emerge from this literature. First, negative affect is the central ingredient in most studies that look for a relationship of illness to personality. Second, a general illness- or disease-prone personality may exist, but the notion of specific personalities predicting specific diseases does not receive substantive support.

KEY TERMS

alcoholic personality
alcoholism,
    and high-risk
    driving
biotypes
bipolar depression
cancer-prone
    personality
coronary, risk
    factors for
depression
depression-prone
    personality
disease-prone
    personality
dispositional theory
extraversion

hypertensive
    personality
introversion
locus of control,
    health behavior
locus of control,
    external
locus of control,
    internal
personality, definition
positive assortative
    mating
psychoanalytic
    theory
psychological
    hardiness
psychosomatic

self-concept
self-esteem, and stress
smoking, and
    personality
somatopsychic
state anxiety
test anxiety
trait anxiety
trait theory
Type A behavior
    pattern
Type A, and anger
Type A, and coronary
    risk
typology
Western Collaborative
    Group Study

REFERENCES

Abella, R., & Heslin, R. (1984, May). *Health locus of control, values, and the behavior of family and friends: An integrated approach to understanding preventive health behavior.* Paper presented at the Midwestern Psychological Association Conference, Chicago.

Alexander, F. (1939). Emotional factors in essential hypertension. *Psychosomatic Medicine, 1,* 173–179.

Alexander, F. (1950). *Psychosomatic medicine: Its principles and applications.* New York: Norton.

Allport, G. W. (1961). *Pattern and growth in personality.* New York: Holt, Rinehart & Winston.

Allred, K., & Smith, T. W. (1989). The hardy personality: Cognitive and physiological responses to evaluative threat. *Journal of Personality and Social Psychology, 56,* 257–266.

Alterman, A. I., & Tarter, R. E. (1983). The transmission of psychological vulnerability: Implications for alcoholism etiology. *The Journal of Nervous and Mental Disease, 171,* 147–154.

Angell, M. (1985). Disease as a reflection of the psyche. *The New England Journal of Medicine, 312,* 1570–1572.

Apao, W. K., & Damon, A. M. (1982). Locus of control and the quantity-frequency index of alcohol use. *Journal of Studies on Alcohol, 43,* 233–239.

Averill, J. R. (1973). Personal control over aversive stimuli and its relationship to stress. *Psychological Bulletin, 80,* 286–303.

Barofsky, I. (1981). Issues and approaches to the psychosocial assessment of the cancer patient. In C. K. Prokop & L. A. Bradley, (Eds.), *Medical psychology: Contributions to behavioral medicine* (pp. 55–65). New York: Academic Press.

Blumenthal, J. A., Barefoot, J., Burg, M. M., & Williams, R. B. (1987). Psychological correlates of hostility among patients undergoing coronary angiography. *British Journal of Medical Psychology, 60,* 349–355.

Booth, G. (1969). General and organ–specific object relationships in cancer. *Annals of the New York Academy of Sciences, 164,* 568–577.

Booth-Kewley, S., & Friedman, H. S. (1987). Psychological predictors of heart disease: A quantitative review. *Psychological Bulletin, 101,* 343–362.

Boyd, D. P., & Begley, T. M. (1987). Assessing the Type A behavior pattern with the Jenkins Activity Survey. *British Journal of Medical Psychology, 60,* 155–161.

Byrne, D. G., & Whyte, H. M. (1983–1984). State and trait anxiety correlates of illness behavior in survivors of myocardial infarction. *International Journal of Psychiatry in Medicine, 13,* 1–9.

Campbell, J. M., Amerikaner, M., Swank, P., & Vincent, K. (1989). The relationship between the Hardiness Test and the Personal Orientation Inventory. *Journal of Research in Personality, 23,* 373–380.

Contrada, R. J. (1989). Type A behavior, personality hardiness, and cardiovascular responses to stress. *Journal of Personality and Social Psychology, 57,* 895–903.

Cunningham, A. J. (1985). The influence of mind on cancer. *Canadian Psychology, 26,* 13–29.

Dattore, P. J., Shontz, F. C., & Coyne, L. (1980). Premorbid personality differentiation of cancer and noncancer groups: A test of the hypothesis of cancer proneness. *Journal of Consulting and Clinical Psychology, 48,* 388–394.

Dembroski, T. M., & Costa, P. (1987). Coronary prone behavior: Components of the Type A pattern and hostility. *Journal of Personality, 55,* 211–235.

Dimsdale, J. E. (1988). A perspective on Type A behavior and coronary disease. *The New England Journal of Medicine, 318,* 110–112.

Donham, G. W., Ludenia, K., Sands, M. M., & Holzer, P. D. (1983). Personality correlates of health locus of control with medical inpatients. *Psychological Reports, 52,* 659–666.

Donovan, D. M., Marlatt, G. A., & Salzberg, P. M. (1983). Drinking behavior, personality factors and high-risk driving: A review and theoretical formulation. *Journal of Studies on Alcohol, 44,* 395–428.

Eysenck, H. J. (1987). Anxiety, learned helplessness, and cancer: A causal theory. *Journal of Anxiety Disorders, 1,* 87–104.

Ferguson, W. E. (1981). Gifted adolescents, stress, and life changes. *Adolescence, 16,* 973–985.

Fleming, J. S., & Courtney, B. E. (1984). The dimensionality of self–esteem: II. Hierarchical facet model for revised measurement scales. *Journal of Personality and Social Psychology, 46,* 404–421.

Friedman, H. S., & Booth-Kewley, S. (1987). The "disease-prone personality": A meta-analytic view of the construct. *American Psychologist, 42,* 539–555.

Friedman, M., & Rosenman, R. H. (1974). *Type A behavior and your heart.* New York: Knopf.

Garron, D. C., & Leavitt, R. (1983). Chronic low back pain and depression. *Journal of Clinical Psychology, 39,* 486–493.

Glass, D. C. (1977). Stress, behavior patterns, and coronary disease. *American Scientist, 65,* 177–187.

Goldband, S. (1980). Stimulus specificity of physiological response to stress and the Type A coronary-prone behavior pattern. *Journal of Personality and Social Psychology, 39,* 670–679.

Goldstein, I. B. (1981). Assessment of hypertension. In C. K. Prokop & L. A. Bradley (Eds.), *Medical psychology: Contributions to behavioral medicine* (pp. 37–54). New York: Academic Press.

Greer, S., & Morris, T. (1975). Psychological attributes of women who develop breast cancer: A controlled study. *Journal of Psychosomatic Research, 19,* 147–153.

Grimm, L. G., & Yarnold, P. R. (1984). Performance standards and the Type A behavior pattern. *Cognitive Therapy and Research, 8,* 59–66.

Hall, R. L., Hesselbrock, V. M., & Stabenau, J. R. (1983). Familial distribution of alcohol use: I. Assortative mating in the parents of alcoholics. *Behavior Genetics, 13,* 361–372.

Hannah, T. E. (1988). Hardiness and health behavior: The role of health concern as a moderator variable. *Behavioral Medicine, 14,* 59–63.

Hannah, T. E., & Morrissey, C. (1987). Correlates of psychological hardiness in Canadian adolescents. *The Journal of Social Psychology, 127,* 339–344.

Howard, J. H., Cunningham, D. A., & Rechnitzer, P. A. (1976). Health patterns associated with Type A behavior: A managerial population. *Journal of Human Stress, 2,* 24–31.

Irvine, J., Lyle, R. C., & Allon, R. (1982). Type A personality as psychopathology: Personality correlates and an abbreviated scoring system. *Journal of Psychosomatic Research, 26,* 183–189.

Jenkins, C. D., Zyzanski, S. J., & Rosenman, R. H. (1965). *Jenkins Activity Survey.* New York: The Psychological Corporation.

Jones, N. F., Kinsman, R. A., Dirks, J. F., & Dahlem, N. W. (1979). Psychological contributions to chronicity in asthma: Patient response styles influencing medical treatment and its outcome. *Medical Care, 17,* 1103–1118.

Kaptein, A. A. (1982). Psychological correlates of length of hospitalization and rehospitalization in patients with acute, severe asthma. *Social Science and Medicine, 16,* 725–729.

Katz, J., Ackerman, P., Rothwax, R., Sachar, E. J., Weiner, H., Hellman, L., & Gallagher, T. F. (1970). Psychoendocrine aspects of cancer of the breast. *Psychosomatic Medicine, 32,* 1–18.

Kissen, D. M. (1967). Psychosocial factors, personality and lung cancer in men aged 55–64. *British Journal of Medical Psychology, 40,* 29–43.

Kobasa, S. C. (1979a). Personality and resistance to illness. *American Journal of Community Psychology, 7,* 413–423.

Kobasa, S. C. (1979b). Stressful life events, personality and health: An inquiry into hardiness. *Journal of Personality and Social Psychology, 37,* 1–11.

Kobasa, S. C. (1982). Commitment and coping in stress resistance among lawyers. *Journal of Personality and Social Psychology, 42,* 707–717.

Kobasa, S. C., Maddi, S. R., & Puccetti, M. C. (1982). Personality and exercise as buffers in the stress-illness relationship. *Journal of Behavioral Medicine, 5,* 391–404.

Kuller, L., Neaton, J., Caggiula, A., & Falvo-Gerard, L. (1980). Primary prevention of heart attacks: The Multiple Risk Factor Intervention Trial. *American Journal of Epidemiology, 112,* 185–199.

Kutash, I. L., Schlesinger, L. B., & Associates (Eds.). (1980). *Handbook on stress and anxiety.* San Francisco: Jossey-Bass.

Lambert, C. E., & Lambert, V. A. (1987). Hardiness: Its development and relevance to nursing. *Image: Journal of Nursing Scholarship, 19,* 92–95.

Leak, G. K., & Williams, D. E. (1989). Relationship between social interest, alienation, and psychological hardiness. *Individual Psychology, 45,* 369–375.

Lefcourt, H. M. (1976). *Locus of control: Current trends in theory and research.* Hillsdale, NJ: Lawrence Erlbaum Associates.

Levy, S. M., & Wise, B. D. (1987). Psychosocial risk factors, natural immunity, and cancer progression: Implications for intervention. *Current Psychological Research and Reviews, 6,* 229–243.

Liebert, R. M., & Spiegler, M. D. (1982). *Personality: Strategies and issues.* Pacific Grove, CA: Brooks/Cole.

Lloyd, G. G., & Cawley, R. H. (1983). Distress or illness? A study of psychological symptoms after myocardial infarction. *British Journal of Psychiatry, 142,* 120–125.

Lovallo, W. R., & Pishkin, V. (1980). A psychophysiological comparison of Type A and B men exposed to failure and uncontrollable noise. *Psychophysiology, 17,* 29–36.

Ludenia, K., & Donham, G. W. (1983). Dental outpatients: Health locus of control correlates. *Journal of Clinical Psychology, 39,* 854–858.

Matthews, K. A., Glass, D. C., Rosenman, R. H., & Bortner, R. W. (1977). Competitive drive, Pattern A and coronary heart disease: A further analysis of some data from the Western Collaborative Group Study. *Journal of Chronic Diseases, 30,* 489–498.

Millon, T. (1982). On the nature of clinical health psychology. In T. Millon, C. Green, & R. Meagher (Eds.), *Handbook of clinical health psychology* (pp. 1–27). New York: Plenum.

Mitchell, R. E., Cronkite, R. C., & Moos, R. H. (1983). Stress, coping, and depression among married couples. *Journal of Abnormal Psychology, 92,* 433–448.

Morrison, F. R., & Paffenbarger, R. A. (1981). Epidemiological aspects of biobehavior in the etiology of cancer: A critical review. In S. M. Weiss, J. A. Herd, & B. H. Fox (Eds.), *Perspectives on behavioral medicine* (pp. 135–161). New York: Academic Press.

Mueser, K. T., Yarnold, P. R., & Bryant, F. B. (1987). Type A behaviour and time urgency: Perception of time adjectives. *British Journal of Medical Psychology, 60,* 267–269.

Nagy, S., & Nix, C. L. (1989). Relations between preventive health behavior and hardiness. *Psychological Reports, 65,* 339–345.

Neiman, L. (1988). A critical review of resiliency literature and its relevance to homeless children. *Children's Environments Quarterly, 5,* 17–25.

Nerviano, V. J., & Gross, H. W. (1983). Personality types of alcoholics on objective inventories: A review. *Journal of Studies on Alcohol, 44,* 837–851.

Newlin, D. B., & Levenson, R. W. (1982). Cardiovascular responses of individuals with Type A behavior pattern and parental coronary heart disease. *Journal of Psychosomatic Research, 26,* 393–402.

Phares, E. J. (1976). *Locus of control in personality.* Morristown, NJ: General Learning Press.

Pilowsky, I., Spalding, D., Shaw, J., & Korner, P. I. (1973). Hypertension and personality. *Psychosomatic Medicine, 35,* 50–56.

Pollock, S. E. (1989). The hardiness characteristic: A motivating factor in adaptation. *Advances in Nursing Science, 11,* 53–62.

Porjesz, B., & Begleiter, H. (1982). Evoked brain potential deficits in alcoholism and aging. *Alcoholism: Clinical and Experimental Research, 6,* 53–63.

Ragland, D. R., & Brand, R. J. (1988). Type A behavior and mortality from coronary heart disease. *The New England Journal of Medicine, 318,* 65–69.

Rhodewalt, F., & Zone, J. B. (1989). Appraisal of life-change, depression, and illness in hardy and nonhardy women. *Journal of Personality and Social Psychology, 56,* 81–88.

Rich, V. L., & Rich, A. R. (1987). Personality hardiness and burnout in female staff nurses. *Image: Journal of Nursing Scholarship, 19,* 63–66.

Richmond, J. B., & Beardslee, W. R. (1988). Resiliency: Research and practical implications for pediatricians. *Journal of Developmental and Behavioral Pediatrics, 9,* 157–163.

Rosen, T. J., Terry, N. S., & Leventhal, H. (1982). The role of esteem and coping in response to a threat communication. *Journal of Research in Personality, 16,* 90–107.

Rosenhan, D. L., & Seligman, M. E. P. (1989). *Abnormal psychology* (2nd ed.). New York: Norton.

Rosenman, R. H., & Friedman, M. (1961). Association of specific behavior pattern in women with blood and cardiovascular findings. *Circulation, 24,* 1173–1184.

Rosenman, R. H., & Friedman, M. (1974). Neurogenic factors in pathogenesis of coronary heart disease. *Medical Clinics of North America, 58,* 269–279.

Rosenman, R. H., & Friedman, M. (1977). Modifying Type A behaviour pattern. *Journal of Psychosomatic Research, 21,* 323–331.

Rosenman, R. H., Friedman, M., Straus, R., Jenkins, C. D., Zyzanski, S. J., & Wurm, M. (1970). Coronary heart disease in the Western Collaborative Group Study: A follow-up experience of 4½ years. *Journal of Chronic Disease, 23,* 173–190.

Rosenman, R. H., Friedman, M., Straus, R., Wurm, M., Kositcheck, R., Hahn, W., & Werthessen, N. T. (1964). A predictive study of coronary heart disease: The Western Collaborative Group Study. *Journal of the American Medical Association, 189,* 15–22.

Rotter, J. B. (1966). Generalized expectancies for internal versus external control of reinforcement. *Psychological Monographs, 80.*

Rotter, J. B. (1990). Internal versus external control of reinforcement: A case history of a variable. *American Psychologist, 45,* 489–493.

Russell, M. A. H. (1976). Tobacco smoking and nicotine dependence. In R. J. Gibbins, Y. Israel, H. Kalant, R. E. Popham, W. Schmidt, & R. G. Smart (Eds.), *Research advances in alcohol and drug problems* (Vol. 3, pp. 1–47). New York: Wiley.

Schatzkin, A., Jones, Y., Hoover, R. N., Taylor, P. R., Brinton, L. A., Ziegler, R. G., et al. (1987). Alcohol consumption and breast cancer in the epidemiologic follow-up study of the first national health and nutrition examination survey. *The New England Journal of Medicine, 316,* 1169–1173.

Scherwitz, L., Graham, L. E., Grandits, G., & Billings, J. (1987). Speech characteristics and behavior-type assessment in the Multiple Risk Factor Intervention Trial (MRFIT) structured interviews. *Journal of Behavioral Medicine, 10,* 173–195.

Scherwitz, L., Graham, L. E., Grandits, G., Buehler, J., & Billings, J. (1986). Self-involvement and coronary heart disease incidence in the Multiple Risk Factor Intervention Trial. *Psychosomatic Medicine, 48,* 187–199.

Shekelle, R. B., Gale, M., Ostfeld, A. M., & Paul, O. (1983). Hostility, risk of coronary heart disease, and mortality. *Psychosomatic Medicine, 45,* 109–114.

Shekelle, R. B., Schoenberger, J. A., & Stamler, J. (1976). Correlates of the JAS Type A behavior pattern score. *Journal of Chronic Disease, 29,* 381–394.

Sparacino, J., Ronchi, D., Brenner, M., Kuhn, J. W., & Flesch, A. L. (1982). Psychological correlates of blood pressure: A closer examination of hostility, anxiety, and engagement. *Nursing Research, 31,* 143–149.

Spielberger, C. D. (1966). Theory and research on anxiety. In C. D. Spielberger (Ed.), *Anxiety and behavior* (pp. 1–22). New York: Academic Press.

Spielberger, C. D., & Jacobs, G. A. (1982). Personality and smoking behavior. *Journal of Personality Assessment, 46,* 396–403.

Stabenau, J. R., & Hesselbrock, V. M. (1983). Family pedigree of alcoholic and control patients. *The International Journal of the Addictions, 18,* 351–363.

Steele, C. M., & Josephs, R. A. (1990). Alcohol myopia: Its prized and dangerous effects. *American Psychologist, 45,* 921–933.

Strickland, B. (1989). Internal-external control expectancies: From contingency to creativity. *American Psychologist, 44,* 1–12.

Subcommittee on Juvenile Justice. (1985). *Teenage suicide* (Serial No. J-98-143). Washington, DC: U.S. Government Printing Office.

Suinn, R. M. (1975). The cardiac stress management program for Type A patients. *Cardiac Rehabilitation, 5,* 13–15.

Sytkowski, P. A., Kannel, W. B., & D'Agostino, R. B. (1990). Changes in risk factors and the decline in mortality from cardiovascular disease. *The New England Journal of Medicine, 322,* 1635–1641.

Taylor, P., Abrams, D., & Hewstone, M. (1988). Cancer, stress and personality: A correlational investigation of life-events, repression–sensitization and locus of control. *British Journal of Medical Psychology, 61,* 179–183.

United States Department of Commerce, Bureau of the Census. (1979). *Statistical Abstract of the United States* (100th ed). Washington, DC: U.S. Government Printing Office.

van Doornen, L. J. P. (1980). The Coronary Risk Personality: Psychological and psychophysiological aspects. *Psychotherapy and Psychosomatics, 34,* 204–215.

van Egeren, L. F., Fabrega, H., & Thornton, D. W. (1983). Electrocardiographic effects of social stress on coronary-prone (Type A) individuals. *Psychosomatic Medicine, 45,* 195–203.

Waldron, I., Zyzanski, S., Shekelle, R. B., Jenkins, C. D., & Tannebaum, S. (1977). The coronary-prone behavior pattern in employed men and women. *Journal of Human Stress, 3,* 2–18.

Werner, E. E. (1984). Resilient children. *Young Children, 40,* 68–72.

Wright, L. (1988). The Type A behavior pattern and coronary artery disease. *American Psychologist, 43,* 2–14.

Yarnold, P. R., & Grimm, L. G. (1982a, May). *Interpersonal dominance and coronary-prone behavior.* Paper presented at the 3rd Annual Meeting of the Society of Behavioral Medicine, Chicago.

Yarnold, P. R., & Grimm, L. G. (1982b). Time urgency among coronary-prone individuals. *Journal of Abnormal Psychology, 91,* 175–177.

CHAPTER 5

The Physiology of Stress: The Brain, Body, and Immune Systems

IT IS HIGHLY DISHONORABLE FOR A REASONABLE SOUL TO LIVE IN SO DIVINELY BUILT A MANSION AS THE BODY SHE RESIDES IN, ALTOGETHER UNACQUAINTED WITH THE EXQUISITE STRUCTURE OF IT.
ROBERT BOYLE

The body is perhaps the most beautiful and intricate, yet efficient, machine ever devised. The more we come to understand its design, the more we admire its perfection. Still, the more we understand its intricacies, the more mystery seems to unfold. For every door opened in the labyrinth of the body, research discovers more doors that need to be opened.

The next few pages will provide a tour through the body beautiful, the body functioning at its normative best. We will discuss six systems: the nervous, respiratory, endocrine, immune, cardiovascular, and digestive systems. I selected these systems because (1) stress research suggests they play a prominent role in defensive reactions of the body, (2) these are the systems we most frequently abuse through misbehavior, and (3) we can influence these systems through modest behavioral and/or attitudinal lifestyle changes.

MIND, BRAIN, AND BODY: SOME DEFINITIONS

The terms **mind,** *brain,* and *body* will be used frequently in this discussion. The issue of mind/body relationships has been a thorn in the flesh of science for a long time. It is necessary, therefore, to make clear how these terms will be used.

In this book, *mind* will be used to mean all the processes of the brain, whether we are aware of these processes as they occur or not. *Mind* describes what is happening when we remember, make decisions, solve problems, reason, reflect, and observe our own reflections. The *mental system* will refer to the interconnected operations of the mind; for example, perceiving, evaluating, and reflecting on and responding to external stimuli. The term *brain* refers to the mass of neural tissue housed in the skull.

There is no dispute that the brain is a physical organ. Yet the way it behaves and our awareness of this behavior makes the brain difficult to talk about without considering its uniqueness. Terms such as *mind* and *mental process* capture that uniqueness adequately. There is little need to become bogged down in a mind/body dispute that is now centuries old. No one has proposed a satisfactory resolution to this conflict yet. In addition, no empirical data or logic will resolve the issue to everyone's satisfaction. As William Uttal (1978) noted, "in almost all cases, it [the debate] will necessarily be based on softer criteria including ones based on emotion, values, and intuitive and aesthetic judgments of consistency, completeness, or productiveness" (p. 81).

CHARTING THE BACK ROADS OF THE MIND

Tracking the flow of information through a system as complex as the body is not an easy job. The problem is all the more difficult because neural control is maintained through an intricate system of checks and balances, including duplicate pathways and feedback circuits that keep things running smoothly—most of the time. Duplication of pathways (called *redundancy*) makes it possible for one part of the brain or body to communicate with other parts even when one pathway is jammed. Feedback circuits allow the brain to *attenuate* (regulate or modify) new input at different stages of processing. In spite of this complexity, scientists have made exciting progress that moves us closer to understanding the body's most complex organ.

THE BRAIN: ITS ROLE IN STRESS AND HEALTH

The brain still conceals many mysteries. It is among the last frontiers of our quest to understand the body. Details of the brain's structure and functions are remarkably intricate. If we waded into this tangled web without some perspective, we could soon lose our bearings. This is the perennial forest-and-trees problem. Before proceeding, then, a brief example may help.

First, imagine you are taking a walk late in the evening. You round a corner and a mugger jumps out and demands money. In what may seem like an eternity to you, the brain has already invoked thousands of connections. It has tapped relevant experiences and information about muggings. It quickly calculates such things as the size of the mugger; the type of weapon, if any; and even something as subtle as the robber's disposition and seriousness of intent. Meanwhile, your body mobilizes its energy for the emergency. You may feel your heart racing, palms sweating, knees knocking. In a flash, you may consider several possible plans of action. Should I run? Scream? Fight? Talk? Give in without resistance? Just as quickly you may estimate the risk of these various plans.

In broad sweep, here is probably what happened. Under normal conditions, the brain monitors a great amount of data simultaneously. Centers in the old brain (the brainstem region) act in combination with motivational and emotional centers to establish priorities for processing. The sight of a dangerous felon instantly and automatically leads to suspension of voluntary processing to attend to survival needs. At the cognitive level, the brain matches the event to existing schemata, including event scripts that may guide behavior. Personality traits probably also interact with event data to bias the interpretation and the action plans.

At the biologic level, the brain activates descending pathways of neural and hormonal control. The result may be increased output from the pituitary, elevated adrenal flow, increased blood pressure, and increased heart rate. Normally, the neural-hormonal systems that regulate this adaptive reflex operate as negative feedback loops. That is, they feed back data to a brain comparator that recognizes when an adequate adaptive response exists. Then the negative feedback loop inhibits or shuts down further activation. After a time, the body returns to normal arousal levels.

Yet, with chronic stressors this negative feedback loop can malfunction, allowing the biological system to flood itself with its own chemicals. The body's defenses then work continuously at high speed. This can lead to alterations in numerous biologic systems, including the immune system. In the early stages, these bodily changes may go undetected because they are so subtle. Still, the long-term effects can include alterations that affect structural integrity and result in serious physical illness. Later, the body loses its ability to resist added stressors and shows signs of exhaustion. You should recognize this as the General Adaptation Syndrome we discussed in Chapter 1.

The Literal Brain

Earlier in this book, the notion of the literal brain (Pelletier, 1977) was introduced. Simply stated, the brain makes no distinction between actual threat and imagined threat. A thought is just as important to the mind as an external event. To the brain, perceived threat is simply threat. When threat is present, the brain sounds the alert, and the body begins mobilizing defensive reactions. In this way, the brain induces change in life-sustaining functions even when only perceived threat is present. In the next few pages, we will look at the components of this literal brain. In the process, we will detail the ways in which these various components function in stress reactions.

Functional Neuroanatomy: A Primer

The nervous system consists of two divisions, the **central nervous system (CNS)** and the **peripheral nervous system (PNS).** The central nervous system contains the brain and spinal cord. The peripheral nervous system is comprised of two subsystems, the **autonomic nervous system (ANS)** and the **somatic nervous system (SNS).** Finally, the autonomic nervous system has two major parts, the **parasympathetic** and the **sympathetic nervous systems.** Figure 5-1 summarizes these divisions. For this discussion we will confine our attention to the brain and autonomic nervous system, since these systems play the major role in the stress response.

Divisions of the Nervous System

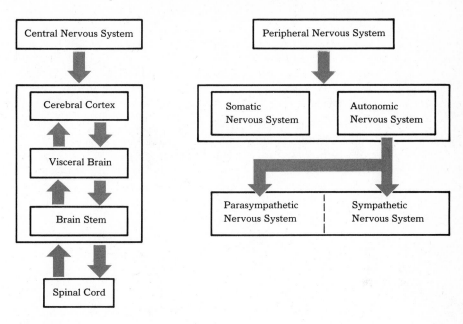

FIGURE 5-1
Major divisions of the nervous system

Neuroanatomists, scientists who specialize in mapping the structure of the brain, now recognize several layers of tissue in the brain. Each layer represents a distinct stage in the brain's development. From old to new, these layers are the brain stem; the visceral brain (comprised of many different parts); and the new brain (neocortex), or cerebral cortex.

The Brain Stem

The **brain stem** is a bulblike outgrowth at the top of the spinal column. It houses control centers that involuntarily regulate vital life functions. The brain stem centers that we will be concerned with include the **medulla** and the **reticular formation (RF).** Figure 5-2 shows these structures.

The medulla is like a neural Grand Central Station. It contains nerve fibers arriving from the body and departing the brain through the spinal cord. Two types of nerve fibers leave the brain through this concourse: the autonomic nerves, which control many visceral activities, and the motor nerves (corticospinal tract), which govern muscle control (Liebman, 1979).

The most important brain stem centers, the *autonomic nuclei,* carry on life-support processes such as respiration, heart action, and digestion. For example, the brain stem respiratory center regulates the rhythmic nature of breathing.

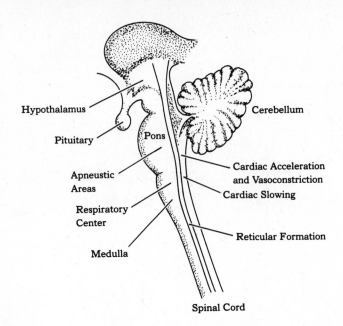

Hypothalamus

Cerebellum

Pituitary

Pons

Apneustic
Areas

Cardiac Acceleration
and Vasoconstriction

Cardiac Slowing

Respiratory
Center

Reticular Formation

Medulla

Spinal Cord

FIGURE 5-2
Brain stem and reticular system with cardiovascular and respiratory control centers

In normal states, breathing occurs at an even pace (about 12 breaths per minute) and with good balance between inspiration and exhalation (about 2 seconds and 3 seconds respectively) (Guyton, 1977).

Stress can alter this balance, as some everyday situations illustrate. Anxiety over public speaking can result in the appearance of being out of breath. If someone runs a red light in front of you, your breathing might stop momentarily; then you would breathe rapidly for a short while. During such stressful events, the cerebral cortex signals the autonomic respiratory nuclei, which in turn signals the respiratory system. Then, the balance of inhalation and exhalation is tipped in the direction of more inhalation, or very deep breathing. This puts more oxygen in the blood than normal. Probably the most common reaction to a stressor is an increase in the rate of breathing.

Anxiety Hyperventilation

A condition called **anxiety hyperventilation** shows what can happen under extreme stress. In hyperventilation, excessive ventilation of the blood supply occurs as it tries to release carbon dioxide. When this happens, the person feels dizzy, perhaps even to the point of blacking out. Shortness of breath occurs, and the heart pounds. The person may experience *parathesia,* a numbness or tingling in parts of the body. This heightens anxiety because people typically perceive these symptoms as an impending heart attack. This is not only uncomfortable, it can be very frightening.

Clinicians regard hyperventilation as a psychogenic reaction. In other words, it is a condition that comes from psychological traits and social circumstances, not from physical pathology. The condition can be relieved in one of two ways. One is to breathe voluntarily at a measured slow pace or to hold the breath for short periods. The other is to breathe into a paper bag and rebreathe the same air. One research group showed that practiced breathing and relaxation is an effective treatment for hyperventilation and resulting chest pain (Hegel et al., 1989).

Control over the activity of the heart also comes from autonomic nuclei in the brain stem. Both the sympathetic and parasympathetic sides of the autonomic system operate to keep the heart pumping smoothly. The sympathetic system drives the heart to higher rates when necessary. Sometimes it can drive the heart to beat as many as 250 beats per minute (normal heart rate is 70 beats per minute). The action of the sympathetic system also increases the strength of the heartbeat. The parasympathetic system moderates the strength of the beat and decreases the rate.

The Reticular Formation

The reticular formation is a bundle of fibers that runs like a great rope through the middle of the brain stem upward into the hypothalamus and thalamus. It may be viewed as the great sentry system of the brain. The work of the RF is threefold: two-way communication between brain and body, selection (gating) of sensory information for processing by the cerebral cortex, and vigilance or arousal.

Brain-body communication   The reticular formation is a major two-way path for communication between the brain and the rest of the body.[1] The descending pathway relays signals from the hypothalamus to several organs controlled by the autonomic system. It also relays involuntary motor impulses to voluntary muscles.

The brain signals the presence of psychosocial stressors via the descending pathway and the hypothalamic-pituitary pathway. (Figure 5-3 shows these connections.) In this way, nonphysical stressors can lead to major changes in physical systems. The most important changes occur in the cardiovascular, glandular, and immune systems. With prolonged stress, these changes may produce undesirable effects.

The second pathway, the ascending RF, signals the brain that physical stressors exist, such as extreme temperatures and injury to the body. These stressors may be translated into a variety of emotional states that produce psychological discomfort and tension. The reticular formation, combined with thalamic centers, controls the awareness of pain. Because pain usually produces

---

[1]The term *reticular formation* (RF) emphasizes the brain structure. An alternate term that emphasizes process is the *reticular activating system* (RAS). Either term, RF or RAS, refers to the same system.

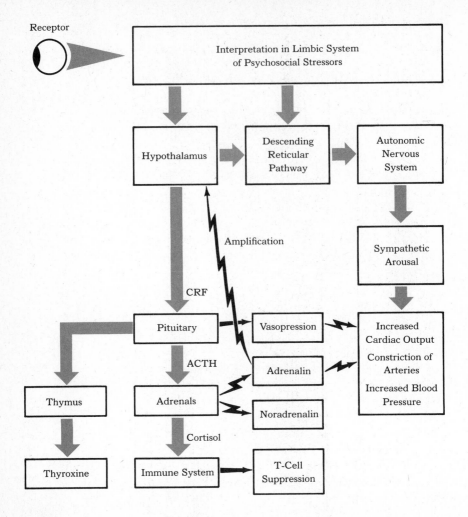

FIGURE 5-3
Effects of prolonged stress in the hypothalamic-pituitary-adrenal complex and autonomic systems

negative emotions, an amplification effect may occur that increases sensitivity to the pain itself. Still, this signal system leads to activation of normal healing processes. The body can even produce its own analgesic-like substances, opiates, to reduce the level of pain experienced while healing is in process. More will be said about this later in this chapter.

Gating   The RF receives input either directly or indirectly from each sensory system. In turn, it can influence receptor sensitivity and alter the state (open or closed) of sensory relay stations. The general outcome of this changing sensitivity is to help the flow of information through one sensory channel while restricting the flow in another. Because of this, a great amount of information initially sent to the brain is lost or distorted. This may not seem like an efficient way of doing business, but it ensures that vital information gets to its destination.

To borrow some terms from communication theory, the RF works to increase the ratio of signal to noise. If every bit of sensory data entered the brain, the brain would simply be overwhelmed. Think of what it would be like to have every radio and TV in your home running full blast while every member of your family talks at once. That is noise! When you turn the radios and TVs down to background level, the sound of only one person talking is signal. By being selective in what gets through, the brain can operate more efficiently.

One important question is "How does the RF know what information is important and what is not?" Only the most general answer can be given. The RF receives input from almost every part of the brain, including centers responsible for motivation, emotion, attention, and associative processes. Changes in any of these internal states bias the way in which the RF selects information. An example may help illustrate this point.

Imagine a parent who puts his or her baby down for a nap and then takes a brief nap also. The TV is on, and there is moderate street noise. In spite of this, the parent rests comfortably, somehow effectively blocking out the noise. Then the baby whimpers softly. Its cry is not as loud as the other sounds, but the parent gets up and immediately attends to the child's needs. Since the baby's cry typically has higher motivational strength than street noise or TV talk, the RF permits this signal to get through and awaken the sleeping parent.

Vigilance and arousal   The third function of the RF, vigilance or arousal, is very important to the way in which the higher brain centers work. The RF looks for important information reaching the senses. Then it provides an alerting signal to higher centers of the brain: "Get ready, I have something important for you." Evidence for this notion comes from surgical procedures that isolate the cortex from the RF and from clinical observations of patients with damage to the RF. When damage occurs to the RF in a certain region, the result is depressed cortical activity, and in extreme cases, coma.

The Visceral Brain

The **visceral brain** is a complex set of structures in the center of the brain. The name comes from its extensive connections with the **hypothalamus,** which controls visceral systems involved in fight-or-flight reactions. Because this group of structures plays a primary role in interpreting potentially emotional stimuli, it is crucial to any explanation of how the brain responds to stress. The most important structures of the visceral brain are the **thalamus,** the hypothalamus-pituitary complex, and other centers associated with the **limbic system.** These structures are illustrated in Figure 5-4.

The thalamus   The thalamus contains several nuclei that are the major relay centers for every sensory system except the sense of smell. It is in an

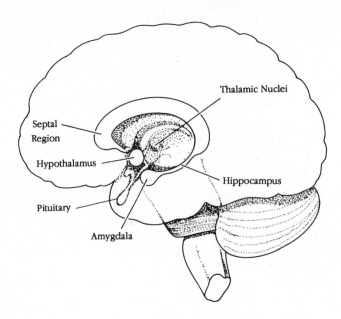

FIGURE 5-4
Cross section of the cerebral cortex showing the major motivational and emotional control centers associated with the "visceral brain"

excellent position to evaluate the emotional content of information the senses provide. The first clinical observations supporting this view came from observing patients who had physical damage to the thalamus. Such people overreact to emotional stimuli. Some patients also showed uncontrollable weeping or laughing without any accompanying subjective experience (Grossman, 1973).

One interesting recent discovery is the role the thalamus plays in the perception of pain. Pain researchers commonly identify three types of pain. Pricking pain comes from a knife cut or a needle, for example. Burning pain is the second type, and aching pain is a deep muscle or bone pain (Guyton, 1977). Each specialized pain pathway terminates in the thalamus. Burning and aching pain also have connections to the RF.

There is some evidence that we can exercise cognitive control over the perception of pain. This might occur by shutting neural gates that are part of the pain pathway (Melzack & Wall, 1965). Another possibility is that cognitive processes might increase the level of **endorphins** (literally the "morphine within") in the pain region. Scientists do not understand these mechanisms well enough to say exactly how pain can be cognitively mediated. Still, they have taken promising steps to provide therapies for people with chronic pain. For example, stimulation techniques act on pain gateways; these techniques have enabled terminally ill patients to control pain levels without drugs.

The limbic system   The limbic system is the part of the primitive brain concerned with survival. It includes the thalamus, hypothalamus, **amygdala,**

hippocampus, and septum. Again, you can refer to Figure 5-4 for details. The functions most often associated with the limbic system include anger, aggression, punishment, reward, sexual arousal, and pain.

For example, damage to the amygdala typically results in greatly increased appetite. Damage to the septum may result in extreme irritability or even rage responses with unprovoked aggression. The amygdala produces the opposite type of reaction, suggesting that these two centers balance aggressive tendencies: the amygdala starting, and the septum moderating, aggressive tendencies. The septum and the hypothalamus also may serve as major reward or pleasure centers in the brain.

Damage to the hippocampus can cause deficits in long-term memory and may slow down or block several types of learning. Most often, these are learning processes that require some kind of avoidance or discrimination response. The hippocampus has extensive connections with the emotional-motivational complex. This suggests that the hippocampus may contribute to distortions in memory for emotionally loaded content.

The hypothalamus The general location of the hypothalamus is just above the roof of the mouth, toward the back. It connects directly to the **pituitary gland,** the **master gland** of the body. Through this connection, the hypothalamus powerfully affects nearly every visceral system in the body. Another measure of the hypothalamus' significance is that nearly every area of the brain interacts with the hypothalamus in some fashion. For example, the hypothalamus has elaborate connections with the RF and the limbic system. Sexual behavior originates in the limbic region but depends on the hypothalamus for control.

Because of this intricate linkage system, the hypothalamus can respond to psychosocial and emotional stimuli. It responds to cognitive stressors that originate from associative thinking or obsessional ruminations. The limbic system can also influence the operation of the autonomic system through this linkage. For example, sleep is co-controlled by centers in the hypothalamus and the RF. Finally, the hypothalamus is very richly supplied with blood, and it monitors the level of nutrients in the blood and body-fluid volume. The hypothalamus also monitors concentrations of hormones originating in other parts of the body. As part of a complex negative-feedback loop, it is crucial to mediating stress reactions.

Still, the role of the hypothalamus in stress is most clearly revealed in four specific functions. These are (1) initiating activity in the autonomic nervous system; (2) stimulating the secretion of **adrenocorticotrophic hormone (ACTH)** from the anterior pituitary; (3) producing antidiuretic hormone **(ADH),** or **vasopressin,** and (4) stimulating the thyroid glands to produce **thyroxine.** To perform these tasks, the hypothalamus has two dedicated centers. One center stimulates sympathetic activity and the production of pituitary stress hormones.[2]

---

[2]This center is called the posterior medial center, which means toward the back and middle of the hypothalamus.

The other center slows down sympathetic activity[3] and inhibits the production of pituitary stress hormones. Understanding these four functions is central to understanding how the stress response begins.

The Autonomic Nervous System

The autonomic nervous system is the primary control system for three different types of tissues: cardiac muscle, most of the glands, and all smooth muscle (Liebman, 1979). The ANS controls heart activity, blood pressure, digestion, urinary and bowel elimination, and many other bodily functions. Control of the ANS comes from the brain stem, the hypothalamus, and the spinal cord.

The ANS is comprised of two parts, the parasympathetic nervous system and the sympathetic nervous system. These two systems exist in a state of dynamic but antagonistic tension. When one is active, the other is quiet or passive, and vice versa. It is not possible for both systems to work at a high level simultaneously.

The parasympathetic nervous system is in control when we are quiet and relaxed. Most of the positive reconstructive processes occur with parasympathetic dominance. Blood concentrates in central organs for such important work as digestion and storage of energy reserves. Breathing is typically slow and balanced. Heart rate slows, and blood pressure drops. Body temperature also drops, and muscle tension decreases.

The sympathetic nervous system is the fight-or-flight system. It springs into action during emergencies or during states of heightened emotionality. The alarm signal itself originates within the hypothalamus. Guyton (1977) identified eight effects of sympathetic arousal. Paraphrased, these are as follows:

1. Increased blood pressure
2. Increased blood flow to support large active muscles, coupled with decreased blood flow to internal (for example, digestive) organs not needed for rapid activity
3. Increased total energy consumption
4. Increased blood glucose concentration
5. Increased energy release in muscles
6. Increased muscle strength
7. Increased mental activity
8. Increased rate of blood coagulation (pp. 600–601)

When the emergency is past, the hypothalamus recalls the parasympathetic system. Thus, the body begins to repair destructive effects from the emergency period.

You may have heard that you should not eat while angry and should engage only in pleasant conversation while eating. This is because anger changes salivary

---

[3]This center is called the anterior lateral center, which means to the front and side of the hypothalamus.

and digestive processes. Indigestion can occur because during aroused emotional states, the body diverts blood from the stomach to support muscle tension. Other undesirable effects of prolonged sympathetic arousal include elevated blood pressure and ulcers.

The Master Gland

The master gland, or pituitary gland, secretes six important hormones (among numerous hormones) from its anterior region and two from its posterior section. The hypothalamus controls these hormonal secretions through its own secretions. One hormone, the **corticotropin-releasing factor (CRF),**[4] tells the anterior pituitary to release ACTH. Release of ACTH activates the adrenal glands. Almost any kind of stress, physical or psychosocial, will lead to a swift rise in the level of ACTH. One psychosocial stressor that typically triggers ACTH release is the death of a spouse or other loved one.

Shortly after ACTH release, the adrenals secrete several hormones, including **cortisol (hydrocortisone), epinephrine,** and **norepinephrine.** Cortisol provides more energy to the body through conversion of body stores into glucose. Recent research suggests that hypersecretions of cortisol play a prominent role in suppressing the **immune system.** Immune suppression reduces the number and effectiveness of lymphocytes, at least in response to acute stressors (Dantzer & Kelley, 1989). Then the body has less resistance to infections and disease. Another major concern is that immune suppression increases vulnerability to cancer (Riley, 1981). These issues will be discussed in detail later. Figure 5-5, which shows interactions within this system, provides an example of a biological negative-feedback system enmeshed in a hierarchical system. The hierarchical components of this system are external systems and cognitive-perceptual systems that influence its activity.

The other two major hormones secreted by the adrenal glands are epinephrine (also called **adrenaline**) and norepinephrine (also called **noradrenaline**), which have the same general effect as the sympathetic nervous system. This output of the adrenal glands thus amplifies actions of the sympathetic nervous system. Epinephrine and norepinephrine levels vary with intensity of stimulation. Under conditions of severe stress, the body can be flooded with epinephrine and norepinephrine.

Epinephrine has a powerful effect on the heart. It increases both the rate and strength of the heart's contractions and raises blood pressure. By a feedback loop to the hypothalamus, epinephrine can increase secretions of ACTH and other hormones to even higher levels. This amplifies the effect of changes in other visceral systems and increases the level of activity in its own loop. This is why activation of the hypothalamic-pituitary-adrenal complex can have such powerful effects under conditions of prolonged stress.

---

[4]This is called corticotropin-releasing hormone (CRH) in some sources.

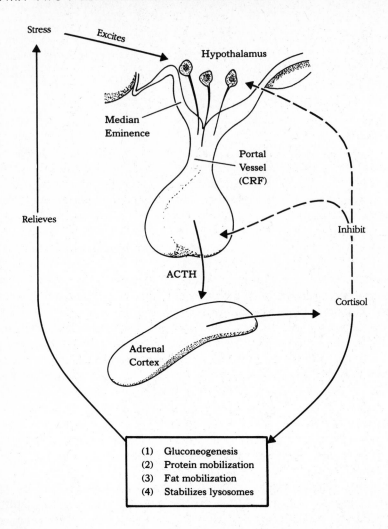

FIGURE 5-5
Stress excitation and adrenal inhibition in the hypothalamic-pituitary-adrenal complex
SOURCE: Guyton (1977).

The brain is also extremely sensitive to the presence of another group of hormones called *adrenocorticosteroids*. These hormones can produce alterations in mental function, which in turn raise adrenocorticosteroid levels even higher. Under these conditions, people become more vulnerable to stress because they cannot deal effectively with daily problems (Riscalla, 1983).

For a short time, some psychologists believed they could link specific emotions to specific physical processes. In this view, love might be a specific neural-hormonal pattern that is the same for any person feeling love. Another emotion—for example, happiness—might be associated with a different neural-hormonal pattern. Up to now, the only consistent evidence of an association between a neural-hormonal pattern and a specific emotion involves epinephrine and norepinephrine. Epinephrine is present in greater amounts when fear occurs, whereas norepinephrine is present in greater amounts when anger occurs (Ax, 1953).

Recent research clarifies the roles of epinephrine and norepinephrine in stress reactions. Early work led researchers to believe that psychological stressors, such as mental arithmetic, continued vigilance, and public speaking were all associated with increased levels of epinephrine in the bloodstream. Further, researchers suspected that norepinephrine increases with physical stressors such as physical restraint or immobilization (Tanaka et al., 1983), submersion in ice water (Aslan, Nelson, Carruthers, & Lader, 1981), isometric stress, and physical exercise. However, the evidence supporting this distinction, epinephrine-psychological stress, norepinephrine-physical stress, was often inconclusive, if not contradictory. More recent research has confirmed that this distinction is correct.

Ward and his team of Stanford researchers (1983) used a very sophisticated, continuous blood-sampling technique and a high-power statistical procedure called *time-series analysis* to do this. They also discovered the reason for the early confusing results. The researchers concluded that the two hormones behave very differently in their speed of reaction and the speed at which they clear out of the bloodstream. Epinephrine is fast-acting and leaves the bloodstream quickly. Norepinephrine clears out of the bloodstream much more slowly. When investigators mixed mental and physical tasks in testing procedures, norepinephrine was still present, especially when mental tasks came later. Thus, norepinephrine logically seemed related to mental stressors. But if the mental and physical stressors are tested at different times, it is clear that epinephrine increases with mental stressors and norepinephrine increases with physical stressors.

Research by Richard Dienstbier (1989) showed that exposure to intermittent stressors leads to a host of interrelated changes in the arousal complex. Dienstbier called these changes, which have positive effects for the organism, **physiological toughness,** a term adapted from Neal Miller's work. The first positive effect of these changes is to reduce the base rate for sympathetic operations. Remember that the usual outcome of stress is to activate or increase the level of the sympathetic system's operation. Dientsbier's research suggests that, after experience with intermittent stress, the body does not work as hard as before because of the reduced base rate for sympathetic nervous system activity.

A second positive effect is that the sympathetic-adrenal-medullary complex can react more swiftly and strongly to challenge or threat. Third, brain catecholamines are not depleted as rapidly as when sympathic nervous system activity is high. This is significant because depletion of catecholamines undermines mental and physical performances. The resulting deficits could be critical to successful coping with stress. Further, catecholamine depletion may be one of the mechanisms involved in depression, and depression may complicate coping efforts in numerous ways. Finally, experience with intermittent stressors suppresses the pituitary- adrenal-cortical response. This can enhance immune-system function because an active pituitary-adrenal-cortical response typically increases cortisol levels and suppresses immune function.

Gold and his colleagues argue, however, that the catecholamine-depletion notion is too simplistic (Gold, Goodwin, & Chrousos, 1988a, 1988b). They showed that stressors can produce a long-term kindling and sensitization of neuronal response, thus impairing the normal feedback restraint on CRF. In their view, this lack of restraint on CRF leads to hypercortisolism, which leads to increased anxiety and other mood/behavioral disturbances commonly associated with depression. Taylor and Fishman (1988) concur with this position. They showed that CRF is a "central integrating signal" in the stress response.

Vasopressin

Vasopressin (ADH) is one of two major hormones produced in the hypothalamus but released by the posterior section of the pituitary gland. It regulates fluid loss through the urinary system. Most significantly, vasopressin influences heart activity and blood pressure. Receptors that feed information to the hypothalamus monitor both the volume and pressure of blood in the venous cavities of the heart. With low volume and pressure, vasopressin production increases. With high volume and pressure, vasopressin production decreases. In this way, the hypothalamic-pituitary system regulates the heart's output. Further, when blood pressure is low, vasopressin constricts arteries, thus causing blood pressure to increase. Traumatic injury is a severe biologic stressor that includes loss of blood volume. When traumatic injury occurs, ADH production increases immediately and dramatically to preserve pressure and restore volume. In addition, vasopressin can directly affect vasoconstriction. During severe stress, ADH can elevate already high blood pressure caused by other neural and hormonal processes (Blessing, Sved, & Reis, 1982).

Thyroid Glands and Thyroxine

Physical and psychological stress can have powerful effects on the rate of metabolism, the rate at which the body burns fuel. Changes in the metabolic rate influence mood, energy, nervous irritability, and mental alertness. Regulation of these changes is a three-step sequence. First, when psychosocial stress or strenuous physical exercise places a demand on the system, the hypothalamus releases a neural hormone called **thyrotropin-releasing factor (TRF).** Release of TRF stimulates the pituitary gland; then the pituitary signals the thyroid, which releases the hormone thyroxine. Second, as demand increases, TRF output increases, thus accelerating metabolic rate. Third, a negative-feedback circuit exists, though, that enables the hypothalamus to adjust the level of TRF. When demand is past, TRF output decreases and metabolism reverts to normal.

A side effect of this sequence is that high levels of thyroxine make the system more responsive to adrenaline. Thus, another amplification effect occurs. The prevailing notion is that adrenaline is a short-term stress hormone, whereas thyroxine is a long-term stress hormone.

Other behavioral effects stem from high thyroxine levels. Mental activity heightens, and the person typically feels more nervous and anxious, always feeling tired, yet achieving sleep only with great difficulty. Blood flow increases greatly, resulting in higher blood pressure. Usually, respiratory rate and intensity also increase. Finally, elevated secretions of gastric juices and stomach motility occur, with resulting diarrhea. These may be recognized as symptoms that occur during periods of stress.

NATURAL DEFENSES: THE IMMUNE SYSTEM

The immune system is among the most sophisticated of body systems. Its one basic function is to help the body resist disease. *Immunity* is "the power of an individual to resist or overcome the effects of a particular disease or other harmful agent" (Memmler & Wood, 1977, p. 281). **Immunocompetence** is the degree to which the immune system is active and effective. When foreign agents (for example, poisons, germs, or toxic substances) invade the body, it defends itself by producing **antibodies** to attack and destroy the invaders. The body may also use its inherited immunity to fight battles against other agents, such as bacteria, viral infections, and blood poisons.

The immune system produces two types of cells to provide immunity, the **T cell** and the **B cell.** The thymus gland, sometimes called the "master organ" of the immune system, produces T cells. They provide cellular immunity, fight bacterial infections (such as tuberculosis), and combat some viral infections. T cells also attack cancer cells, fungi, and cells from transplanted organs. B cells derive from bone marrow. They are responsible for antibody formation and can neutralize foreign agents (Nossal, 1987).

Until recently, scientists regarded the immune system as an autonomous system, operating only to recognize what is self and what is not-self. The immune system's sole purpose was to attack and kill what is not-self. In his review of scientific literature, Robert Ader (1983) argued that "the immune system is integrated with other physiological systems and, like all such systems operating in the interests of homeostasis, is sensitive to regulation or modulation by the brain" (p. 251). Ader provided convincing evidence for (1) the influence of conditioning on the immune function; (2) the relation between psychosocial factors, such as life stress and immunocompetence; and (3) the relationship between use of psychoactive drugs and immunocompetence.

A new scientific discipline, **psychoneuroimmunology,** reflects the importance of this view. Psychoneuroimmunology seeks to uncover the intricate relations between psychosocial stressors and neural-immunologic systems that govern adaptive biologic response to stress (Jemmott, 1985).

Stress and the Immune System

Uncovering the processes that link stress and immunity has not been easy for scientific sleuths. Jemmott and Locke (1984), in their extensive review of the literature, noted that work has moved beyond retrospective psychodynamic speculation into the arena of sober empiricism. Research on the relationship between stress and immunity now suggests that stress alters the way in which the immune system operates (Baker, 1987; Jemmott & Locke, 1984; Locke, 1982). Initially, researchers concluded that stress lowers the body's resistance to disease by suppressing the number of disease-fighting cells available. The net outcome for the person presumably would be an increase in the frequency or intensity of afflictions. Lowered resistance could also slow down recovery from existing disease.

In particular, animal research showed that numerous stressors suppressed T cell circulation (Irwin & Livnat, 1987; Keller et al., 1981). One research team also showed that genetic factors influence immune response to stress, but the exact role is not yet well understood (Irwin & Livnat, 1987). Abrupt changes in social contact increased tumor growth in laboratory mice (Sklar & Anisman, 1980). Observations of human reactions to stress generally confirm this result (Locke, Hurst, Heisel et al., 1978). Plaut and Friedman (1981), for example, showed that stress increased risk for contracting infectious diseases, allergic reactions, and autoimmune disease in humans. Another project showed that antibody response is lower on days with high negative mood and higher on days with high positive mood (Stone et al., 1987). Other researchers showed that grief after the death of a spouse (Bartrop et al., 1977) and after an abortion (Assael et al., 1981) can lower the number of lymphocytes available to fight disease. In sum, these results present a substantive argument for a stress–immune response interaction.

The research on grief and immune suppression must be viewed with some caution. If suppression is present, it may result in a change in morbidity only, not in mortality as early research suggested. A large-scale epidemiologic study looked at mortality in a group of parents whose sons died in war or in auto accidents (Levav, Friedlander, Kark, & Peritz, 1988). Death rates of this group of bereaved parents were no different from those of the general population. In fact, fathers who lost sons in war had lower mortality rates than those who lost sons in accidents.

Robert Dantzer and Keith Kelley (1989) suggested that the immunosuppression view is far too simplistic. They believe that immune-system interactions with stressors are part of a long-loop regulatory feedback system that includes reciprocal influences. Dantzer and Kelley see this as a "true mechanism for communication between physiologic systems" as opposed to a fortuitous indirect effect. Included in this complex network are brain catecholamines, endogenous opioids, and pituitary hormones. Because stress also can enhance immune function, it is important to understand the conditions under which either suppression or facilitation may occur.

Dantzer and Kelley pointed out that the influence of stressors on the immune system depends on the nature, duration, and frequency of stressor events.

In addition, the stressor event interacts with a dynamic immune system. Because the system's status varies over time, the timing of stressors is important. The pituitary growth hormone is one endogenous chemical that may be involved in positive, restorative immunoregulation. This is still somewhat speculative, but there is some evidence to support this notion.

Finally, Dantzer and Kelley discussed the complex relationship of mood states to immunocompetence. One popular position suggests that depression (helplessness/hopelessness) is the cause, and altered immune function with subsequent cancer onset is the outcome. Dantzer and Kelley pointed out that the relationship may be just the opposite. That is, the manifestation of altered emotional mood may result from altered neural functions, which are themselves the result of altered immune function. Leonard (1988) also concluded that altered immune function can precipitate symptoms of anxiety, depression, and schizophrenia.

The Brain and Immune System

As more evidence accumulates, one major neural-hormonal regulatory system emerges in a central role in influencing the immune system. That is the hypothalamic-pituitary-adrenal system, which Antoni (1987) described as a negative feedback loop. We have already discussed at some length the importance of this system in stress reactions. When stress occurs, the hypothalamic-pituitary system signals the adrenal glands. Output from the adrenal glands (cortisol, aldosterone, and desoxycorticosterone) stimulate the immune system (Comsa, Leonhardt, & Wekerle, 1982). This has the desired effect of initiating defensive reactions, increasing resistance, and speeding recovery.

Unfortunately, some hormones (especially cortisol) secreted by the adrenals tend to suppress or damage both T cells and B cells. Then resistance to many infectious diseases declines, and vulnerability to common ailments such as colds and flu increases. Under conditions of prolonged stress, certain people may be more susceptible to the development of cancer.

One critical question is, How can stress produce a health-promoting response sometimes but a health-defeating response at other times? Kiecolt-Glaser's group showed that relaxation training increased natural killer-cell activity[5] (Kiecolt-Glaser et al., 1985). This suggests that certain coping actions can aid immune response. The biologic mechanism for this is not yet known. As Dantzer and Kelley (1989) noted, though, it may be related to the type of stress confronting the person or to the time course of the stress itself. Comsa and his colleagues also conclude that timing factors are important (Comsa, Leonhardt, & Wekerle, 1982). Another theory is that negative outcomes result from chronic activation of the HPA system, and positive outcomes result from activation of the sympathetic-adrenomedullary system (Antoni, 1987).

[5]We should note that baseline differences in natural killer-cell activity existed between the relaxation group and the social-contact group. These baseline differences were not experimentally or statistically controlled. The increase in natural killer-cell activity appears reliable when compared to the no-contact group but uninterpretable when compared to the social-contact group.

Two other critical factors in the relation of stress to immunity are chronicity and intensity (Ader, 1983). *Chronicity* refers to a condition that goes on seemingly without end. Under conditions of prolonged stress, the health-promoting response becomes fatigued. The body exhausts the vital supply of adrenal hormones, and the immune response weakens. Again, this parallels Selye's (1956) stage concept of alarm, reaction, and exhaustion.

Intensity is the strength or power of a stressful condition. Still, the potency of a stressor depends partly on personal appraisal processes. Recent research reveals that different stressful situations can produce very different neural-hormonal reactions. For example, investigators at the University of California, Los Angeles (UCLA), manipulated the predictability of the stressor (Shavit et al., 1984). They wanted to learn more about the role of **opioid peptides** in stress-related immune deficiency, especially as it related to **natural killer cells.** We must identify these elements before proceeding.

First, neural cells in the brain and pituitary construct opiods, which are concentrated in lower and middle regions of the brain, such as the thalamus and limbic system. Opioids produce analgesia for pain by blocking the transmission of pain signals. Some indication of their potency is that natural opioids produce an analgesic effect roughly comparable to that of morphine (Stephens, 1980).

Natural killer cells are a type of lymphocyte specialized to recognize and kill tumor cells and other foreign bodies. Previous investigations showed that natural killer cells decline in animals exposed to stressors such as surgery, starvation, and transportation. Also, suppression of natural killer-cell activity occurs in college students who have poor coping skills for life-change (Shavit et al., 1984).

In the UCLA study, the investigators used two groups of rats exposed to two different stress (that is, shock) conditions. The crucial difference was that one group received shock on an unpredictable schedule while the other group received shock continuously. Both groups showed an analgesic, or pain blocking, response as expected. Yet the group that received unpredictable shock blocked pain through activation of the natural opioid mechanism in the brain, a stress-induced analgesia.

The results clearly showed suppression of natural killer-cell activity in the opioid-analgesia group but not in the other group. The investigators concluded that the production of opioid peptides is one mechanism that mediates the relation between certain types of stress and suppression of natural killer cells. Further, they suggested that the primary ingredient in the opioid-analgesia group's stressful condition was similar to that in learned helplessness situations. These situations typically contain inescapable punishment, unpredictability, and lack of personal control. Experiments in learned helplessness have shown a similar release of opioids.

The Body at War with Itself

One side effect of the way the immune system works is the development of allergies. **Allergies** may be described as wars between special antibodies and external agents called **allergens.** The warfare results in the rupture of two different white blood cells and the release of toxic materials into the bloodstream. One of these materials is the substance histamine.

Hives and hay fever   The most common allergies are anaphylaxis, urticaria, **asthma,** and **hay fever.** Anaphylaxis, though rare, is extremely serious because it can lead to circulatory shock and death within a few minutes of onset. Urticaria is a type of anaphylaxis localized in the skin. The skin becomes inflamed and swollen, a condition most commonly called "hives." Hay fever occurs when the allergic reaction occurs in the nasal area, leading to increased capillary pressure and rapid fluid leakage into the nose. Physicians commonly prescribe **antihistamines** for both urticaria and hay fever because histamine is the primary cause of the difficulty. Antihistamines are not used for asthma because other products of the allergic reaction are involved.

In Japan, one research group provided evidence for the relation of stress to skin diseases (Teshima et al., 1982). Using a clinical sample, the investigators found that lifestyle changes and substantial daily stress preceded the appearance of urticaria. Lifestyle changes occurred most frequently in schools, residence, type of work, marriage, promotion, and so forth. The stressors most frequently experienced were overwork, interpersonal difficulties, or family difficulties. Autogenic training, a relaxation-imagery method described in Chapter 12, was effective in reducing the levels of histamine in the blood.

Asthma   Asthma is "an intermittent, variable, and reversible obstruction of bronchial airways" (Pinkerton, Hughes, & Wenrich, 1982, p. 234). Asthma has received more attention than the other allergies, probably because of the sheer number of its victims and the cost of treatment. Asthma afflicts about 4% of the population at any given time and costs several billion dollars each year for treatment and care.

Many clinicians have speculated that psychological factors contribute to the etiology of allergic reactions such as urticaria and asthma. We discussed evidence on this issue in Chapter 4. Clinical studies suggested that hypnosis is useful in relieving these conditions, which supports the psychogenic argument (Hall, 1982–1983). There is still no convincing evidence, though, that either family stress or personality is important in the origin of asthma. Psychosocial factors might play a role in the day-to-day intensity of reaction. Evidence also shows that conditioning can affect the immune system. This might, then, produce an asthmatic attack. Again, there is no proof that such a mechanism exists. More importantly, behavioral treatment programs have had little or no success in treating asthma. Perhaps the most important observation is that lifestyle serves to intensify symptoms and/or defeat medical treatment. This suggests that psychological factors are mediators, not precipitators of asthma.

Acquired immune deficiency syndrome   No health issue of the 1980s has demanded more attention than **acquired immune deficiency syndrome (AIDS).** Batchelor (1984) called AIDS "a modern-day black plague." In a special issue of *American Psychologist,* Stephen Morin (1988) wrote that AIDS was a three-stage epidemic that started with the insidious and silent onset of the disease. It continued with intense case surveillance, and it persists in sociocultural reactions to the epidemic. Although current numbers may pale in comparison to plagues of the past, the toll in human life and suffering has grown at an alarming rate. Through early 1986, there were nearly 19,000 adult cases in the United States (Bakeman, Lumb, Jackson, & Smith, 1986). These figures did not include cases in Haiti and Africa (Kreiss et al., 1986). By late 1988, there were 65,000 cases. The Centers for Disease Control estimated there could be as many as 1.4 million cases in America and 5 million cases worldwide (Batchelor, 1988). Uganda reported 8000 cases, but some fear that as many as 10,000 new cases could surface each month (Goodgame, 1990).

The Centers for Disease Control referred to AIDS as a syndrome "characterized by opportunistic infections and malignant diseases in patients without a known cause for immunodeficiency" (cited in Seligman et al., 1984, p. 1286). Intensive research uncovered the cause of AIDS, the HTLV-III/LAV virus. Following recommendation of an international committee, the virus is now called the *human immunodeficiency virus,* or HIV (Coffin et al., 1986). The virus does not destroy the immune system, as one unfortunate myth suggested. It selectively attacks the T4 lymphocyte, a white blood cell that is key to immune response (Burny, 1986). The side effects are numerous and include CNS abnormalities that may lead to an AIDS dementia complex. Recent research showed that even persons with asymptomatic HIV infection manifest subclinical signs of neurologic impairment (Koralnik, et al., 1990).

In the United States, AIDS attacks specific at-risk groups, including male homosexuals, intravenous drug abusers, and African-American and Hispanic men (Batchelor, 1988). These three groups constituted 90% of the cases. Figure 5-6 shows the distribution of AIDS in these high-risk groups. In spite of this predominant pattern, there is evidence that AIDS can be transmitted through heterosexual contact as well (Calabrese, & Gopalakrishna, 1986). In addition, once HIV prevalence exceeds 10% in a community, the utility of identifying risk groups decreases (Goodgame, 1990).

At the outset, many fears about AIDS were based largely on ignorance of modes of transmission. Now substantial evidence exists that members of a family with an AIDS victim have little or no risk of infection (Friedland et al., 1986). Further, epidemiological and clinical studies show that routine, nonsexual contact in offices, restaurants, or medical facilities does not transmit the virus. The virus is fragile and is easily killed by soaps and bleaches (Batchelor, 1988).

The common modes of AIDS transmission involve few but crucial high-risk behaviors. This suggests that AIDS is a behavioral disease that may respond to behavioral interventions. The modes of transmission are evident in the lifestyles of the high-risk groups: high-risk sexual behavior and sharing needles. One ingredient receiving additional attention is alcohol use. It contributes to indiscriminate sexual activity that increases the risk of contracting and transmitting the disease. Behavioral interventions are largely educational and target lifestyle changes to reduce the inherent dangers. Unfortunately, current data do not provide much help to centers trying to structure behavioral strategies.

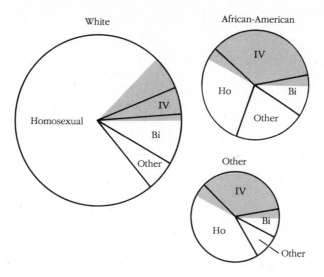

FIGURE 5-6

Proportion of AIDS cases represented by various risk groups in the United States, shown separately for Whites, Blacks, and other nonwhites (92% of whom are Hispanic). The circles are proportional to the number of cases reported for the three racial or ethnic groups. The group at risk because of intravenous (IV) drug use is indicated by shading in order to show the overlap between it and the homosexual (Ho) and bisexual (Bi) groups. (Data based on the 18,907 adult cases of AIDS reported to the Centers for Disease Control as of April 7, 1986).

SOURCE: Bakeman et al. (1986), p. 192.

The most encouraging note from the early data is that risk can be reduced (des Jarlais & Friedman, 1988; Peterson & Marín, 1988; Stall, Coates, & Hoff, 1988).

In addition to the life-threatening nature of AIDS, AIDS victims experience extreme forms of psychosocial stress. Members of the gay community, for example, suffer from heightened anxiety, panic attacks, loss of self-esteem, fear of isolation from friends and loved ones, and loss of self-sufficiency (Morin, Charles, & Malyon, 1984). Extensive publicity, combined with widespread antigay sentiment, almost isolates gays. Even gays diagnosed and found free of AIDS experience high levels of stress. They are among the "worried well." They have no disease, but excessive worry leads them to engage in behaviors that hurt their physical or mental well-being. These behaviors include extremes of denial and repression or obsessional thinking about the bad things that are about to happen. The long-term impact on health may be nearly as detrimental as if the person had contracted AIDS. Herek and Glunt (1988) called this "an epidemic of stigma."

Research on psychosocial processes in immune function is also relevant. Kiecolt-Glaser and Glaser (1988) suggested that positive psychosocial factors may reduce the impact of the virus. Conversely, negative psychosocial factors (for example, the perception of high risk and lack of social support) may intensify the effect of AIDS. In such cases, a type of social victimization may be in process that subjects a person to negative consequences due largely to being part of one of society's less favored groups.

THE CARDIOVASCULAR SYSTEM

The heart is a miracle organ by any standard. It works day and night, seldom missing a beat as it pumps life-giving blood through the entire body. The pulse rate of a newborn child is around 120 to 140 beats per minute. In the mature adult, the heart beats 60 to 70 times per minute. At this rate, the average heart beats 3900 times per hour, or 93,600 beats each day. During light exercise, the pulse rate can rise to around 100, and in strenuous exercise it can go much higher. Astronauts have pulse rates around 140 beats per minute during the most stressful periods of liftoff and reentry.

Stress and the Heart

Biomedical research has devoted much attention to the physical origins of heart failure. Now, more attention has shifted to psychosocial factors and lifestyle forces that contribute to cardiovascular problems. The major focuses are on stress, personality, diet, exercise, and abstinence or temperance from the use of addictive drugs.

We have already discussed several pathways the brain uses to influence other organs. Events interpreted as stressful or emotionally loaded can produce changes in the rate, intensity, or balance of processes in several physical systems including the cardiovascular (Gliner, Bedi, & Horvath, 1979), respiratory, and digestive systems. We have traced this influence from the limbic system through the HPA complex and the sympathetic division of the autonomic nervous system. This should provide convincing evidence that stress has powerful effects on the cardiovascular system.

Hypertension

Hypertension is an elevation in blood pressure above accepted levels, no matter what produced it. This is the usual diagnosis given when systolic blood pressure exceeds 160 and diastolic exceeds 120. Yet even slight increases in blood pressure over 140/90 predict increased risk of premature death (Taylor & Fortmann, 1983). Serious danger exists when systolic pressure reaches 200.[6] **Essential hypertension** is the term given to hypertension of unknown origins. It may be due to higher peripheral resistance or increased cardiac output (Taylor & Fortman, 1983). Activation of the sympathetic nervous system, as in stress-anxiety reactions, increases cardiac output, resulting in an increase in blood pressure. Under normal circumstances this condition will last only a matter of hours. With continued sympathetic arousal and prolonged constriction of the arteries supplying the kidneys, long-term hypertension may appear.

---

[6]Blood pressure measured at peak heart output is the *systolic* pressure, and measured at the resting phase of the heart is *diastolic* pressure. In the normal heart, these pressures are 120/80 respectively.

In addition to sympathetic arousal, control from the HPA complex initiates release of epinephrine and norepinephrine, along with renin from the kidneys. In addition to increasing cardiac output and elevating blood pressure, adrenaline and noradrenaline speed up the rate of damage to the arteries. Renin is a chemical that stimulates production of a peptide called *angiotensin,* "the most potent vasoconstrictor known" (Guyton, 1977, p. 231). The presence of these three hormones duplicates and amplifies the effect of sympathetic arousal. Thus, cardiac output and blood pressure can increase to even higher levels than with sympathetic arousal alone.

Taylor and Fortmann (1983) suggested that hypertension should be viewed in a systems context. This position suggests that single-cause models of hypertension are inadequate given ample evidence of multiple biologic systems that interact in different ways to produce high blood pressure.

Research also has considered how genetic/constitutional factors influence hypertension and stress reactions. In one study, people with a family history of hypertension showed higher resting systolic and diastolic blood pressure compared with those with no family history of hypertension (Jorgensen, & Houston, 1989). These investigators also observed higher systolic blood pressure and diastolic blood pressure under conditions of laboratory stress. The link to life-event stress, though, was different for men and women. Men showed higher resting systolic pressure with more negative stress events. Women showed higher resting systolic pressure with fewer negative events. Catherine Stoney and her colleagues reviewed several studies that point to a sex difference linking physiological reactivity to stress and coronary heart disease (Stoney, Davis, & Matthews, 1987). Greenberg and Shapiro (1987) showed that stressors combined with caffeine had an additive effect in raising blood pressure that was not dose-dependent. Systolic pressures were higher in subjects from families with a history of hypertension, but this did not change in response to caffeine.

The medical treatment of hypertension typically follows a stepped-care, antihypertensive medication program. Patients also make lifestyle changes that include diet, weight control, and relaxation methods designed to offset stress (Taylor & Fortmann, 1983). McCaffrey and Blanchard (1985) reviewed stress management approaches to the treatment of essential hypertension. They concluded that pharmacotherapy is clearly superior to stress management therapy. Despite the usefulness of stress management therapy, few would ever consider treating essential hypertension in isolation from pharmacological interventions.

Atherosclerosis

In medical terms, **atherosclerosis** is a disease of the large arteries "in which yellowish patches of fat are deposited, forming plaques that decrease the size of the [opening]" (Memmler & Wood, 1977, p. 299). The yellowish patches of fat, called *arterial plaques,* are deposits of cholesterol and other lipids. A variety of factors, including genetic risk, diet, lack of exercise, and stress, can all contribute to the formation of arterial plaques. Rosenman and Friedman (1974) were among the first to note the relation between stressful events and the appearance of cholesterol. They reported that tax accountants in the two weeks before the April 15 income tax deadline had greatly increased serum cholesterol levels compared with levels in either February or March.

Behavioral interventions to reduce coronary risk may be effective in both young and old. Heather Walter and her colleagues conducted a five-year school-based intervention with a large sample of children in and around New York City (Walter, Hofman, Vaughan, & Wynder, 1988). They found that changes in dietary intake and health knowledge occurred during the study. The positive effects on blood cholesterol were small but significant in one school system, and favorable but not significant in the other school system. Further research suggested there is some benefit to lowering cholesterol even after myocardial infarction (Rossouw, 1990). Patients with symptoms of coronary disease have a relative risk five to seven times higher than those without signs of coronary disease. Although prevention of coronary disease in the normal population is important, this research program suggested that risk factors are equally modifiable before and after myocardial infarction.

Another effect of stress and sympathetic arousal is the increase of the tendency for blood to coagulate. Even when no injury has occurred, the effect in the bloodstream is the same. There is a buildup of blood platelets (also called *thrombocytes*), which become part of the arterial plaques. Because plaques reduce the physical space that blood has to pass through, pressure increases. Plaques also cause a breakdown in the wall of the artery itself. The body then tries to repair this breakdown. The platelets, rather than helping in this process, contribute to the problem by making the plaques even thicker. At this point, it is mostly irrelevant how the plaques got there. Stress only adds to the problem.

In the later stages of atherosclerosis, fibrous cells also infiltrate the plaques and add to the scar tissue on the artery wall. Calcium deposits further harden the cell walls and narrow the corridor. Blood must be squeezed through a much smaller space than normal, and the heart must work even harder to produce blood flow. Just as a weight lifter develops larger muscles with increasing workouts, heart muscle also grows as it works harder. Unfortunately, the muscle grows faster than the supply network grows to keep blood flowing to the heart. The muscle that pumps blood to the rest of the body does not have enough of its own resource to stay healthy, a condition called *myocardial ischemia.* Rozanski's (1988) research group observed irregular ventricular-wall motion during mental-stress tasks. They concluded that personally relevant stress may precipitate myocardial ischemia in coronary-artery–disease patients.

THE DIGESTIVE SYSTEM AND ULCERS

One of the early conclusions of Selye's stress research was that stress can have disastrous effects on the digestive system, including perforated ulcers and death. The executive-monkey study convincingly showed this. Many other observations support the notion that psychosocial factors contribute to the origin of

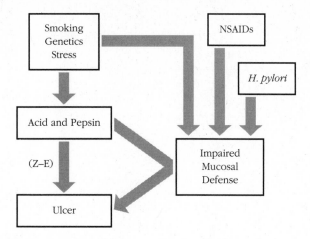

FIGURE 5-7
Model of the pathogenesis of peptic ulcer
SOURCE: Soll (1990).

ulcers: urban populations have a higher prevalence of ulcers than rural populations; also, the prevalence of ulcers increases in wartime. Certain occupational groups with higher levels of psychological stress, such as air-traffic controllers, are also more prone to ulcers (Pinkerton, Hughes, & Wenrich, 1982).

There are several different types of ulcers. **Peptic ulcers** occur when excess amounts of gastric juices are used to digest food. Figure 5-7 shows how a peptic ulcer originates and devleops. In the absence of neutralizing secretions, these juices attack the stomach lining. The result is irritation, bleeding, and in severe cases, a break in the stomach wall itself. In sum, peptic ulcers result when acidity and peptic activity overpower mucosal defense (Soll, 1990).

Peptic ulcers may be acute, the so-called stress ulcer, or chronic. There are probably several physical causes for the stress ulcer. The most likely include excess production of hydrochloric acid and pepsin under control of the parasympathetic system, and excess secretion of adrenal hormones under the control of the HPA complex. Nonsteroidal anti-inflammatory drugs (NSAIDs) irritate the stomach lining; but aspirin is probably the worst barrier breaker (Soll, 1990).

Gastric ulcers are deeper erosions in the stomach lining. They occur most frequently on the bottom curved surface of the stomach, just below the outlet to the intestines. They can be caused by excessive use of aspirin and alcohol. They may also result from chronic anxiety and depression (Stephens, 1980).

SUMMARY

In this chapter, we have seen how the brain translates emotional or stressful stimuli into specific physical processes. The process begins when the older visceral brain interprets an external stimulus as emotionally loaded. Resulting output from the brain via the autonomic system and the hypothalamic-pituitary-adrenal complex mobilize the body's natural defenses to fight the stress. The physical response is a general state of arousal with increased cardiac volume, higher blood pressure, faster formation of arterial plaques, and accelerated wear and tear on the heart. Other effects include altered respiratory response and suppression of the immune system. These physical changes in organ or system function can have negative consequences for the organism if maintained over a long time.

KEY TERMS

acquired immune deficiency syndrome (AIDS)
adrenocorticotrophic hormone (ACTH)
allergens
allergies
amygdala
antibodies
antihistamines
anxiety hyperventilation
asthma
atherosclerosis
autonomic nervous system (ANS)
B cell
brain stem
central nervous system (CNS)
corticotropin-releasing factor (CRF)

cortisol (hydrocortisone)
endorphins
epinephrine (adrenaline)
essential hypertension
gastric ulcers
hay fever
hippocampus
hypertension
hypothalamus
immune system
immunocompetence
limbic system
medulla
mind
natural killer cells
neuroanatomists
norepinephrine (noradrenaline)
opioid peptides

parasympathetic nervous system
peptic ulcers
peripheral nervous system (PNS)
physiological toughness
pituitary gland (master gland)
psychoneuro-immunology
reticular formation (RF)
somatic nervous system (SNS)
sympathetic nervous system
T cell
thalamus
thyrotropin-releasing factor (TRF)
thyroxine
vasopressin (ADH)
visceral brain

REFERENCES

Ader, R. (1983). Developmental Psychoneuroimmunology. *Developmental Psychobiology, 16,* 251–267.

Antoni, M. H. (1987). Neuroendocrine influences in psychoimmunology and neoplasia: A review. *Psychology and Health, 1,* 3–24.

Aslan, S., Nelson, L., Carruthers, M., & Lader, M. (1981). Stress and age effects on catecholamines in normal subjects. *Journal of Psychosomatic Research, 25,* 33–41.

Assael, M., Naor, S., Pecht, M., Trainin, N., & Samuel, D. (1981). *Correlation between emotional reaction to loss of loved object and lymphocyte response to mitogenic stimulation in women*. Paper presented at the Sixth World Congress of the International College of Psychosomatic Medicine, Quebec, Canada.

Ax, A. F. (1953). The physiological differentiation of fear and anger in humans. *Psychosomatic Medicine, 15*, 433–442.

Bakeman, R., Lumb, J. R., Jackson, R. E., & Smith, D. W. (1986). AIDS risk-group profiles in whites and members of minority groups. *The New England Journal of Medicine, 315*, 191–192.

Baker, G. H. B. (1987). Invited review: Psychological factors and immunity. *Journal of Psychosomatic Research, 31*, 1–10.

Bartrop, R. W., Lazarus, L., Luckhurst, E., Kiloh, L. G., & Penny, R. (1977). Depressed lymphocyte function after bereavement. *Lancet, 1*, 834–836.

Batchelor, W. F. (1984). AIDS: A public health and psychological emergency. *American Psychologist, 39*, 1279–1284.

Batchelor, W. F. (1988). AIDS 1988: The science and limits of science. *American Psychologist, 43*, 853–858.

Blessing, W. W., Sved, A. F., & Reis, D. J. (1982). Destruction of noradrenergic neurons in rabbit brainstem elevates plasma vasopressin, causing hypertension. *Science, 217*, 661–663.

Burny, A. (1986, May). More and better trans-activation. *Nature, 321*, p. 378.

Calabrese, L. H., & Gopalakrishna, K. V. (1986). Transmission of HTLV-III infection from man to woman to man. *The New England Journal of Medicine, 314*, 987.

Coffin, J., Haase, A., Levy, J. A., Mautagnier, L., Oroszlan, S., Teich, N., et al. (1986). What to call the AIDS virus? *Nature, 321*, 10.

Comsa, J., Leonhardt, H., & Wekerle, H. (1982). Hormonal coordination of the immune response. In R. H. Adrian et al. (Eds.), *Reviews of physiology, biochemistry and pharmacology, 92*, 115–191.

Dantzer, R., & Kelley, K. W. (1989). Stress and immunity: An integrated view of relationships between the brain and the immune system. *Life Sciences, 44*, 1995–2008.

des Jarlais, D. C., & Friedman, S. R. (1988). The psychology of preventing AIDS among intravenous drug users: A social learning conceptualization. *American Psychologist, 43*, 865–870.

Dienstbier, R. A. (1989). Arousal and physiological toughness: Implications for mental and physical health. *Psychological Review, 96*, 84–100.

Friedland, G. H., Saltzman, B. R., Rogers, M. F., Kahl, P. A., Lesser, M. L., Mayers, M. M., & Klein, R. S. (1986). Lack of transmission of HTLV-III/LAV infection to household contacts of patients with AIDS or AIDS-related complex with oral candidiasis. *The New England Journal of Medicine, 314*, 344–349.

Gliner, J. A., Bedi, J. F., & Horvath, S. M. (1979). Somatic and non-somatic influences on the heart: Hemodynamic changes. *Psychophysiology, 16*, 358–362.

Gold, P. W., Goodwin, F. K., & Chrousos, G. P. (1988a). Clinical and biochemical manifestations of depression: Relation to the neurobiology of stress [First of two parts]. *The New England Journal of Medicine, 319*, 348–353.

Gold, P. W., Goodwin, F. K., & Chrousos, G. P. (1988b). Clinical and biochemical manifestations of depression: Relation to the neurobiology of stress [Second of two parts]. *The New England Journal of Medicine, 319*, 413–420.

Goodgame, R. W. (1990). AIDS in Uganda—Clinical and social features. *The New England Journal of Medicine, 323*, 383–388.

Greenberg, W., & Shapiro, D. (1987). The effects of caffeine and stress on blood pressure in individuals with and without a family history of hypertension. *Psychophysiology, 24*, 151–156.

Grossman, S. (1973). *Essentials of physiological psychology.* New York: Wiley.

Guyton, A. C. (1977). *Basic human physiology: Normal function and mechanisms of disease.* Philadelphia: Saunders.

Hall, H. R. (1982–1983). Hypnosis and the immune system: A review with implications for cancer and the psychology of healing. *American Journal of Clinical Hypnosis, 25,* 92–103.

Hegel, M. T., Abel, G. G., Etscheidt, M., Cohen-Cole, S., & Wilmer, C. I. (1989). Behavioral treatment of angina-like chest pain in patients with hyperventilation syndrome. *Journal of Behavior Therapy and Experimental Psychiatry, 20,* 31–39.

Herek, G. M., & Glunt, E. K. (1988). An epidemic of stigma: Public reactions to AIDS. *American Psychologist, 43,* 886–891.

Irwin, J., & Livnat, S. (1987). Behavioral influences on the immune system: Stress and conditioning. *Progress in Neuro-Psychopharmacology and Biological Psychiatry, 11,* 137–143.

Jemmott, J. B. (1985). Psychoneuroimmunology: The new frontier. *American Behavioral Scientist, 28,* 497–509.

Jemmott, J. B., & Locke, S. E. (1984). Psychosocial factors, immunologic mediation, and human susceptibility to infectious diseases: How much do we know? *Psychological Bulletin, 95,* 78–108.

Jorgensen, R. S., & Houston, B. K. (1989). Reporting of life events, family history of hypertension, and cardiovascular activity at rest and during psychological stress. *Biological Psychology, 28,* 135–148.

Keller, S. E., Weiss, J. M., Schleifer, S. J., Miller, N. E., & Stein, M. (1981). Suppression of immunity by stress: Effect of a graded series of stressors on lymphocyte stimulation in the rat. *Science, 213,* 1397–1400.

Kiecolt-Glaser, J. K., & Glaser, R. (1988). Psychological influences on immunity: Implications for AIDS. *American Psychologist, 43,* 892–898.

Kiecolt-Glaser, J. K., Glaser, R., Williger, D., Stout, J., Messick, G., Sheppard, S., et al. (1985). Psychosocial enhancement of immunocompetence in a geriatric population. *Health Psychology, 4,* 25–41.

Koralnik, I. J., Beaumanoir, A., Häusler, R., Kohler, A., Safran, A. B., Delacoux, R., et al. (1990). A controlled study of early neurologic abnormalities in men with asymptomatic human immunodeficiency virus infection. *The New England Journal of Medicine, 323,* 864–870.

Kreiss, J. K., Koech, D., Plummer, F. A., Holmes, K. K., Lightfoote, M., Piot, P., et al. (1986). AIDS virus infection in Nairobi prostitutes. *The New England Journal of Medicine, 314,* 414–418.

Leonard, B. E. (1988). Stress, the immune system and psychiatric illness. *Stress Medicine, 4,* 207–213.

Levav, I., Friedlander, Y., Kark, J. D., & Peritz, E. (1988). An epidemiologic study of mortality among bereaved parents. *The New England Journal of Medicine, 319,* 457–461.

Liebman, M. (1979). *Neuroanatomy made easy and understandable.* Baltimore: University Park Press.

Locke, S. E. (1982). Stress, adaptation, and immunity: Studies in humans. *General Hospital Psychiatry, 4,* 49–58.

Locke, S. E., Hurst, M. W., Heisel, J. S., et al. (1978, April). *The influence of stress on the immune response.* Annual Meeting of the American Psychosomatic Society, Washington, DC.

McCaffrey, R. J., & Blanchard, E. B. (1985). Area review: Hypertension. *Annals of Behavioral Medicine, 7,* 5–12.

Melzack, R., & Wall, P. (1965). Pain mechanisms: A new theory. *Science, 50,* 971–979.

Memmler, R. L., & Wood, D. L. (1977). *The human body in health and disease* (4th ed.). Philadelphia: Lippincott.

Morin, S. F. (1988). AIDS: The challenge to psychology. *American Psychologist, 43,* 838–842.

Morin, S. F., Charles, K. A., & Malyon, A. K. (1984). The psychological impact of AIDS on gay men. *American Psychologist, 39,* 1288.

Nossal, G. J. V. (1987). The basic components of the immune system. *The New England Journal of Medicine, 316,* 1320–1325.

Pelletier, K. (1977). *Mind as healer, mind as slayer: A holistic approach to preventing stress disorders.* New York: Dell.

Peterson, J. L., & Marín, G. (1988). Issues in the prevention of AIDS among black and Hispanic men. *American Psychologist, 43,* 871–877.

Pinkerton, S. S., Hughes, H., & Wenrich, W. W. (1982). *Behavioral medicine: Clinical applications.* New York: Wiley.

Plaut, S. M., & Friedman, S. B. (1981). Psychosocial factors, stress, and disease processes. In R. Ader (ed.), *Psychoneuroimmunology* (pp. 3–29). New York: Academic Press.

Riley, V. (1981). Psychoneuroendocrine influences on immunocompetence and neoplasia. *Science, 212,* 1100–1109.

Riscalla, L. M. (1983). A holistic concept of the immune system. *Journal of the American Society of Psychosomatic Dentistry and Medicine, 30,* 97–101.

Rosenman, R. H., & Friedman, M. (1974). Neurogenic factors in pathogenesis of coronary heart disease. *Medical Clinics of North America, 58,* 269–279.

Rossouw, J. E. (1990). The value of lowering cholesterol after myocardial infarction. *The New England Journal of Medicine, 323,* 1112–1119.

Rozanksi, A., Bairey, C. N., Krantz, D. S., Friedman, J., Resser, K. J., Morell, M., et al. (1988). Mental stress and the induction of silent myocardial ischemia in patients with coronary artery disease. *The New England Journal of Medicine, 318,* 1005–1012.

Seligman, M., Chess, L., Fahey, J. L., Fauci, A. S., Lachmann, P. J., L'Age-Stehr, J., et al. (1984). AIDS--an immunologic reevaluation. *The New England Journal of Medicine, 311,* 1286–1292.

Selye, Hans. (1956). *The stress of life.* New York: McGraw-Hill.

Shavit, Y., Lewis, J. W., Terman, G. W., Gale, R. P., & Liebeskind, J. C. (1984). Opioid peptides mediate the suppressive effect of stress on natural killer cell cytotoxicity. *Science, 223,* 188–190.

Sklar, L. S., & Anisman, H. (1980). Social stress influences tumor growth. *Psychosomatic Medicine, 42,* 347–365.

Soll, A. H. (1990). Pathogenesis of peptic ulcer and implications for therapy. *The New England Journal of Medicine, 322,* 909–916.

Stall, R. D., Coates, T. J., & Hoff, C. (1988). Behavioral risk reduction for HIV infection among gay and bisexual men: A review of results from the United States. *American Psychologist, 43,* 878–885.

Stephens, G. J. (1980). *Pathophysiology for health practitioners.* New York: Macmillan.

Stone, A., Cox, D. S., Valdimarsdottir, H., Jandorf, L., & Neale, J. M. (1987). Evidence that secretory IgA Antibody is associated with daily mood. *Journal of Personality and Social Psychology, 52,* 988–993.

Stoney, C. M., Davis, M. C., & Matthews, K. A. (1987). Sex differences in physiological responses to stress and in coronary heart disease: A causal link? *Psychophysiology, 24,* 127–131.

Tanaka, M., Kohno, Y., Nakagawa, R., Ida, Y., Takeda, S., Nagasaki, N., & Noda, Y. (1983). Regional characteristics of stress-induced increases in brain noradrenaline release in rats. *Pharmacology, Biochemistry and Behavior, 19,* 543–547.

Taylor, A. L., & Fishman, L. M. (1988). Corticotropin-releasing hormone. *The New England Journal of Medicine, 319,* 213–222.

Taylor, C. B., & Fortmann, S. P. (1983). Essential hypertension. *Psychosomatics, 24,* 433–448.

Teshima, H., Kubo, C., Kihara, H., Imada, Y., Nagata, S., Ago, Y., & Ikemi, Y. (1982). Psychosomatic aspects of skin diseases from the standpoint of immunology. *Psychotherapy and Psychosomatics, 37,* 165–175.

Uttal, W. R. (1978). *The psychobiology of mind.* Hillsdale, NJ: Lawrence Erlbaum Associates.

Walter, H., Hofman, A., Vaughan, R. D., & Wynder, E. L. (1988). Modification of risk factors for coronary disease: Five-year results of a school-based intervention trial. *The New England Journal of Medicine, 318,* 1093–1100.

Ward, M. M., Mefford, I. N., Parker, S. D., Chesney, M. A., Taylor, C. B., Keegan, D. L., & Barchas, J. D. (1983). Epinephrine and norepinephrine responses in continuously collected human plasma to a series of stressors. *Psychosomatic Medicine, 45,* 471–486.

PART THREE

SOCIAL SYSTEMS AND STRESS

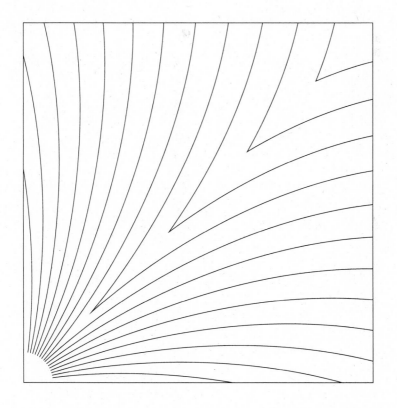

CHAPTER 6

Stress in the Family: Adjustment, Conflict, and Disruption

MOST OF THE COMPLAINTS ABOUT THE INSTITUTION OF HOLY MATRIMONY ARISE
NOT BECAUSE IT IS WORSE THAN THE REST OF LIFE, BUT BECAUSE IT IS NOT IN-
COMPARABLY BETTER.
JOHN LEVY AND RUTH MUNROE

The night of November 16, 1982, was a night that would bring the Richard Jahnke family national notoriety. That night, 16-year-old Richard Jahnke, Jr., shot and killed his father with six blasts from a shotgun loaded with deer slugs. He apparently had planned the killing for some time. That fateful night, his parents' anniversary, Richard hid in the garage waiting for them to return from their celebration outing. This may sound like a story of cold-blooded murder by a psychopathic criminal. Still, when Richard revealed his motives, there were pleas for Richard to be absolved of responsibility for the crime.

Richard revealed that his mother and his 17-year-old sister, Deborah, were victims of a brutal man who knew little of affection and even less of human decency. The man frequently beat Richard's mother, sexually molested Richard's sister, and abused Richard. Richard became terrified of his father and anguished about what he saw happening to his sister and mother. The social service agency contacted earlier did nothing to stop the abuse. Therefore, Richard concluded that he was the only one who could stop it.

Family stress does not always come from this extreme end of the continuum. Still, family stress is a problem of substantial proportions. This chapter provides a perspective on what we know about stress in the family and about family coping strategies. First, some working definitions will be presented, followed by the description of a comprehensive theory of family stress. Later, stress from marital disruption, child abuse, and sexual abuse will be discussed. Finally, this chapter will present some coping and problem-solving strategies for the family.

FOCUS ON THE FAMILY

Most research on stress and health has focused on the variety and quality of *individual* reactions to stressors. It is now apparent, however, that this approach has limits. The equation of stress involves the family in both destructive and constructive ways. Stress is seldom, if ever, an isolated event affecting only one person in one remote situation. Stress spills over from the job, children bring it home from the classroom, and social events produce stress that ends up at home.

A search for the sources of stress in the family is a search for the interplay of forces between the family unit and its members. The appearance of stress in any family member is likely to alter a family's functioning during the time stress is present. On the other hand, the way a family unit responds to stress affects the burden each family member carries. Consider a family that has suffered severe economic loss. Ideally, family leaders keep their emotions in check and use rational problem-solving behavior. However, some leaders may display hysterical, irrational, and "catastrophizing" behavior instead (Ellis, 1962). The rest of the family may then interpret the situation as being much worse than it really is. More vulnerable family members, such as young children, may develop feelings of anxiety and insecurity. Worse yet, they may learn that this is the "adult" way to respond to stressors and carry the style with them into adult life.

The family is a fertile ground for the emergence of stress as well as for stress-spillover effects. The family cycle has distinct phases—mate selection, marital adjustment, family planning, childbearing, child rearing, career decline, and retirement. Each phase has its unique joys and sorrows, harmony and stress, from the first breath of commitment to the dying breath of a spouse. Later in this chapter, I will outline some of these stage stressors. For the interested reader, I have included references that provide thorough coverage of stress in marriage and the family (Curran, 1987; Hobbs & Cole, 1976; Menaghan, 1982; Rollins & Feldman, 1970; Russell, 1974).

Finally, attempts to resolve stress normally occur first at home. People usually do not seek outside help until after personal resources fail and the home no longer provides solace and solution. The normal course is for a spouse or parent to serve as confidant to the stressed member. Unfortunately, the person under stress may "unload" problems in an emotional outburst. In other cases, the person cannot open up about the internal conflict, but he or she carries the burden so visibly that it affects other family members.

Involvement in one member's stress may consume so much energy and family resources that the entire family becomes distressed and maladjusted. When this happens, it is unlikely that anyone can obtain the support needed to bear the strain and resolve feelings of helplessness, guilt, loneliness, neglect, or anger. The long-term effects of stress in the family are exemplified by what has been happening recently in farm families.

A CASE STUDY IN FAMILY STRESS

For many American farmers, the past several years have seen frustration, unsteady prices for commodities, increasing production costs, staggering indebtedness for many, foreclosures for others, and death of the family farm. Projections in one state suggested that 40% of its farmers could lose their farms. While the economic load carried by the head of the family is immense, the emotional load apparently can be unbearable. The prospect of loss is more than just economics. It is psychological and social, a personal failure witnessed by the entire extended family. Many farms have been "in the family" for years. Loss of the farm signifies a separation, an enforced detachment, from all that has carried family pride and tradition for years. In one Iowa community of 8000, three farmers committed suicide within 18 months because of despair over the prospect of losing their farms (Turkington, 1985).

Family members suffer emotionally as well. Some members, especially the children, have little or no direct control over the situation and no responsibility for the origins of the difficulty. They become victims of the family disruption. The incidence of depression, poor schoolwork, and suicide among children of farm families has increased with pressures on the family. The problems described here, though, are not necessarily confined to the farm family. The type of stressors varies from rural to suburban families, but the general outcome is much the same.

One body of evidence supports the notion that stress in the family increases vulnerability of individual members to physical and emotional distress (Bloom, Asher, & White, 1978). On the other hand, numerous factors unique to the family increase resistance to distress. One benefit found in a family's support for its members is the **social buffer** it provides against the storms and stresses of daily life (Cobb, 1976). Early theory suggested that the presence of social buffers might have a direct, positive effect on coping. More recent analyses suggest that lack of social support is the key factor because its absence interferes with adjustment (Walker, 1985). Which occurs, vulnerability or resistance, depends on the psychosocial traits of family members, the dynamics of family interactions and communications, and the problem-solving strategies established by the family.

FAMILY STRESS: PROBLEMS IN DEFINITION

To this point, I have not used the term **family stress** as some authors have used it (McCubbin et al., 1980) because the previous definition of stress is not wholly appropriate when referring to groups. A group of people cannot experience stress the same way an individual does. Qualitative differences exist that require different levels of analysis and different intervention strategies.

Personal versus Family Stress

First, it seems intuitively acceptable to say that a family is under stress. Everyday language frequently uses just this type of expression. One example came from the 17-day ordeal following the hijacking of TWA Flight 847 from Athens, Greece. Televised interviews with families who had husbands or brothers still held hostage amply documented the fear, torment, frustration, and anger many of the families felt. In a similar vein, studies of families who lost loved ones, homes, or investments through natural catastrophes show the terrible stress families

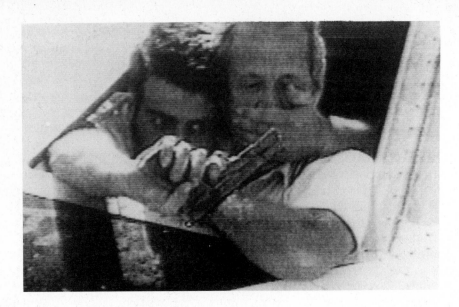

Captain John Testrake under the gun of a hijacker, while the world, including families
of the crew and passengers, watched
SOURCE: AP/Wide World Photo.

sometimes have to endure. Few would quibble with the notion that families in
any of these situations are families under stress.

Still, a problem exists when we use the concept of stress this way. To put
it simply, we speak of families under stress, but it is really individuals who grieve
and become depressed, frustrated, or angry. Family-stress theory thus straddles
a fence between "the hazard of blatant reductionism to the level of individual
behavior" and "the hazard of assuming that groups have the properties of individuals" (Klein, 1983, p. 93). We need to shift our focus, then, from the personal system to the **family as a system,** a set of connected elements that
function as a whole, that can be disrupted.

Family is a descriptive term that refers to a unique social cluster of people
who enjoy a special relationship through love, mutual commitment, and reciprocal dependence. Traditionally, families have formed through marriage and
extended through procreation, but nontraditional families share many features
of traditional families. Families share common goals and values. They work
cooperatively to realize their goals and usually become more closely united when
threats to family integrity appear.

To meet family needs, the system has adult leaders and child followers.
There is a parallel division of teachers and learners. Usually, some division of
labor exists for productive earning and household management. Stress on the
family may cause the system to malfunction, disrupting harmony and destroying the organization of the family. Family leaders may experience more difficulty managing family resources. Earning productivity may decrease, and the

child's socialization may stop. When this happens, the family system is a maladaptive system. On the other hand, a family that functions as an organized, coherent, and integrated unit is an adaptive system.

To summarize, family stress is qualitatively different from personal stress. Where individuals experience emotional distress, families suffer a loss of harmony. Where individuals suffer from lack of concentration and loss of fluid thinking, families have reduced resources for collective problem solving. Where individuals suffer from ulcers or migraine, families break up in separation or divorce. For individuals stress is an insult to a biopsychological system. For families, stress is an insult to a social system.

Stressors, Stress, and Crises

Several authors use stress definitions that recognize this difference between personal and family stress. McCubbin and Patterson (1983, p. 8) define **stressor** as "a life event or transition impacting upon the family unit which produces, or has the potential of producing, change in the family social system." The death of a parent, long-term hospitalization of a family member, loss of income, or imprisonment of a family member qualify as stressors in this view.

The same authors define stress in terms of the family's response to an event. That reponse depends on how the family interprets or assigns meaning to the event and on the seriousness of the threat. Finally, McCubbin and Patterson define a **crisis** or **distress** as the disorganization or incapacity that results from the family's lack of resources and problem-solving skills to manage the stress.

A TRANSACTIONAL THEORY OF FAMILY STRESS

Although numerous family-stress theories exist, Reuben Hill (1949) provided one of the most comprehensive. To its credit, the model is still highly respected today. The theory's sterile title obscures its content—the **ABCX model.** The ABCX theory states the following: some *event* (A) interacts with the family's *resources* for meeting crises (B) and the family's *definition* of the event (C) to produce a *crisis* (X). David Klein (1983) refers to this and related theories as **stress-crises-coping (SCC)** theories.

It is interesting to note parallels between the ABCX model and the cognitive-transactional model of personal stress proposed by Richard Lazarus. While Hill did not choose to call his theory transactional, the preceding summary suggests it is a transactional theory. McCubbin and Patterson (1983) also noted this similarity. In the family, a stressor exists only if the family has appraised (defined) the event as threatening and the family's resources (secondary appraisal) are inadequate to meet the demands. Table 6-1 lists the essential features of this theory and compares it to other theories introduced later in this chapter, a systems theory and a cognitive-contextual theory.

TABLE 6-1
Summary of Three Theories of Family Stress

Stress model	Definition of stress	Source(s) of stress	Model's strengths	Model's weaknesses
ABCX model	An event that inter-acts with resources and appraisals to produce a crisis	Various events that require fam-ily adjustment	Parallels the inter-actional model Some empirical support Potential to be a com-prehensive theory	Still largely in the theoretical/speculative mode Difficult to give terms opera-tional reference Concept of family appraisal is very problematic Arbitrary definition of stressor
Systems theory	No definition given	Family violence and marital conflict	Indirect but large body of supporting evidence Compatible with other more comprehensive theories	Primarily developed to ex-plain family violence Limited in scope Difficult to give terms opera-tional reference
Cognitive-contextual theory	No definition given	Parental conflict	Parallels and com-plements the interac-tional model	Primarily developed for one type of family stress Limited in scope

Components of Family Stress and Coping

Two ideas are central to Hill's ABCX model. One is the *amount of change* induced by the stressor event. The second is the **family's vulnerability** to stress. Figure 6-1 shows the general model. Amount of change is the extent to which the event necessitates family adjustment. Death of the major wage earner produces a substantial change in the family structure, as does divorce. Less dramatic but still powerful is the change produced when the major wage earner takes a new company assignment that involves relocating the family to a new city. On the other hand, imprisonment of a family member might be welcomed if it removes a child molester or spouse beater from the home. Thus, the influence of change is still dependent on how the family appraises or defines the change.

Family vulnerability In Hill's model, family vulnerability is the most complex and crucial factor contributing to family stress. Stressors interact with family vulnerability to produce a crisis. Assuming that vulnerability is constant, the more threatening an event is, the more likely the family will have a crisis on its hands. Similarly, holding threat constant, the more vulnerable the family, the more likely the family will experience stress. This relationship holds true when the event produces short-term or acute stress. Still, small stressors can pile up, or one stressor can become chronic. This may be likened to the proverbial "straw that broke the camel's back." Then, the effect is the same as that of a severe short-term stressor.

Family appraisals Numerous factors contribute to family vulnerability. As Figure 6-1 shows, the family's definition, or **appraisal,** of the seriousness of the change, combined with family integration and adaptability, lead to

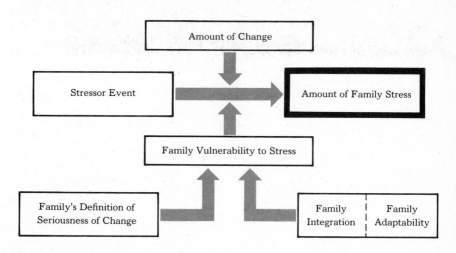

FIGURE 6-1
Modified Hill ABCX model of family stress
SOURCE: Adapted from McCubbin & Patterson (1983).

vulnerability.[1] The family's definition of seriousness combines personal assessments (what the change means to each person individually) and group assessments (what the change means to the family as a social unit). The actual stress felt by any member probably depends on his or her personal awareness of the implications of the change. In addition, individual stress may depend on the extent to which the person can influence or help alter the course of the stressor event or reduce the impact of the change.

Family resources   Another factor contributing to family vulnerability is the family's resources for meeting the demands of the stress event. Family resources are a combination of **personal resources** possessed by the individual family members and resources that are part of the family system. Family-stress research has focused on four personal resources. These are financial status or economic well-being, health status or physical well-being, psychological resources (usually assessed as personality variables), and educational level. Educational level is an indirect measure of cognitive skills, which presumably aid realistic appraisals and contribute to problem-solving ability.

Family decision making and problem solving   Perhaps the most significant family resource is the family's pattern of decision making and competence in problem solving. David Klein (1983; Klein & Hill, 1979) wrote extensively on this topic and addressed several issues in family problem solving. One issue is the way the family addresses stress. Another is how the family socializes children to become competent problem solvers and mature adults who can withstand stress.

Karl Weick (1971) identified 11 aspects of family problem solving that distinguish families from other problem-solving groups. David Klein (1983) summarized these as follows:

1. Families work at solving problems when energy levels are low (such as at the beginning or end of the day).
2. Family members tend to "mask" expert power and allocate responsibility for problem solving based on legitimate power.
3. Distribution of necessary knowledge for family problem solving is uneven among family members as is investment in the outcome; the most informed member values acceptance more than the outcome quality and, therefore, can selectively control the flow of information to maximize acceptance at the expense of quality.
4. Affection in families is mostly noncontingent. Family problem solving, thus, is independent of learning through reinforcement.
5. Discussion of family problems often occurs in "cascading" fashion. One problem "hitchhikes" with another. This suggests that family members

[1]Burr (1983) detailed eight factors related to vulnerability, including family definition, integration, and adaptability. The other five variables are (1) amount of positional influence of the family, (2) amount of personal influence (discussed briefly in the text), (3) externalization of blame for change, (4) amount of time changes anticipated, and (5) amount of anticipated socialization. Space does not permit a full discussion of each factor.

may be more interested in releasing emotional tension than in instrumentally or rationally resolving concerns.

6. Families have both a voluntary (psychic) and involuntary (biological, legal) membership component; psychic withdrawal is a potential threat and, thus, an instrument of power.

7. Family problem solving is "embedded" in ongoing activity. It is not readily separated in the fashion of a council meeting, and thus, it is difficult to know when problem solving is occurring.

8. Family problem solving occurs in relative isolation from outside influences. It is therefore likely to become stylistically rigid within a given family group.

9. Many family problems contain a "developmental confound"; that is, they are best left untreated and relegated to "normal, natural trouble" that will pass with time.

10. Families carry over large amounts of "unfinished business," and members lack consensus on criteria of satisfactory problem resolution; thus presumed solutions to one problem evoke new problems.

11. The ecology of families is disorderly and gestural, and body cues are cryptic at best. (pp. 511–512)

Coping with Family Stress

McCubbin and his colleagues (McCubbin et al., 1980) specified four general hypotheses of how family coping actions work to protect the family from stress. The first is the notion that coping behaviors reduce family vulnerability. Consider a family member who is emotionally disturbed or one who threatens to leave the family unit after conflict. The family needs to allocate time and energy to these matters. Dealing with issues satisfactorily may remove the threat, thus restoring balance to the family and reducing vulnerability. Second, coping actions may strengthen or maintain family cohesiveness and organization. Third, coping may reduce or eliminate stressor events. Fourth, coping may actively operate on the environment to change it.

Investigators acknowledge that faulty coping can produce stress for the family. Some coping strategies are inferior, misguided, or non–reality oriented. According to McCubbin's analysis, coping efforts can damage the family system in at least three ways. First, coping may produce indirect harm to the family unit or members of the family. One example McCubbin gives is when the family compensates for inflation by cutting back on health care. Second, coping efforts may produce direct damage to the family, as when a family member abuses alcohol or attempts suicide as a way out of current problems. Third, coping may increase family risks by retarding adaptive behaviors. This is most obvious when the family engages in denial or refuses to accept reality. For example, when a child becomes ill, possibly terminally ill, the family may reorganize realistically or unrealistically. When the latter is the case, the long-term picture is usually bleak.

Stages in Family Coping

In studies of families with fathers missing in action in Vietnam, the McCubbin group observed three stages in the family's adjustment (McCubbin et al., 1980). These were resistance, restructuring, and consolidation. The initial reaction of most family members was resistance as they tried to deny or avoid the reality forced on them. As the family began to acknowledge this unalterable reality, members began to reorganize their lives around the notion of a partial family. They redefined family roles. Children assumed more of the responsibilities for day-to-day maintenance of the household, and the mother looked for employment. In addition, the mother became more independent while exercising a stronger authority in the family. One interesting note was that the extended family (for example, in-laws) frequently had difficulty adjusting to this new strength in the mother. They expressed disapproval, which only served to increase her stress. Finally, the family consolidated its gains by making the reorganization permanent, and used this growth as a springboard for more changes in family life. Part of this final stage included new meanings assigned to the crises and a newly structured lifestyle for the entire family.

Criticism of the ABCX Model

In spite of the appeal of this model, it is subject to criticism. Alexis Walker (1985) discussed weaknesses of Hill's model at length. Walker noted that Hill arbitrarily identified a stressor at a given point. Yet a stressor may result from a cumulative history of factors. In other words, Hill ignored process in favor of a time-anchored event. Second, Walker contends that family resources are not adequately defined. Third, the family's definition (appraisal) is problematic. Each family member probably has his or her personal representation of the event. It is unlikely that there is a "family mind" that formulates a unitary definition of the event.

Walker argued that family-stress theory should be contextual and systems oriented. Stress must be viewed in sociohistorical context. This includes understanding the way external systems (social networks, communities, and agencies) influence the family. It also entails understanding how changes in family support systems alter the family process for better or for worse. Unfortunately, Walker does not provide a testable contextual-systems model.

TRANSITIONAL STRESS

We noted earlier that transitions create stress for family systems. Transitions are normative to some extent. That is, transitions are part of the natural history of every family. Although some transitions occur frequently, they are not normative according to society's standards; for example, divorce occurs frequently, but it is not normative. Society believes divorce is incompatible with the value of a stable family unit. For this discussion, we will use Fosson's (1988) scheme.

Fosson identified five major family transitions that are likely to produce stress. These are formation of a new family unit, addition of new family members, separation of members from the family unit, loss of a family member, and disintegration of the family unit. Disintegration will be covered in more detail later in this chapter when we discuss separation and divorce. For now, we will discuss only Fosson's first four transitions.

Creation of a New Family Unit

Society customarily creates new family units through legal or religious ritual or by recognizing reciprocal commitment between two people. In so doing, the unit is distinguished in a special way from other social units. Family members take on new roles and responsibilities that differ from those they had before. The family dyad has an implicit or explicit understanding about sharing emotional support and keeping exclusive intimacy. They divide obligations in some equitable fashion, and they negotiate patterns of communication and mechanisms for decision making and financial management. When two people share similar histories, values, and patterns of decision making, the transition probably will be smooth. The more pronounced their differences are, the more likely they are to encounter stress.

Adding a New Family Member

The birth of a baby or adoption of a child also requires adjustment in roles and responsibilities. The new roles of father and mother alter the exclusive companionship of husband and wife. The infant demands time and attention, which changes the pattern of interaction for the parents. These interactions are important to the parents' sense of fulfillment or frustration. Husbands may feel deprived of companionship. Wives as primary caregivers may feel that they do not control their time. These interactions also begin to establish patterns of reciprocity and autonomy in the child. Discord may occur when the couple do not share common child-rearing values. When either parent sees the child as a rival for the spouse's affection or time, or when the child's demands seem to compete with career goals, stress may result. Additional stress occurs when boundaries between parents and grandparents are fluid and the child receives mixed messages about standards and conduct.

Separation of a Family Member

When members leave their nuclear families, alignments among family members also change. Support systems for both parents and children are disrupted. Siblings may be left without their best friend. Parents may lose a sense of closeness to their child. When the child leaves for college, family resources may be taxed.

If the child is ill prepared for college life, he or she may return pressure to the family by introducing emotionality and uncertainty to family interactions.

The effect of separation may be even more traumatic when it comes under duress. Teenagers may leave because of conflict with family values. They may engage in antisocial behavior that leads to jail or be pressed into military duty. The family may go through a type of grieving process under these circumstances.

A common separation stress is the "empty nest" syndrome, when the last child leaves and the parents are again a dyad. Parents may miss the excitement and structure that revolved around helping their children reach maturity. At this time, they may find it necessary to reassess mutual and individual goals and establish new ways of interacting.

Loss of a Family Member

Separations of the type mentioned in the preceding paragraphs retain the clear hope and expectation that continued interaction is possible. The death of a family member provides no such hope. The loss of a young family member is usually more traumatic than the loss of an older family member. A sudden loss is usually more difficult than loss following chronic illness. The grieving process may be difficult, but as Fosson (1988) noted, the family system does not change greatly and stress is usually not insurmountable. Events of this nature may draw family units together, making them even closer knit and stronger.

SEPARATION AND DIVORCE

Living in a family unit where everything goes smoothly engenders enough day-to-day tensions. No matter how devoted two people are to each other, there will be disagreements at times. Even the most loving of brothers and sisters fight occasionally. Family members also have many different needs and wants that can put pressure on the family budget. A study based on a large Chicago sample (Pearlin & Schooler, 1978) found that the one family stressor most consistently identified was financial pressures on the family. Curran (1987) also lists economic issues of budget and finance as the number one stressor in the healthy family.

If life is this way in families that are presumably close knit, think what it must be like in families where quarreling and fighting are the rule rather than the exception; where alternating periods of separation and reconciliation keep everyone off guard; when one never knows when Dad will walk out the door next or whether it will be the last time before divorce breaks the family up for good. Research, starting with the work of Holmes and Rahe (1967) on life-change, shows that the three most potent family stressors are death of a spouse, divorce, and marital separation. These events can produce both emotional and physical health problems in the family, including adjustment problems for the children (Grych & Fincham, 1990).

In 1976 there were 2,133,000 marriages and 1,077,000 divorces. The rate of divorce dropped by about 6% between 1979 and 1984 (Heatherington, Stanley-Hagan, & Anderson, 1989). In spite of this, 40% of the children born in the 1970s and 1980s are still likely to experience divorce (Grych & Fincham, 1990). Part of the decline in the divorce rate may be related to changing ideas about marriage itself: more people establish homes now without the legal sanction of marriage. Still, alarm exists about the trend to end marriages frequently, even casually, making little effort to salvage the relationship. Many social scientists are now trying to discover the factors that contribute to marital conflict and divorce (Amato & Keith, 1991; Grych & Fincham, 1990). The hope is not just to stop the rush to divorce but to reduce the toll on victims of divorce.

Personal Traits and Divorce

Bernard Bloom's team from the University of Colorado carried out a comprehensive review of stress and **marital conflict** (Bloom, Asher, & White, 1978). They reported that divorced and separated people contribute disproportionately to the numbers of psychiatric patients, whereas married people are underrepresented. In addition, based on statistics supplied by the National Center for Health Statistics (1970), divorced, separated, or widowed persons had substantially higher rates of illness and disability than married or never-married persons. If one research team is correct, people who have serious difficulty with their health are less likely to marry, have more problems maintaining their marriages, and are less likely to remarry (Carter & Glick, 1976). Divorced and separated groups also have a higher rate of alcoholism. One obvious question is whether the reported difficulties follow marital disruption or cause marital disruption. The evidence suggests that the problems were present before marriage and contributed to marital disruption; marital disruption probably intensified the problems.

Sluggers, Attackers, and Threateners

Suzanne Steinmetz (1977) conducted a revealing study on how people deal with conflict in marriage. She obtained responses from 78 college students and their older friends. The results indicated that fully 30% of young families had used some type of physical violence to resolve marital conflicts. Steinmetz identified four approaches to conflict in marriage. *Screaming sluggers* were the couples who made both verbal and physical attacks on each other. The *silent attackers* avoided quarreling at first, but soon released pent-up anger through physical assault. Then there were *threateners,* the ones who attacked each other verbally and threatened violence but never followed through with their threats. Finally, there were the *pacifists,* those who could resolve their marital conflicts without the use of either verbal or physical attacks.

The Aftermath of Marital Disruption

Disruption in marital relations produces numerous additional problems. Divorced people more frequently commit suicide and homicide. Compared to married people, they also have a higher incidence of specific diseases, such as cancer (Kitagawa & Hauser, 1973). Divorced people are involved in motor vehicle accidents more frequently, and they average about three times the death rate from auto accidents than married people do (National Center for Health Statistics, 1970). Table 6-2 summarizes divorce as a family stressor along with two other stressors, single-parenting and violence in the family.

THE SINGLE-PARENT FAMILY

When marital conflict ends in divorce or separation, the troubles are often only beginning, especially for the partner who retains custody of the children. Schlesinger (1969) studied a group of single parents, 90% of whom were women. These parents reported a set of common problems in their struggles to keep the family intact. These included difficulty in managing the children, having to go to work, financial problems, difficulties with sexual expression, and feelings of failure and shame. Most often, mothers and children could stay in the original home, retaining some sense of continuity and stability. On the other hand, fathers most often had to abandon those same homes, homes they had worked hard to provide. This appeared to contribute to fathers' feelings of isolation and rootlessness immediately after divorce.

Nancy Colletta (1983) compared low-income families with moderate-income families and found that low income presented the major problem. Low-income mothers had more difficulty related to child-rearing practices, baby-sitters, and health crises. These problems did not occur in moderate-income families, where stress was lower for both mother and child. Unfortunately, Colletta did not assess the families' educational levels; this could also have influenced the reported stress levels.

Single-parent families tend to be more disorganized, which increases stress on individual members (Heatherington, Cox, & Cox (1976). Divorced parents felt more anxious, angry, rejected, and depressed than did married parents (Heatherington, Cox, & Cox, 1977). Kessler and Essex (1982) advanced the theory that married people show less depression than single people because they are less emotionally damaged by stressful experiences. Single parents may be both psychologically and physically vulnerable. Kiecolt-Glaser and her colleagues found evidence that marital disruption suppresses the immune system, which increases vulnerability to illness and even death (Kiecolt-Glaser et al., 1985).

Children in the Single-Parent Family

Just as divorced parents experience great stress while adjusting to the single-parent reality, so do children. According to statistics compiled by the Bureau

TABLE 6-2
Summary of Major Family Stressors

Family stressors	Contributing factors	Possible consequences
Separation and divorce	Physical illness or disability	Increased physical illness
	Mental illness or emotional instability	Increased anxiety, tension, and/or mental illness
	Alcoholism	Suicide
		Homicide
		Increased motor vehicle accidents and deaths
Single-parenting	Family disorganization	Increased feelings of guilt, shame, and failure
	Postdivorce conflict	
	Time management and work	Increased anxiety
	Financial pressures	Frustrated expectations for child
	Child care	
	Interpersonal conflict with extended family and ex-spouse	
	Intrapsychic conflict	
	Adult responsibility placed on children	
Family violence and abuse	*Historical variables:* Developmental history of family violence and abuse	Damaged self-image and self-esteem
	Parental rejection	Poorer long-term emotional stability and adjustment
	Modeled aggression	
	Failure to learn how to parent effectively	Feelings of failure and incompetence
	Current variables: Family disorganization	Feelings of helplessness and hopelessness
	Life-change stress	Failure to thrive
	Traumatic bonding or co-dependencies	Instrumental but maladaptive acts to restore balance
	Premature, difficult, or unhealthy baby	
	Child misbehavior	
	Tacit or explicit support for sibling abuse	

of the Census (1982), the number of children living in single-parent homes doubled in the last decade. Further, the number of children living with mothers who never married has increased fourfold. Probably 40% to 50% of children born in the 1970s and 1980s will spend about five years in a single-parent home (Heatherington, Stanley-Hagan, & Anderson, 1989). Many children must take on adult responsibility at the expense of time for enjoying their childhood. Avis Brenner (1984) noted that children may enjoy the signs of adult status, but they still miss the privileges of being children.

Another problem is that children of divorce and separation may create as much stress as they suffer. Single mothers tend to have more difficulty with their sons, whereas single fathers tend to have more difficulty with their daughters (Heatherington, Stanley-Hagan, & Anderson, 1989). Because women head roughly 90% of the single-parent families, the difficulties encountered more frequently result from problems in dealing with a son. This appears to increase the mother's anxiety and feelings of helplessness and incompetence. The long-term cycle may be one of escalating tensions between the two, eroding the relationship and resulting in the mother's loss of self-confidence.

One of the most frequent problems for children is the continued hopes and dreams that Mommy and Daddy will get back together again. It appears that this dream is especially unshakable, lasting for years in some children (Heatherington, Stanley-Hagan, & Anderson, 1989). It takes a gentle but persistent effort to help the children accept reality without adding greatly to their inner turmoil.

This problem can carry over into postdivorce and remarriage as well. All too often, adults expect children to accept remarriage as a blessing. What many adults do not realize is that remarriage shatters their child's dreams of reconciliation. In addition, the child has little time to mourn the death of the dream when the parent remarries. Single parents intending to remarry would do well to consider this source of stress for their children. One solution is to include children as much as possible in the decision process. This might also help them put to rest any hopes that still existed for the dissolved marriage.

Postdivorce Conflict and Stress

Even after divorce, many factors force the separate families to interact, beginning with visitation rights and schedules. In joint custody arrangements, parents must arrange for moving the children from one home to another. Both partners usually share continued interest in the children's development. There are the father's financial obligations and the mother's concern when payments are inconsistent. These continued contacts may represent new opportunities for old conflicts to surface.

One research team (Cline & Westman, 1971) identified five patterns that seem to mark postdivorce conflict. These are listed with explanatory comments.

1. *Hostilities over parenting.* Recent research shows that fathers' parenting styles tend to change more than mothers'. This may contribute to conflict. Single fathers are more easygoing (Smith & Smith, 1981), and they spend more time with their children after obtaining custody than single mothers do (Orthner, Brown, & Ferguson, 1976).

2. *Hostilities over matters unrelated to the children.* For example, parents may carry over bitterness and acrimony about the cause of the divorce. Parents may also harbor anger over perceived injustices in the divorce settlement.

3. *Pressure from the children to maintain contact between mother and father.* This pressure is largely due to the child's continued dream that the parents will reunite.

4. *Tugs-of-war, choosing sides, and shifting alliances.* A parent may use one or more of the children as pawns to wage a war of nerves against the other parent. This pattern can be especially destructive to everyone. More often than not, the children are the real losers. Research shows that children of divorce fare best where the parents can maintain an amicable relationship (Rofes, 1982), share the children with warmth and regard for each other's rights (Wallerstein & Kelly, 1980), and help the children understand that the love of both parents is not dependent on a marriage contract alone.

5. *Continued interaction caused by grandparents and the extended family.* One forgotten aspect of divorce is that divorce does not just shatter the dreams of the nuclear family; it shatters the dreams of members of the extended family as well. Parents of the divorced couple have to explain to their friends why their son's or daughter's marriage failed. They may perceive their child's divorce as their parenting failure. In addition, they have vested interest in their grandchildren and frequently want to retain some contact. Making arrangements for this can be a source of stress to both the mother and father.

VIOLENCE IN THE FAMILY

Of the family stressors receiving attention today, none rate higher than **spouse abuse and child abuse.** Recent statistics reveal that family quarrels or ongoing patterns of family violence lead directly to many physical injuries and deaths. Unfortunately, counting just the physical scars ignores the real toll: the lifelong emotional scars that abused people carry wherever they go. At the least, abused children tend to suffer a damaged self-image; poorer emotional adjustment, if not mental disturbance; more disturbed family relationships; lower impulse control; and inferior coping skills (Hjorth & Ostrov, 1982).

Violence in the family is not a modern innovation, and it may not even be as rare as some like to think. One investigative team takes the position that violence is *normal.* They based this judgment on the sheer frequency of violence in the family. The team also suggests that conflict is "an inevitable and necessary part of social relationships," although physical violence is not (Gelles, 1985; Gelles & Straus, 1979). Police records do not help dispel this notion, as nearly 20% of homicides are a direct result of family violence (Emery, 1989).

Stress and Child Abuse

The National Center on Child Abuse and Neglect (1981) conducted a study on child abuse from May 1979 to June 1980. They defined child abuse and **neglect** as follows:

> A child maltreatment situation is one where, through purposive acts or marked
> inattention to the child's basic needs, behavior of a parent/substitute or other
> adult caretaker caused foreseeable and avoidable injury or impairment to a
> child or materially contributed to unreasonable prolongation or worsening
> of an existing injury or impairment. (p. 4)

Ignoring instances of abuse or neglect caused by siblings or institutional staff,
the study reported a total of 652,000 maltreated children. Of this group, 207,000
had been physically assaulted, 138,400 had been emotionally abused, and 1000
had been killed.

Add to this toll another 329,000 children whose treatment meets the criterion of neglect. There are many formal definitions of neglect. Still, Brenner
(1984) described it best when he said that "children live with caretakers who
are unwilling or unable to become involved with them and who are emotionally and sometimes physically absent" (p. 115). Brenner's description of the
neglected child is almost nauseating, but it reveals the silent and insidious tragedy
of neglect.

> Households . . . cluttered with garbage, piles of clothing, excrement, dirty
> dishes, and stained mattresses lacking sheets and blankets. Drugs, liquor,
> poisons, and matches are discarded wherever they have been used last. It
> is not unusual to find a baby lying naked in a crib covered with feces and
> next to it a bottle of soured milk. (p. 117)

I have witnessed many of these things and more (for example, chickens perched
on a baby's crib, adding excrement to human feces). Unfortunately, mere words
cannot convey the magnitude of the horror.

Attempts to identify the factors that contribute to abuse and neglect recently
turned up some leads. Still, there are few constructive plans for preventing child
and spouse abuse. For the moment, consider the following major contributors
to abuse and neglect (Belsky, 1980).

Abuse and Developmental History

First, parents who maltreat their children often have a developmental history
that predisposes them to do so. Both retrospective and prospective studies confirm this conclusion. This does not mean that all abusive parents were themselves
abused as children. Suffering personal abuse or neglect as a child is only one
factor that sets the stage for becoming an abusive parent.

Another factor is the powerful influence of observing aggression. Albert
Bandura's (1973) classic work on modeled aggression supports the idea that
parents' reciprocal aggression may contribute to children becoming abusive in
adult life. Further, being rewarded for aggressive actions within the family contributes to becoming abusive in adult relationships.

Parental rejection also may be a key factor that contributes to becoming
an abusive parent. The evidence suggests that abusive parents are looking for
the love and acceptance from their children that they did not receive from their

parents (Rohner, 1975). In effect, abusive parents create a role reversal in which the parents are the "cared-for" and the children are the longed-for "caregivers." When the parents do not receive the care they expected from their children, they may turn to abuse.

Lack of developmental experiences that enable children to pass into adulthood with suitable parenting values and skills is equally important. This includes experience with child care during childhood and adolescence. Blumberg's (1974) research suggests that parents who abuse their children are woefully ignorant of the most rudimentary information on the sequence and timing of a child's growth and maturation. Without this knowledge, it may be difficult for parents to comprehend that the way a child thinks and behaves is natural and is not contrived expressly to irritate. Theodore Dix (1991) believes that emotional expression and control are at the core of parental competence. On the one hand, emotional sensitivity to the child's needs contributes to effective parenting. On the other hand, inappropriate expression or control of emotions in the parent serves to undermine effective parenting.

Life-Change, Stress, and Abuse

Many adults who were abused as children raise their children with love, sensitivity, and regard. This shows that development history alone cannot account for being abusive as an adult. Other forces must interact with developmental influences. One suspect in this equation is family stress. Abuse of a spouse or child creates extreme stress, especially when the attack was unexpected. This suggests that stress is only an outcome of maltreatment.

Is it possible that stress may also cause abuse? Several investigators have addressed this issue. Life changes such as a spouse's death, divorce, loss of a job, and economic hardships correlate strongly with child abuse and neglect *when the developmental history described earlier is also present* (Conger, Burgess, & Barrett, 1979; Smith, 1984). Stress as a cause of maltreatment may begin a vicious cycle in which abuse creates more stress, which then perpetuates abuse.

One of the most powerful family stressors is marital conflict. Studies of the relationship between marital conflict and abuse show that conflict is high in families where child abuse is present (Smith & Hanson, 1975). We must be careful with interpretations because it is not always clear whether the conflict preceded or followed the child abuse. Yet Steinmetz (1977) showed that spouses who use physical and verbal aggression in resolving marital conflict also use the same tactics in disciplining their children. Finally, the transition to parenthood may create stress. For some parents, birth of a child is a disruption. In addition, they lack preparation for the responsibilities of parenting, and this may be enough to tip some over the edge into child abuse. This is especially true when the first child is premature or abnormal (Lowenthal, 1987).

Conflict between parents also relates to diminished skills in mothers' feeding of young infants. A worst case scenario begins with problems in feeding the baby that lead to stomach upsets and colic. The baby grows more uncomfortable and more vocal about its displeasure. On the other side, the mother's confidence in her ability begins a slow downward spiral. The father helps erode the mother's confidence by directly questioning the mother's skills while threatening drastic action if the child cannot be silenced. The mother feels trapped between a husband with little patience for the baby's disrupting influence and a baby who seems ungrateful for the mother's efforts. In this climate, either parent, or both, may turn on the child, scapegoating frustrations and venting anger against the most helpless family member.

Finally, family disorganization may be related to a pattern of abuse. Disorganization disables family coping capacity, which usually leads to increased stress. Among the most powerful disorganizing influences are unemployment and economic privation. Research in both the United States and Great Britain shows that unemployment is probably the most important factor related to abuse and neglect (Light, 1973).

Children as Causes of Stress and Abuse

Another factor that has received attention is the role the child plays in raising levels of tension and stress in the family (Smith, 1984). According to this view, infants are still innocent, unwitting provocateurs. Older children may be both less than innocent and partially aware of what they are doing. Based on this notion, investigators looked for patterns of physical and/or psychological traits of children that might be linked to aggression in adults.

First, evidence exists that many maltreated children are premature babies (Klein & Stern, 1971). Premature and maltreated infants often lack social responsiveness (Egeland & Brunquell, 1979). Parents may see this as a source of mild irritation at first. Should this pattern continue, parents may feel rejected and begin to question their competence as parents. Soon, a parent may feel a strong sense of frustration followed by anger and ultimately aggression. Another line of evidence shows that some parents find their premature babies' crying and appearance aversive and disagreeable (Frodi et al., 1978; Lowenthal, 1987). As Jay Belsky (1980) pointed out, "child maltreatment must be considered an interactive process; although children may play a role in their own abuse or neglect, they cannot cause it by themselves" (p. 324). In Belsky's view, the interaction is between the parent's traits and the child's characteristics.

Older children may prompt abuse through misbehavior. Studies of family interactions reveal that when parents punish or discipline a child, the child probably will react with more coercive actions toward the parent (Patterson, 1977). The interaction may deteriorate into "a war of wills" as each combatant seeks to control or resist control with escalating punitiveness and counteraggression. This may end only when the more powerful adult physically attacks the less powerful child.

Sibling Abuse

An overlooked aspect of child abuse is physical injuries caused by siblings. We now recognize that sibling rivalry can take on sinister twists, producing traumas equaling those that parents inflict. Tooley (1971) described children abused by siblings as "weaponless and without safe refuge" in their homes (p. 26). One study found that sibling abuse had occurred in over half the families studied (Straus, Gelles, & Steinmetz, 1980). Because the National Center on Child Abuse and Neglect specifically ignored sibling abuse, we must consider their estimates of abuse to be conservative.

One sinister aspect of sibling abuse is that it can occur in the presence of parents. Tooley described three different parental patterns that suggest how sibling abuse can occur. First, some parents simply choose to ignore or deny that abuse is going on. Second, some parents apparently are unable to manage a violent child, or the child intimidates an inadequate parent. The parent, then, may indulge the child, allowing attacks on the other children to occur without interference. Third, some parents may encourage sibling aggression to act out their own violent impulses.

A Systems Model of Family Violence

In a thoughtful review of family violence, Robert Emery (1989) noted both conceptual and methodological problems in family violence research. He also advanced a theory of the child's reaction to parental conflict. Emery suggested that current definitions of abuse are social value judgments rather than operational definitions. This makes it difficult to assess the true incidence and severity of abusive acts. Further, it is difficult to construct credible theories of process and outcomes. This in turn undermines efforts to design effective interventions to prevent abuse and to offset the effects of abuse.

The theory Emery advances is brief. First, he points out that even 1-year-old children show distress in response to displays of anger between their parents. They show negative emotions, such as crying and aggression, even when the anger does not include them. Second, distress motivates instrumental acts by the child to reduce or offset the distress. These acts may include diverting attention to other problems or directly intervening to protect a parent. Third, the function of the child's instrumental act is crucial. In Emery's view, the child acts to preserve order, homeostasis, in the family system. The child may act as a scapegoat—a personally maladaptive response, but a response that is adaptive for the family system. Emery noted that this theory is very new, but a substantial body of evidence supports it.

After an extensive literature review of marital conflict and child adjustment, John Grych and Frank Fincham (1990) proposed a **cognitive-contextual theory** for understanding children's reactions to marital conflict. (See Figure 6-2 and also compare this theory to other theories summarized in Table 6-1.) In this

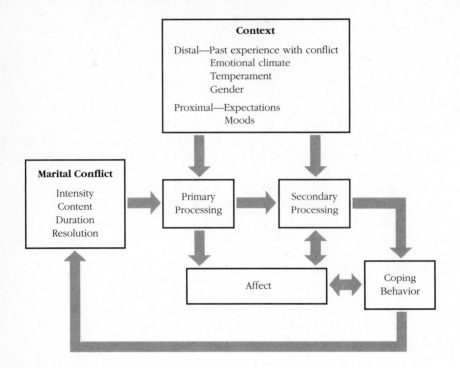

FIGURE 6-2
A cognitive-contextual analysis of children's reactions to and appraisals of marital conflict
SOURCE: Grych & Fincham (1990).

model, parental conflict is a stressor that places adaptive demands on children. Children try to make sense of conflict through an appraisal process that combines cognitive and affective elements. Qualities of the conflict, such as intensity, directly affect the child's first appraisal. In the second stage, the child assigns causal attributions for the events. They may assign blame to a parent. Worse yet, they may assume personal responsibility for the conflict. Coping efforts, if successful, reduce tension and negative emotions. On the other hand, failures in coping may both add to family tension and increase the child's distress. Historical factors relating to the child's experiences in the family and to the family system itself will influence the child's appraisal.

BATTERED WIVES

Spouse abuse involves many of the factors that contribute to child abuse. For example, abusive men and battered women are likely to come from families with patterns of violence already established (San Francisco Family Violence Project, 1980). Further, the more often a woman was struck as a child, the more likely she was to be in a violent intimate relationship (Straus, 1977).

One issue of concern is why an abused adult will not only tolerate abuse but will also keep coming back for more. Children may be forced to stay in abusive homes because they are dependent on adults for basic biological needs. No such necessity exists for most adults. Adults presumably can act to protect themselves. Yet, time and again, adults stay in abusive relationships at great risk to personal safety until a traumatic event breaks the bond.

Traumatic Bonding and Battered Women

Don Dutton and Susan Painter (1981) believe the answer to this paradox is **traumatic bonding.** There is no simple definition of traumatic bonding; it is a complex process in which personal, familial, and social forces operate in consort and collusion to lock the woman into the abusive union. In the interest of brevity, only an outline of the process appears here.

First, as Dutton and Painter noted, domestic violence is more often than not a series of events in which periods of quarreling and abuse alternate with almost equally passionate attempts by the abusive male to make amends. This pattern may beguile women to think the abuse is an exceptional part of the relationship or to ignore it altogether (Rounsaville, 1978). Many clinical and laboratory studies with both human and animal subjects support the argument that alternating abuse and passion increases the chance of traumatic bonding. Rajecki's group reviewed emotional bonding in infants. They concluded that inconsistent treatment by the source of affection (punishment by a parent who also bestows love) intensifies the child's attempts to become closer to the parent (Rajecki, Lamb, & Obmascher, 1978).

A second factor involved in traumatic bonding is the power imbalance between the abuser and the abused. This imbalance may mask mutual dependency needs in which the abused identifies with the abuser and gains some sense of power. On the other hand, the abuser needs the partner's submission to his needs (Dutton & Painter, 1981).

SEXUAL ABUSE OF CHILDREN

Sexual abuse of a child may be the most despicable violation of the trust given to parents as guardians of their children. In 1981 there were 17,880 reports of sexually abused children, all under the age of 12 years. More than 2000 of this group were under the age of 5!

Most instances of sexual abuse take place within the family. Recent statistics show that nearly 80% of child abuse cases involve the stepfather (30%), father (28%), mother's lover (11%), or mother (10%). When this is not true, the offender is usually someone from the extended family or a friend or acquaintance of the family. Offenders appear to operate from one of three motives: they are seeking tenderness, they are exercising power not available in other aspects of their life, or they are venting sadistic rage (Groth & Burgess, 1977).

Physical and Psychological Symptoms of Sexual Abuse

Investigators report numerous physical and psychological problems in sexually abused children. These include sleep disturbances with nightmares; general restlessness, sometimes hyperactivity; eating problems that may include stomachaches and vomiting; and a **failure-to-thrive syndrome.**[2] The child may experience genital irritation, painful discharge of urine, or bed-wetting and soiling. Avis Brenner (1984) summarized the long-term psychological effects of sexual abuse as follows:

1. Poor self-concept
2. Poor social skills
3. Depression
4. Hostility and suicidal feelings
5. Inability to get along with family
6. Inability to trust others
7. Inability to experience sex as satisfying (p. 131)

Hostility, guilt, and low self-esteem often result in suicidal thoughts, if not actions. This appears true of children victimized by parental sexual abuse as well.

Major Warning Signs of Sexual Abuse

The following is a composite of behaviors that children may display after sexual abuse.

1. Appearance of new and strong fears, such as fear of the dark, of being alone, of sleeping alone, of strangers, or of men.
2. Insistence on having mother nearby and refusal to go to formerly favored places.
3. Changes in emotionality such as increased irritability, worry about staying clean, withdrawal from normal activities and circle of friends, crying, and sleep disturbances.
4. Changes in habitual behaviors, such as occurrence of bed-wetting, loss of appetite, and excessive bathing.
5. Appearance of more "adultlike" behaviors, including overt interest in and expressions of sexuality, seductive talk and actions, and so on. This may include intense acting-out behaviors, including sexual acting-out such as promiscuity or prostitution.
6. Sudden changes in school performance, inability to concentrate, failing grades, and indirect attempts to divulge sexual actions and fears.
7. Major changes in relationships with parents, such as parents (or the perpetrator) becoming overprotective, jealous of other friends, inordinate

---

[2]Failure-to-thrive syndrome generally refers to a state in which the child is listless, disinterested, lacking energy and initiative, and also shows signs of despondency and lack of joy in living.

attention and control by a parent. Such changes may be a clue to the offender's identity.

8. Appearance of clandestine contacts between the perpetrator and the child, such as contriving to be alone and being secretive.

These signs do not all appear in any given child. The most important and easily detected signs are physical injury, irritation, bruises, and swelling and bleeding in the genital region. Signs of venereal disease reveal sexual contact. Beyond these physical signs, the most important clues include marked changes, usually for the worse, in behaviors or performances that children normally display.

Effects on the Family

Repercussions in the family are countless. The most basic include strains in familial relationships, changes in natural family roles, and distortion in patterns of affection (Muldoon, 1979). Unhealthy alliances frequently shift the balance of power to the abused daughter, especially when she is old enough to recognize the power she wields. Mary de Young (1982) pointed out that the daughter holds power over the offender because his security depends on her willingness to keep silent. The offender also may resort to a variety of forms of bribery or threat to keep the victim silent. This may include increased attempts to buy the child's loyalty and silence through gifts of money, trips, favors, and clothes. The perpetrator may try to interpret morality and reality for the child to prevent the child from developing a sense that the sexual activities are wrong. The child usually lacks mature cognitive structures to interpret the meaning of the interaction; this only aids the success of the deceit (Orzek, 1985). The cognitive deficit also may contribute to the child's self-blame and feelings of guilt and shame.

The child's psychological problems carry over into the adult years. Victims of child sexual abuse often experience disturbances in marital relationships, perhaps looking for the father figure they never had as a child. They continue to harbor negative—at best, confused—feelings toward their family. They feel a mixture of hate, sympathy, understanding, and faint affection mixed with strong ambivalence for the father. Surprisingly, 38 (79%) of the victims in de Young's study felt more strongly negative toward their mothers than toward their fathers. de Young (1982) concluded that

> the origin of these commonly noted negative feelings toward the mothers is in the recognition that the mothers, above anyone else, had the power to stop the incest from continuing or to prevent it from occurring in the first place. Most of the mothers of the victims in the clinical sample chose not to exercise that power. Therefore, feelings of anger toward the offending father or stepfather ("How could he do this to me?") are easily transferred to the nonparticipating mother ("How could she *let* him do this to me?"). (p. 58)

POSITIVE COPING IN THE FAMILY

There are positive and constructive aspects of coping in the family. Because the family is a social system, it provides a variety of intimate contacts and supports not routinely available in society. In this sense, the family serves as a major source of **social support.**

The Family as a Social Support System

A major moderator of stress is the extent of social support available. Social support may be defined as help given by spouses, parents, and friends. Pearlin's group suggested that social support is "access to and use of individuals, groups, or organizations in dealing with life's vicissitudes" (Pearlin, Lieberman, Menaghan, & Mullan, 1981, p. 340). Gerald Caplan's team looked at social support as attachments to individuals and groups that reduce vulnerability to stress and improve the person's ability to cope with "short-term challenges, stresses, and privations" (Caplan & Killilea, 1976, p. 41).

Social support functions at two levels in the family. First, the family is a social support network for family members. Second, families are embedded in a community. The extent to which that community provides a social support network for the family is important in moderating stress. Unfortunately, some communities function as sources of stress instead of as support networks.

Sidney Cobb (1976) provided a systematic theory of social support. According to Cobb's analysis, social support conveys three types of information to a person. First, social support leads a person to a sense of being cared for and loved. Second, social support leads a person to a sense of being esteemed and valued by other people. Third, social support leads a person to a sense of belonging to a communication network with mutual obligations.

Cobb's analysis can be extended to the gamut of social systems. Social support groups exist at every stage of the life cycle. They wax and wane in importance as personal needs shift. There is a time, for example, when the teenage peer group is the teenager's most important, perhaps only, support network. As the young adult looks for employment and seeks to become a respected member of the community, the social network will consist of bosses, work associates, and community leaders. Thus, many different social groups may provide support to moderate the effects of stress.

Research shows that social support is important to early development, recovery from surgical procedures, and to health. For example, Forssman, and Thuwe (1966) conducted a study of children born after their mothers had requested an abortion. The researchers showed that unwanted children were more likely to have trouble with the law. Also, these children were more likely to require psychiatric treatment in their youth than were matched control children who were presumably "wanted" by their parents.

There are health implications of social support as well. Children experience less stress from hospital procedures when parents and staff can provide a warm supportive environment. This is why many hospitals now allow parents to stay with their children. Parents now have the legal right to stay with their infant or young child (Brenner, 1984).

In addition to social support, a child's acceptance of hospital procedures may depend on cognitive expectations. Children can be prepared for their hospitalization through presurgical visits in which they meet their hospital caregivers. They can view films in which similar-aged and same-sex children model the hospital procedure (Melamed & Siegel, 1975). When this occurs at the child's level of cognitive development, he or she can deal more adequately with the anxiety of hospitalization or outpatient surgical procedures. However, this may depend on other psychological characteristics of the child (Saile, Burgmeier, & Schmidt, 1988). Some children may be sensitized by modeling procedures. In addition, prior experience with hospitals and medical procedures influences children's response to modeling.

An extensive study of 10,000 men with angina pectoris showed the importance of support in the marital relationship. Men with a satisfying love relationship were significantly less likely to present symptoms of angina, even when physical risk factors were present (Medalie & Goldbourt, 1976). Social support is also important in compliance with medical prescriptions and treatment programs. One review (Baekeland & Lundwall, 1975) looked at 19 projects that studied social support. All 19 studies observed that social isolation and/or lack of affiliation related strongly to dropping out of treatment. Other research shows that social support is crucial to minimizing the impact of stress from job loss (Cobb, 1974), long-term illness and recovery, grief after the loss of a loved one, and retirement (Shapiro, 1983). Finally, social support may moderate the effects of essential hypertension, increase the chances of surviving a heart attack, and increase the expected length of survival in cancer patients (Turner, 1983).

SUMMARY

Family stress is defined as pressure that disrupts or changes the family system. Family stress reduces harmony and resources for collective problem solving. Reuben Hill's ABCX model of family stress states that an event interacts with the family's resources for meeting crises and the family's definition of the event to produce a crisis.

We discussed several types of family stress, including separation and divorce, the single-parent family, family violence, and abuse. Single-parent families tend to be more disorganized, and children in such families tend to be placed in a position of conflict in which they are neither truly child nor adult. These children also tend to maintain hopes that their parents will reunite, a hope that is dashed when one parent remarries.

Abuse occurs most in families where the parents have a developmental history that predisposes them to neglect or abuse. The parents may have been abused themselves, or they may have witnessed abuse. Stress in the family increases the likelihood that abuse will occur. When the wife is abused, there may be a traumatic bonding that serves to keep the abused person in the family in spite of the suffering.

When the family functions in its intended way as a sensitive social support system, many outside stressors may be minimized. Families can structure problem solving to avoid common pitfalls and increase the chances of finding useful solutions.

KEY TERMS

ABCX model

child abuse

child neglect

cognitive-contextual

theory

crisis

distress

failure-to-thrive

syndrome

family appraisals

family as system

family resources

family stress

family vulnerability

life-change and abuse

marital conflict

personal resources

social buffer

social support and

family stress

spouse abuse

stress-crises-coping

(SCC) theories

stressors

systems model

(Emery's) of

family violence

traumatic bonding

REFERENCES

Amato, P. R., & Keith, B. (1991). Parental divorce and the well-being of children: A meta-analysis. *Psychological Bulletin, 110,* 26–46.

Baekeland, F., & Lundwall, L. (1975). Dropping out of treatment: A critical review. *Psychological Bulletin, 82,* 738–783.

Bandura, A. (1973). *Aggression: A social learning analysis.* Englewood Cliffs, NJ: Prentice-Hall.

Belsky, J. (1980). Child maltreatment: An ecological integration. *American Psychologist, 35,* 320–335.

Bloom, B. L., Asher, S. J., & White, S. W. (1978). Marital disruption as a stressor: A review and analysis. *Psychological Bulletin, 85,* 867–894.

Blumberg, M. (1974). Psychopathology of the abusing parent. *American Journal of Psychotherapy, 28,* 21–29.

Brenner, A. (1984). *Helping children cope with stress.* Lexington, MA: Lexington Books.

Bureau of the Census. (1982). *Marital status and living arrangements: March 1982* (Population Characteristics Series P-20, No. 380). Washington, DC: U.S. Government Printing Office.

Caplan, G., & Killilea, M. (1976). *Support systems and mutual help: Multidisciplinary explorations.* New York: Grune & Stratton.

Carter, H., & Glick, P. C. (1976). *Marriage and divorce: A social and economic study.* Cambridge, MA: Harvard University Press.

Cline, D. W., & Westman, J. C. (1971). The impact of divorce on the family. *Child Psychiatry and Human Development, 2,* 135–139.

Cobb, S. (1974). Physiological changes in men whose jobs were abolished. *Journal of Psychosomatic Research, 18,* 245–258.

Cobb, S. (1976). Social support as a moderator of life stress. *Psychosomatic Medicine, 38,* 300–314.

Colletta, N. D. (1983). Stressful lives: The situation of divorced mothers and their children. *Journal of Divorce, 6,* 19–31.

Conger, R., Burgess, R., & Barrett, C. (1979). Child abuse related to life change and perceptions of illness: Some preliminary findings. *Family Coordinator, 28,* 73–78.

Curran, D. (1987). *Stress and the healthy family.* San Francisco: Harper & Row.

de Young, M. (1982). *The sexual victimization of children.* Jefferson, NC: McFarland.

Dix, T. (1991). The affective organization of parenting: Adaptive and maladaptive processes. *Psychological Bulletin, 110,* 3–25.

Dutton, D., & Painter, S. L. (1981). Traumatic bonding: The development of emotional attachments in battered women and other relationships of intermittent abuse. *Victimology: An International Journal, 6,* 139–155.

Egeland, B., & Brunnquell, D. (1979). An at-risk approach to the study of child abuse: Some preliminary findings. *Journal of the American Academy of Child Psychiatry, 18,* 219–235.

Ellis, A. (1962). *Reason and emotion in psychotherapy.* New York: Stuart.

Emery, R. E. (1989). Family violence. *American Psychologist, 44,* 321–328.

Forssman, H., & Thuwe, I. (1966). One hundred and twenty children born after application for therapeutic abortion refused. *Acta Psychiatry Scandinavia, 42,* 71–88.

Fosson, A. (1988). Family violence. In S. Fisher & J. Reason (Eds.), *Handbook of life stress, cognition, and health* (pp. 161–174). New York: Wiley.

Frodi, A., Lamb, M., Leavitt, C., Donovan, W., Neff, C., & Sherry, D. (1978). Fathers' and mothers' responses to the faces and cries of normal and premature infants. *Developmental Psychology, 14,* 490–498.

Gelles, R. J. (1985). Family violence. *Annual Review of Sociology, 11,* 347–367.

Gelles, R. J., & Straus, M. A. (1979). Determinants of violence in the family: Toward a theoretical integration. In W. R. Burr, R. Hill, F. I. Nye, & R. L. Reiss (Eds.), *Contemporary theories about the family* (Vol. 1, pp. 549–581). New York: Free Press.

Groth, A. N., & Burgess, A. W. (1977). Motivational intent in the sexual assault of children. *Criminal Justice and Behavior, 4,* 253–264.

Grych, J. H., & Fincham, F. D. (1990). Marital conflict and children's adjustment: A cognitive-contextual framework. *Psychological Bulletin, 108,* 267–290.

Heatherington, E. M., Cox, M., & Cox, R. (1976). Divorced fathers. *Family Coordinator, 25,* 417–428.

Heatherington, E. M., Cox, M., & Cox, R. (1977). The aftermath of divorce. In J. H. Stevens, Jr., & M. Matthews (Eds.), *Mother-child, father-child relations* (pp. 149–176). Washington, DC: National Association for the Education of Young Children.

Heatherington, E. M., Stanley-Hagan, M., & Anderson, E. R. (1989). Marital transitions: A child's perspective. *American Psychologist, 44,* 303–312.

Hill, R. (1949). *Families under stress.* New York: Harper & Row.

Hjorth, C. W., & Ostrov, E. (1982). The self-image of physically abused adolescents. *Journal of Youth and Adolescence, 11,* 71–76.

Hobbs, D., & Cole, S. P. (1976). Transition to parenthood: A decade replication. *Journal of Marriage and the Family, 38,* 723–731.

Holmes, T. H., & Rahe, R. H. (1967). The social readjustment rating scale. *Psychosomatic Medicine, 11,* 213–218.

Kessler, R. C., & Essex, M. (1982). Marital status and depression: The importance of coping resources. *Social Forces, 61,* 484–507.

Kiecolt-Glaser, J. K., Fisher, L. D., Ogrocki, P., Stout, J. C., Speicher, B. S., & Glaser, R. (1985). Marital quality, marital disruption, and immune function. *Psychosomatic Medicine, 40,* 13–34.

Kitagawa, E. M., & Hauser, P. M. (1973). *Differential mortality in the United States: A study in socioeconomic epidemiology.* Cambridge, MA: Harvard University Press.

Klein, D. M. (1983). Family problem solving and family stress. *Marriage and Family Review, 6,* 85–112.

Klein, D. M., & Hill, R. (1979). Determinants of family problem-solving effectiveness. In W. R. Burr, R. Hill, F. I. Nye, & I. L. Reiss (Eds.), *Contemporary theories about the family* (Vol. 1, pp. 493–548). New York: Free Press.

Klein, M., & Stern, L. (1971). Low birth weight and the battered child syndrome. *American Journal of Diseases of Childhood, 122,* 15–18.

Light, R. (1973). Abuse and neglected children in America: A study of alternative policies. *Harvard Educational Review, 43,* 556–598.

Lowenthal, B. (1987). Stress factors and their alleviation in parents of high risk pre-term infants. *The Exceptional Child, 34,* 21–30.

McCubbin, H. I., Joy, C. B., Cauble, A. E., Comeau, J. K., Patterson, J. M., & Needle, R. H. (1980). Family stress and coping: A decade review. *Journal of Marriage and the Family, 42,* 855–871.

McCubbin, H. I., & Patterson, J. M. (1983). The family stress process: The double ABCX model of adjustment and adaptation. *Marriage and Family Review, 6,* 7–37.

Medalie, J. H., & Goldbourt, U. (1976). Angina pectoris among 10,000 men: II. Psychosocial and other risk factors as evidenced by a multivariate analysis of a five year incidence study. *American Journal of Medicine, 60,* 910–921.

Melamed, B. G., & Siegel, L. J. (1975). Reduction of anxiety in children facing surgery by modeling. *Journal of Consulting and Clinical Psychology, 43,* 511–521.

Menaghan E. (1982). Assessing the impact of family transitions on marital experience. In H. I. McCubbin, A. E. Cauble, & J. M. Patterson (Eds.), *Family stress, coping and social support* (pp. 90–108). Springfield, IL: Charles C Thomas.

Muldoon, L. (Ed.). (1979). *Incest: Confronting the silent crime.* St. Paul, MN: Minnesota Program for Victims of Sexual Assault.

National Center for Health Statistics. (1970). *Mortality from selected causes by marital status* (Series 20, Nos. 8A & 8B, USDHEW). Washington, DC: U.S. Government Printing Office.

National Center on Child Abuse and Neglect. (1981). *Study findings: National study of the incidence and severity of child abuse and neglect* (OHDS 81-30325). Washington, DC: U.S. Government Printing Office.

Orthner, D. K., Brown, T., & Ferguson, D. (1976). Single-parent fatherhood: An emerging family life style. *The Family Coordinator, 25,* 429–437.

Orzek, A. M. (1985). The child's cognitive processing of sexual abuse. *Child and Adolescent Psychotherapy, 2,* 110–114.

Patterson, G. (1977). A performance theory for coercive family interaction. In R. B. Cairns (Ed.), *The analysis of social interactions: Methods, issues, and illustrations* (pp. 119–162). Hillsdale, NJ: Lawrence Erlbaum.

Pearlin, L., Lieberman, M., Menaghan, E., & Mullan, J. (1981). The stress process. *Journal of Health and Social Behavior, 22,* 337–356.

Pearlin, L. I., & Schooler, C. (1978). The structure of coping. *Journal of Health and Social Behavior, 19,* 2–21.

Rajecki, P., Lamb, M., & Obmascher, P. (1978). Toward a general theory of infantile attachment: A comparative review of aspects of the social bond. *The Behavioral and Brain Sciences, 3,* 417–464.

Rofes, E. E. (Ed.). (1982). *The kids' book of divorce: By, for and about kids.* New York: Vintage Books.

Rohner, R. (1975). Parental acceptance-rejection and personality: A universalistic approach to behavioral science. In R. W. Brislin, S. Bochner, & W. J. Lonner (Eds.), *Cross-cultural perspectives on learning* (pp. 251–269). New York: Halsted.

Rollins, B. C., & Feldman, H. (1970). Marital satisfaction over the family life cycle. *Journal of Marriage and the Family, 32,* 20–28.

Rounsaville, B. (1978). Theories of marital violence: Evidence from a study of battered women. *Victimology: An International Journal, 3,* 11–31.

Russell, C. (1974). Transition to parenthood: Problems and gratifications. *Journal of Marriage and the Family, 36,* 294–302.

Saile, H., Burgmeier, R., & Schmidt, L. R. (1988). A meta-analysis of studies on psychological preparation of children facing medical procedures. *Psychology and Health, 2,* 107–132.

San Francisco Family Violence Project Handbook (1980).

Schlesinger, B. (1969). The one-parent family in perspective. In B. Schlesinger (Ed.), *The one-parent family: Perspectives and annotated bibliography* (pp. 3–12). Toronto, Canada: University of Toronto Press.

Shapiro, J. (1983). Family reactions and coping strategies in response to the physically ill or handicapped child: A review. *Social Science and Medicine, 17,* 913–931.

Smith, R. M., & Smith, C. W. (1981). Child rearing and single-parent fathers. *Family Relations, 30,* 411–417.

Smith, S. L. (1984). Significant research findings in the etiology of child abuse. *Social Casework, 65,* 665–683.

Smith, S. M., & Hanson, R. (1975). Interpersonal relationships and childrearing practices in 214 parents of battered children. *British Journal of Psychiatry, 127,* 513–525.

Steinmetz, S. K. (1977). The use of force for resolving family conflict: The training ground for abuse. *The Family Coordinator, 26,* 19–26.

Straus, M. A. (1977). Sociological perspective on the prevention and treatment of wifebeating. In M. Roy (Ed.), *Battered women: A psychosociological study of domestic violence* (pp. 194–239). New York: Van Nostrand Reinhold.

Straus, M. A., Gelles, R. J., & Steinmetz, S. K. (1980). *Behind closed doors: Violence in the American family.* Garden City, NY: Doubleday/Anchor.

Tooley, K. M. (1977). The young child as victim of sibling attack. *Social Casework, 58,* 25–28.

Turkington, C. (1985, April). Farmers strain to hold the line as crisis uproots mental health. *APA Monitor, 16,* pp. 1, 26, 27, 38.

Turner, R. J. (1983). Direct, indirect, and moderating effects of social support on psychological distress and associated conditions. In H. B. Kaplan (Ed.), *Psychosocial stress: Trends in theory and research* (pp. 105–155). New York: Academic Press.

Walker, A. (1985). Reconceptualizing family stress. *Journal of Marriage and the Family, 47,* 827–837.

Wallerstein, J. S., & Kelly, J. B. (1980). *Surviving the breakup: How children and parents cope with divorce.* New York: Basic Books.

Weick, K. E. (1971). Group processes, family processes, and problem solving. In J. Aldous et al. (Eds.), *Family problem solving: A symposium on theoretical, methodological, and substantive concerns* (pp. 3–32). Hinsdale, IL: Dryden Press.

CHAPTER 7

Job Stress: Dissatisfaction, Burnout, and Obsolescence

MANY . . . HAVE REACHED THE TOP OF THE SUCCESS LADDER BUT ARE BEGINNING TO SUSPECT IT MAY BE LEANING AGAINST THE WRONG WALL.
SAM KEEN

Sunday, May 19, 1985: headlines in the *New York Times* business section read "Warren Anderson: A Public Crisis, A Personal Ordeal." These headlines introduced the inside story of a corporation and its chief executive officer struggling to deal with a tragedy of immense proportions (Diamond, 1985). For both Union Carbide and Warren Anderson, it was a period of intense, unyielding stress. Half the story described the public, legal, and corporate pressure on Union Carbide Corporation following the Bhopal tragedy. The accident tarnished the company's image worldwide, contributed to plummeting stock, slowed the pace of company expansion, and produced multibillion-dollar lawsuits.

The rest of the story, more intimate and personal, concerned Anderson's dramatic changes in lifestyle. Though Anderson was not directly involved in the events that led to spilling toxic gases, he had to take ultimate responsibility as the company's chief executive officer. Immediately after news reports revealed the immensity of the tragedy, he assembled technical and medical experts to help at Bhopal. In Bombay, he met two of Union Carbide's Indian officials. Upon arrival in Bhopal, police arrested and jailed all three. Anderson spent several hours in jail before flying to New Delhi, but his Indian colleagues spent nine days in jail. Anderson's wife, Lillian, said the few days he was in India were filled with more terror for her than she had known during her entire life.

When Anderson returned to his Connecticut office, he devoted attention only to matters related to Bhopal. He left day-to-day operations to junior officers. Anderson said that he felt "like I'm taking tests all the time. You know there is going to be a grade on everything you do and say" (p. 8F).

Meanwhile, Lillian kept a doctor on call for fear that her husband might collapse from the stress. All the while, she kept her worries secret lest she add to the load he carried. The Andersons felt they were prisoners of Bhopal, a private jail they carried wherever they went. Reading the paper, watching the news, or going out for an evening dinner might bring unwelcome reminders of what had happened. They lay down at night with "lumps in [their] chests," and both experienced difficulty sleeping. Always regarded as a low-profile couple, their lifestyle became almost reclusive.

DIMENSIONS OF JOB STRESS

This case study highlights important aspects of **job stress.** First, work stress generally involves both the organization and its employees. Job stress is not a private matter for the employee to deal with alone and in isolation. Employees may transport personal and family problems to the job, but work problems also spill over to the home (Rousseau, 1978).

Second, job stress produces negative effects for both the company and the employee. For the organization, the results are disorganization, disruption in normal operations, lowered productivity, and lower margins of profit. For the employee, the effects are threefold: increased physical health problems, psychological distress, and behavioral changes. Problems with health may not be so much related to the onset of a specific disease but to the quiet and gradual loss of health. Psychological distress usually comes with loss of job satisfaction and several related negative emotions. The resulting changes in behavior tend to affect both productivity within the company and lifestyle outside the workplace.

Third, job stress requires both organizational and personal solutions (Ivancevich, Matteson, Freedman, & Phillips, 1990). Employee assistance programs that focus solely on the employee perpetuate the myth that job stress is the worker's problem and the worker's fault. Removing job stress also requires some intervention and change in the organization. Until this happens, personal coping strategies are little more than Band-Aids that help the employee survive from one crisis to the next. We will discuss several organizational and personal intervention strategies later in this chapter.

DEFINING JOB STRESS

One definition suggests that job stress results from job features that pose a threat to the individual (Caplan et al., 1975). Threat may be due to either excessive job demands or insufficient supplies to meet employees' needs. When the job requires too much work in too short a time, job overload exists. Supply deficits concern things employees expect from their jobs: adequate salary, job satisfaction, and promotion or growth in the job.

Terry Beehr and John Newman (1978) reviewed numerous definitions of job stress. They concluded that job stress is the interaction of work conditions with worker traits that changes normal psychological or physiological functions or both. Their definition also provides for stress that improves performance. This is important for both industry and employees. For the purposes of this chapter, *job stress* will be defined as work demands that exceed the worker's coping ability. This definition is consistent with the cognitive-transactional theory presented earlier in this book.

THE COSTS OF WORK STRESS

A preeminent concern is the immense economic loss from job stress and from unsafe conditions on the job. The cost of work stress has to be calculated across a spreading network of accounts from personal to family, to business, to society. Based on studies of many occupations, the federal government estimates that 100,000 workers die each year from job-related diseases, and another 390,000 develop some type of job-related illness. In addition, 14,000 workers die each year from accidents on the job. Another 2.2 million suffer some type of disabling injury (Institute of Medicine, 1979). Acute reactive stress probably contributes to accidents (Green, 1985).

Based on data from a 1976 survey by the Bureau of Labor Statistics, Robert Veniga and James Spradley (1981) estimated that American workers lose 3.5% of their total work hours through absenteeism. Further, they estimated that one in every three workers, on any given day, called in sick because of stress-related problems. The cost is millions of dollars in unpaid wages annually.

Business loses over $32.8 billion annually from lost productivity. An analysis by James Greenwood (cited in Everly & Girdano, 1980) suggested that job stress adds up to billions of dollars in direct and indirect costs every year. He calculated the direct costs of *executive* stress at $19.7 billion per year. The indirect costs are difficult to calculate but may be as large as or larger than the direct costs. Training an employee who subsequently must be let go or quits because of job dissatisfaction costs about $5000 for blue-collar laborers and support staff. For executives, the loss may exceed $100,000 (Adams, 1981).

SYMPTOMS OF WORK STRESS

Mere monetary computation of losses overlooks the most important outcomes of work stress. Adults spend roughly half their waking life on the job. Because more wage earners now work overtime or hold two jobs simultaneously, that figure may be an underestimate. Conditions at work thus contribute significantly to lifestyle and health. The effects may spread, either positively or negatively, to all facets of life.

Terry Beehr and John Newman (1978) reviewed many job stress studies and concluded that three negative personal outcomes result from work stress: psychological health symptoms, physical health symptoms, and behavioral symptoms. The following paragraphs summarize symptoms that reveal the onset of work stress. The list will probably change in the future as we increase our knowledge of work stress.

Psychological Symptoms of Work Stress

Psychological disorders bear an important relation to occupational conditions. This is evident from the inclusion of an occupational-stress category in the *Diagnostic and Statistical Manual of Mental Disorders,* Third Edition, Revised (DSM-III-R) (American Psychiatric Association, 1987; Sauter, Murphy, & Hurrell, 1990). The following list is typical of findings from job stress research in various occupational settings.

1. Anxiety, tension, confusion, and irritability
2. Feelings of frustration, anger, and resentment
3. Emotional hypersensitivity and hyperreactivity
4. Suppression of feelings
5. Reduced effectiveness in communication
6. Withdrawal and depression
7. Feelings of isolation and alienation
8. Boredom and job dissatisfaction
9. Mental fatigue and lower intellectual functioning
10. Loss of concentration
11. Loss of spontaneity and creativity
12. Lowered self-esteem

Perhaps the most predictable consequence of job stress is job dissatisfaction. The employee feels little motivation to go to work, to do a good job while at work, or to stay on the job. Other symptoms occur at different stages on the road to job dissatisfaction and vary from one person to another. Current research on workplace motivation is beginning to integrate systems variables with human factors to obtain a better balance between job demands and job satisfaction (Katzell & Thompson, 1990).

Anxiety, tension, anger, and resentment are among the more commonly reported symptoms. Some people find job pressure so great they increase psychological distance and gradually become depressed. This may occur after the employee tried but failed to correct the stress situation. When this occurs often, the outcome may be *learned helplessness,* which prevents the employee from making changes even when it is within his or her power to do so. On the other hand, some employees probably never try because they bring a load of learned helplessness to the job.

Physical Symptoms of Work Stress

The major physical symptoms of work stress are shown in the following list.

1. Increased heart rate and blood pressure
2. Increased secretions of adrenaline and noradrenaline
3. Gastrointestinal disorders such as ulcers

4. Bodily injuries
5. Physical fatigue
6. Death
7. Cardiovascular disease
8. Respiratory problems
9. Increased sweating
10. Skin disorders
11. Headaches
12. Cancer
13. Muscular tension
14. Sleep disturbances

Adequate research exists to verify the effects of work stress on the cardio-vascular and gastrointestinal systems. Physical fatigue, bodily injuries, and sleep disturbances are also well established. The remaining disorders are not as reliably established as resulting from work stress.

Stress also comes from unsafe work environments. The National Institute for Occupational Safety and Health (NIOSH) lists the ten leading work-related diseases or injuries as follows: occupational lung diseases; musculoskeletal injuries; occupational cancers; severe occupational traumatic injuries; cardiovascular disease; disorders of reproduction; neurotoxic disorders; noise-induced loss of hearing; dermatologic conditions; and psychological disorders (Levi, 1990). Poor lighting, unclean shop areas that create hazards, high-intensity noise levels, and inadequate ventilation may contribute to a variety of physical health problems.

Obvious examples of unsafe work environments are plants that produce toxic chemicals or materials using unsafe methods. Kenneth Pelletier (1984) summarized the results of studies by several federal agencies that have linked hazardous chemicals to on-the-job diseases. Asbestos, the most common of these chemicals (Cullen, Cherniack, & Rosenstock, 1990), causes white-lung disease and cancer. Benzene causes leukemia and aplastic anemia. Coal dust causes black-lung disease. Radiation causes cancer, leukemia, and genetic damage. Lead causes kidney disorders, anemia, central nervous system damage, sterility, and birth defects. NIOSH estimates that 1 million of the 16 million working women of childbearing years work in jobs with the potential for exposure to hazards that could produce birth defects or miscarriages (Institute of Medicine, 1979). Behavioral methods may be effective in reducing exposure (Hopkins et al., 1986), but the need to alter unsafe production environments is still evident.

One problem in making the work-stress-health connection is that employees bring physical health problems to the job. These problems may be related to high-risk behaviors in the social environment. Work conditions may intensify a health problem and make it visible; the job may then be blamed. James House (1987) argues that current research does not provide a strong and convincing picture of the relationship between stress and disease because research fails to consider the etiology of chronic disease. This is due in part to continued reliance on the life-events model, which uses both positive and negative stressors.

House points to the massive body of research showing that affective variables, especially negative affect, are most important to stress and health. But these negative affective variables have not been adequately reflected in job stress research.

Paul Spector and his colleagues also argue that current research uses simple, linear, cause-effect models that do not do justice to complex stress-health relationships (Spector, Dwyer, & Jex, 1988). They suggest that three hypotheses must be entertained when investigating stress-health relationships. First, performance indicators might alter workers' perceptions of stress, a *reverse causality* model. Another is the *reciprocal causation* notion that both outside events and performance outcomes cause perceptions of stress; this in turn feeds back negatively to performance. Finally, there is the *external cause* model, which suggests that some individual dispositional variable is responsible for both performance outcomes and perceptions of stress. Spector's group found little evidence for the dispositional approach. They did, however, find evidence for the reciprocal causation model without ruling out the reverse causality model.

Behavioral Symptoms of Work Stress

Several behavioral symptoms reveal job stress. These include the following:

1. Procrastination and avoidance of work
2. Lowered performance and productivity
3. Increased alcohol and drug use and abuse
4. Outright sabotage on the job
5. Increased visits to the dispensary
6. Overeating as an escape, leading to obesity
7. Undereating as a withdrawal, probably combined with signs of depression
8. Loss of appetite and sudden weight loss
9. Increased risk-taking behavior, including reckless driving and gambling
10. Aggression, vandalism, and stealing
11. Deteriorating relationships with family and friends
12. Suicide or attempted suicide

Procrastination is often disguised as busywork. The comment "just getting organized" may be a mere coverup to avoid doing something bothersome. Work stress frequently combines with other problems such as alcoholism and drug abuse.

Behavioral Symptoms with Organizational Impact

Work stress has a major impact on employee mental and physical health, but it also affects the organization. Randall Schuler (1980) identified several behaviors that have an impact on the organization. Stress is associated with poor job performance, absenteeism, and accident proneness. The employee experiences low job involvement and loses a sense of responsibility to the job. The employee also displays a lack of concern for the organization and for colleagues. The final outcome may be the employee's leaving the job. A cautionary note about absenteeism is necessary. Dan Farrell and Carol Stamm (1988) conducted a meta-analysis of 72 studies on absenteeism to resolve inconsistencies reported in previous studies. They found that the only significant correlates of absenteeism were work environment and organizational variables, including control policies (warnings, incentives, dismissals, and so forth). Demographic and psychological factors did not predict absenteeism.

SOURCES OF WORK STRESS

Attempts to identify the sources of stress on the job disclose many culprits. First, stress is an interaction between the objective work conditions and the perception that skills match job demands. Thus, the sources of job stress noted here are not solely responsible for job stress. Instead, they add potential for stress in combination with worker traits and perceptions. Cary Cooper (1983) gave a complete yet concise list of six sources of work stress. These stressors are summarized in Table 7-1 with both contributing factors and possible consequences. These are job-specific stress, role stress, interpersonal stress, career development, organizational structure and development, and the home-work interface. We will use this list to structure the discussion that follows. Before reading further, it may be instructive to fill out the Work Stress Profile on page 188.

Stress Related to Job Conditions

Specific work conditions that contribute to stress include job complexity, work overload or underload, unsafe physical conditions, and shift work. *Job complexity* is the inherent difficulty of the work to be done. Several factors contribute to job complexity. It may be related to the amount and sophistication of information required to function in the job. Expansion or addition of methods for performing the job may also contribute. Finally, introducing contingency plans for completing a job also create complexity (Everly & Girdano, 1980).

Work overload   Work overload customarily is divided into **quantitative** and **qualitative overload.** Quantitative overload results when the physical demands of the job exceed the worker's capacity. This occurs when the employee must do too much work in too short a time. Some jobs may require physical strength beyond the worker's capacity or set unreasonably high quotas. The assembly line may keep moving no matter how strained or fatigued the worker is. The day may be heavily scheduled, with no downtime. Qualitative overload results when work is too complex or difficult. This occurs when the job taxes either the technical or mental skills of the worker.

TABLE 7-1
Summary of Major Job Stressors

Job stressors	Contributing factors	Possible consequences
Job conditions	Quantitative work overload	Physical and/or mental fatigue
	Qualitative work overload	Job burnout
	Assembly-line hysteria	Increased irritability and tension
	People decisions	
	Physical dangers	
	Shift work	
	Technostress	
Role stress	Role ambiguity	Increased anxiety and tension
	Sex bias and sex-role stereotypes	Lowered performance on the job
	Sexual harassment	Job dissatisfaction
Interpersonal factors	Poor work and social support systems	Increased tension
	Political rivalry, jealousy, or anger	Elevated blood pressure
	Lack of management concern for worker	Job dissatisfaction
Career development	Underpromotion	Lowered productivity
	Overpromotion	Loss of self-esteem
	Job security	Increased irritability and anger
	Frustrated ambitions	Job dissatisfaction
Organizational structure	Rigid and impersonal structure	Lowered motivation and productivity
	Political battles	Job dissatisfaction
	Inadequate supervision or training	
	Nonparticipative decision making	
Home-work interface	Spillover	Increased mental conflict and fatigue
	Lack of support from spouse	Lowered motivation and productivity
	Marital conflict	Increased marital conflict
	Dual-career stress	

SELF-STUDY EXERCISE 7-1

Work Stress Profile

This scale provides some information on work stress. Instructions for scoring and interpreting the scale appear at the end of the questionnaire.

The following statements describe work conditions, job environments, or personal feelings that workers encounter in their jobs. After reading each statement, circle the answer that best reflects the working conditions at your place of employment. If the statement is about a personal feeling, indicate the extent to which you have that feeling about your job. The scale markers ask you to judge, to the best of your knowledge, the approximate percentage of time the condition or feeling is true.

NEVER = not at all true of your work conditions or feelings
RARELY = the condition or feeling exists about 25% of the time
SOMETIMES = the condition or feeling exists about 50% of the time
OFTEN = the condition or feeling exists about 75% of the time
MOST TIMES = the condition or feeling is virtually always present

	NEVER	RARELY	SOMETIMES	OFTEN	MOST TIMES
1. Support personnel are incompetent or inefficient.	1	2	3	4	5
2. My job is not very well defined.	1	2	3	4	5
3. I am not sure about what is expected of me.	1	2	3	4	5
4. I am not sure what will be expected of me in the future.	1	2	3	4	5
5. I cannot seem to satisfy my superiors.	1	2	3	4	5
6. I seem to be able to talk with my superiors.	5	4	3	2	1
7. My superiors strike me as incompetent, yet I have to take orders from them.	1	2	3	4	5
8. My superiors seem to care about me as a person.	5	4	3	2	1
9. There is a feeling of trust, respect, and friendliness between me and my superiors.	5	4	3	2	1

	NEVER	RARELY	SOMETIMES	OFTEN	MOST TIMES
10. There seems to be tension between administrative personnel and staff personnel.	1	2	3	4	5
11. I have autonomy in carrying out my job duties.	5	4	3	2	1
12. I feel as though I can shape my own destiny in this job.	5	4	3	2	1
13. There are too many bosses in my area.	1	2	3	4	5
14. It appears that my boss has "retired on the job."	1	2	3	4	5
15. My superiors give me adequate feedback about my job performance	5	4	3	2	1
16. My abilities are not appreciated by my superiors.	1	2	3	4	5
17. There is little prospect of personal or professional growth in this job.	1	2	3	4	5
18. The level of participation in planning and decision making at my place of work is satisfactory.	5	4	3	2	1
19. I feel that I am over-educated for this job.	1	2	3	4	5
20. I feel that my educational background is just right for this job.	5	4	3	2	1
21. I fear that I will be laid off or fired.	1	2	3	4	5
22. In-service training for my job is inadequate.	1	2	3	4	5
23. Most of my colleagues are unfriendly or seem uninterested in me as a person.	1	2	3	4	5

	NEVER	RARELY	SOMETIMES	OFTEN	MOST TIMES
24. I feel uneasy about going to work.	1	2	3	4	5
25. There is no release time for personal affairs or business.	1	2	3	4	5
26. There is obvious sex/race/ age discrimination in this job.	1	2	3	4	5

> **NOTE:** Complete the entire questionnaire first! Then add all the values circled for → questions 1–26 and enter here.   Total 1–26

	NEVER	RARELY	SOMETIMES	OFTEN	MOST TIMES
27. The physical work environment is crowded, noisy, or dreary.	1	2	3	4	5
28. Physical demands of the job are unreasonable (heavy lifting, extraordinary periods of concentration required, etc.).	1	2	3	4	5
29. My work load is neverending.	1	2	3	4	5
30. The pace of work is too fast.	1	2	3	4	5
31. My job seems to consist of responding to emergencies.	1	2	3	4	5
32. There is no time for relaxation, coffee breaks, or lunch breaks on the job.	1	2	3	4	5
33. Job deadlines are constant and unreasonable.	1	2	3	4	5
34. Job requirements are beyond the range of my ability.	1	2	3	4	5
35. At the end of the day, I am physically exhausted from work.	1	2	3	4	5

	NEVER	RARELY	SOMETIMES	OFTEN	MOST TIMES
36. I can't even enjoy my leisure because of the toll my job takes on my energy.	1	2	3	4	5
37. I have to take work home to keep up.	1	2	3	4	5
38. I have responsibility for too many people.	1	2	3	4	5
39. Support personnel are too few.	1	2	3	4	5
40. Support personnel are incompetent or inefficient	1	2	3	4	5
41. I am not sure about what is expected of me.	1	2	3	4	5
42. I am not sure what will be expected of me in the future.	1	2	3	4	5
43. I leave work feeling burned out.	1	2	3	4	5
44. There is little prospect for personal or professional growth in this job.	1	2	3	4	5
45. In-service training for my job is inadequate.	1	2	3	4	5
46. There is little contact with colleagues on the job.	1	2	3	4	5
47. Most of my colleagues are unfriendly or seem un-interested in me as a person.	1	2	3	4	5
48. I feel uneasy about going to work.	1	2	3	4	5

NOTE: Complete the entire questionnaire first! Then add all the values circled for questions 27–48 and enter here.   →   ☐

Total 27–48

NEVER   RARELY   SOMETIMES   OFTEN   MOST TIMES

49. The complexity of my job
is enough to keep me
interested.   [5]   [4]   [3]   [2]   [1]

50. My job is very exciting.
                                     [1]   [2]   [3]   [4]   [5]

51. My job is varied enough
to prevent
boredom.   [1]   [2]   [3]   [4]   [5]

52. I seem to have lost
interest in my work.   [1]   [2]   [3]   [4]   [5]

53. I feel as though I can
shape my own destiny
in this job.   [5]   [4]   [3]   [2]   [1]

54. I leave work feeling
burned out.   [1]   [2]   [3]   [4]   [5]

55. I would continue to work
at my job even
if I did not need the
money.   [1]   [2]   [3]   [4]   [5]

56. I am trapped in this
job.   [1]   [2]   [3]   [4]   [5]

57. If I had it to do all over
again, I would
still choose this job.   [5]   [4]   [3]   [2]   [1]

NOTE: Now go back and add the values for
questions 1–26. Do the same for questions
27–48. Enter the values where indicated.
Then add all the values circled for   [   ]
questions 49–57.   Total 49–57

Last, enter those sums for each of the following
groups of questions and add them all together to
get a cumulative total.

QUESTIONS:	1–26 Inter-personal	27–48 Physical Condition	49–57 Job Interest	TOTAL 1–57
TOTALS:	[ ] +	[ ] +	[ ] =	[ ]

The first scale measures stress due to problems in interpersonal relationships and to job satisfaction or dissatisfaction, as the case may be. The second scale measures the physical demands of work that wear on the person daily. The third scale measures job interest and involvement. For each of the scales, you can gain some sense of how much job stress you live with relative to the original test group by locating your scores on the scale provided below. On each scale, a high score means more job-related stress. If you are high in one of the areas, say interpersonal stress, it could be of some help to pay attention to the interpersonal aspects of your job.

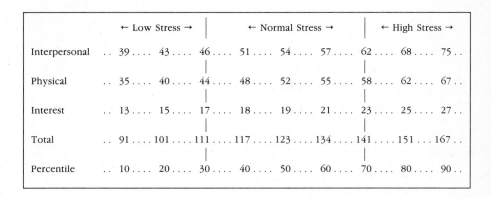

	← Low Stress →	← Normal Stress →	← High Stress →
Interpersonal	.. 39 .... 43 .... 46	51 .... 54 .... 57	62 .... 68 .... 75 ..
Physical	.. 35 .... 40 .... 44	48 .... 52 .... 55	58 .... 62 .... 67 ..
Interest	.. 13 .... 15 .... 17	18 .... 19 .... 21	23 .... 25 .... 27 ..
Total	.. 91 .... 101 .... 111	117 .... 123 .... 134	141 .... 151 ... 167 ..
Percentile	.. 10 .... 20 .... 30	40 .... 50 .... 60	70 .... 80 .... 90 ..

The work stress profile has been tested in a sample of 275 school psychologists. The three scales are virtually identical to those identified in other work stress scales. The reliability of this scale is quite high. For the total scale, the reliability is .921. Reliabilities for the three subscales are .898, .883, and .816, respectively. A reliability of 1.00 indicates perfect reliability. The high reliability shown by this scale may be due in part to the fact that it was tested on a single occupational group. Additional studies with other occupational groups will be needed to determine if the scales are stable across a variety of occupations.

Assembly-line hysteria   Work underload means that the job is not challenging or fails to maintain the worker's interest and attention. George Everly and Daniel Girdano (1980) call this **deprivational stress.** They suggest that understimulation is most frequently found in assembly-line workers and in large bureaucracies. NIOSH described an **assembly-line hysteria** in which victims display symptoms of nausea, muscle weakness, severe headaches, and blurred vision, but no physical basis for these symptoms exists. Instead, the symptoms may be a psychological response to a job that is boring, repetitive, lacking in social interaction on the job, and low in job satisfaction.

Decision making, responsibility, and stress   Qualitative overload may occur when a manager must make decisions that affect company production and the employees' future. Managers may have to plan production schedules, procure materials, evaluate staff, and make recommendations on hiring, firing, and layoffs. When decisions involve only *things* as opposed to *people*, managers may function effectively. When the manager's decision involves responsibility for other people, stress is more likely.

Stress also increases as managers assume more responsibility for their decisions. Conversely, stress declines when management spreads out the responsibility for decisions, as in a committee. A decision that must be made by some deadline can be highly stressful. Some people even try to avoid making deadline decisions. In many jobs, though, there is no time to waste. People working in life-and-death situations, such as emergency service crews, cannot take their ideas to a board room or request a computer simulation showing the likelihood of success for a plan of action. Presidents, military leaders, and pilots of stricken aircraft also fit in this category.

Physical danger   Physical danger is a potential source of job stress, especially when the worker confronts the threat of injury. People in emergency service jobs, such as police officers, miners, fire fighters, soldiers, and bomb disposal squad members, confront this type of stress. Successful coping is closely related to one critical factor: whether the employees feel adequately trained to handle the emergencies. This is consistent with the cognitive view that stress results when demands exceed capacity.

Shift work   **Shift work** requires that workers rotate schedules. This can produce disturbances in sleep patterns, neurophysiological rhythms, metabolic rate, and mental efficiency. These reactions occur because of disturbances in the **circadian rhythm,** a type of internal body clock. Jet lag is one example of this type of problem.

The primary pacemaker for the circadian rhythm is the hypothalamus (Czeisler et al., 1990). This may account for several body processes that change with disturbances in the body clock. For example, in the morning the body secretes only small amounts of the stress hormones, adrenaline and noradrenaline. These secretions increase as the day progresses. Also, some people describe themselves as "morning people." They feel most alert and work most efficiently in the morning. Then they fizzle out by mid- to late afternoon. Other people are "night owls." They never seem to get going until midday and do not hit full stride until even later. They may work late into the night but struggle to get out of bed in the morning.

One circadian rhythm is the 24-hour sleep-waking cycle, with the norm of nighttime sleep and daytime work. Work schedules often force people out of this cycle, though. An extreme example is the graveyard shift. The body's clock is temporarily disturbed when on this schedule. Physical and psychological effects may occur as described earlier. The person may feel out of sync mentally and physically. Irritability may increase, and typical family interactions may be disrupted.

There is evidence that the 24-hour cycle may not be the best for everyone. Some people might be better off on a 23-hour cycle, while others might function best on a 26-hour cycle. Unfortunately, time-based societies do not take circadian rhythms into account when setting work schedules, so the worker suffers while trying to adjust. Research suggests that people can adjust to shift work, but it is not easy. Fast adapters adjust in about one week. Slow adapters require about three weeks. Some people feel that they never do adjust. If the swing shift rotates monthly, the body may never completely adjust before another change occurs. Recent evidence (Czeisler et al., 1990) shows that controlled exposure to bright light and darkness can help night-shift workers adapt in as little as three days.

Role Ambiguity: What Am I Doing Here?

Role ambiguity as a source of work stress is a frequently cited problem, especially in very large and/or ill-structured organizations. The term *role* refers to society's expectations that a person will display certain behaviors when he or she occupies a certain position. Thus, role ambiguity occurs when you do not know what management expects you to accomplish. A *Quality of Employment Survey* (Quinn & Staines, 1979) showed that 52% of workers reported conflicting demands. Role conflict is central to the midcareer crisis. In a midcareer crisis, the employee feels stress from such conditions as overpromotion, underpromotion, lack of job security, and thwarted ambition.

The effects of role ambiguity include low performance and low job satisfaction, high anxiety, tension, and motivation to leave the company (Moch, Bartunek, & Brass, 1979). French and his colleagues showed that women perceive more role ambiguity than men (French, Caplan, & Van Harrison, 1982). They also observed that women had higher levels of life stress compared to men. Among the possible reasons for this are sex-role stereotypes and dual-career families that place more pressure on women (Cramer, Keitel, & Rossberg, 1986). However, Martocchio and O'Leary (1989) conducted a meta-analysis of sex differences in occupational stress and discovered no significant sex differences in experienced and perceived work stress. How this inconsistency will be resolved remains to be seen.

Interpersonal Stress: Does Anyone Care?

Personal relationships on the job are very important to job satisfaction. Broad social networks, including support from workers, management, family, and friends relieve strain (Fisher, 1985). This statement is consistent with Cobb's (1976) findings that social support serves as a buffer against stress. Social support on the job appears to temper physiological stress reactions by reducing the amount of cortisone released, lowering blood pressure, holding down the number of cigarettes smoked, and promoting complete cessation of smoking.

The *Quality of Employment Survey* previously mentioned revealed that 30% of the workers doubted that supervisors cared about their welfare. This concern is often related to leader characteristics and organizational structure. Management style and what the manager believes about employees is also critical.

Career Development: Where Am I Going?

Job stress mirrors the developmental peaks and valleys in the employee's career. According to one national study of work stress, people bring several specific hopes to a job. They hope for rapid, or at least steady, advancement. They hope for some freedom in the job and increased earning power. Preferably, they hope to learn new things and work at new jobs. Finally, they hope to find solutions to certain work problems (Veniga & Spradley, 1981). For some employees, the promotion does not come. The job that once looked so secure may be eliminated. Then they may respond in ways that reveal building stress.

When their hopes and dreams only flicker faintly, employees often lose a sense of accomplishment and self-esteem. Minor irritants they would have casually brushed aside when the dream was fresh now irritate and fester inside. Four factors are closely related to stress in career development: underpromotion, overpromotion (also called the **Peter Principle**), lack of job security, and frustrated ambitions. Contrary to what some managers believe, job insecurity, not increasing production demands, increases stress and generally lowers productivity.

Organizational Structure: What Are They Doing Up There?

The structure of a business can also produce stress. Most often, employees complain about rigid structure, interoffice or intraoffice political squabbles, and inadequate supervision from management. Employees also dislike lack of involvement in decision making and restrictions on their behavior, including lack of support for individual initiative and creativity. Paul Spector (1986) conducted a meta-analysis of studies dealing with autonomy and participative decision making. He found that when *perception* of control is high, workers experience high levels of job satisfaction and low levels of physical symptoms. The same pattern occurred for actual participation in decision making.

The Home-Work Connection: Sanctuaries and Spillover

Most people think of home as a sanctuary, a place that is private and quiet and where one can be alone. It is a retreat that allows rebuilding and regrouping of inner strengths to meet outside demands. When pressure invades that sanctuary, however, it may magnify the effects of stress at work. Denise Rousseau (1978) provided evidence of a **spillover** from events at work to events at home. Rousseau believes that work experiences are positively related to nonwork experiences. If a person has a job that diminishes self-esteem and produces low satisfaction, that person will have similar experiences in social life. Research has discovered spillover in numerous occupations, including logging, manufacturing, and professional work.

Spillover is only one of five models that seeks to explain the home-work connection. *Compensation theory* suggests that positive events in one area compensate for deficits in the other. *Segmentation theory* considers home and work as two independent arenas that do not influence each other. *Instrumental theory* assumes that we use one area to obtain things for the other. Finally, *conflict theory* states that work and home are incompatible and that sacrifices have to be made in one to fulfill obligations in the other (Burke, 1986; Zedeck & Mosier, 1990). This is a situation in which research may not resolve the issue in favor of one theory. There is support for each model, perhaps because each reflects a valid way to link home and work in cognitive schemata. Personal appraisals of job satisfaction and typical stress reactions appear to influence which process is functioning for a given employee.

One example of stress due to the home-work connection is **dual-career stress.** Zedeck and Mosier (1990) report that the once-traditional nuclear family with a working husband, homemaker wife, and children now makes up only 11% of the nation's families. Nearly 40% of the work force now consists of dual-earner couples, and nearly 45% of married women are working outside the home. Even with children under 6, 37% of married women are working. These figures show substantial increases from 1960 figures, which were 31% and 19%, respectively (Cooper, 1983). A recent correlational study of dual-career women showed that coping strategies and marital adjustment combine to protect against stress. Dual-career women use more coping strategies when marital adjustment is good. They also report lower levels of stress compared to women whose marital adjustment is poor (McLaughlin, Cormier, & Cormier, 1988). Unfortunately, we cannot judge from this correlational analysis whether the use of coping strategies is responsible for both better marital adjustment and lower stress or whether other variables are responsible for both.

ARE BOREDOM AND MONOTONY REALLY STRESSORS?

For some time, the popular conception of job stress included the idea that monotonous, repetitive jobs (for example, assembly-line work) are stressful. In support of this notion, research showed that blue-collar workers tend to experience high job **boredom** while professionals tend to experience low boredom (French, Caplan, & Van Harrison, 1982). Three terms often used interchangeably in discussions of job stress are *boredom, monotony,* and *repetition.* It may be more accurate to say that workers perceive repetitive, low-complexity jobs as monotonous. This produces a psychological state of boredom. Using the terms this way keeps job features distinct from subjective feelings.

Boredom does seem to have some bad side effects. For example, monotonous jobs are associated with low self-esteem, job dissatisfaction, and low life satisfaction (Johansson, Aronsson, & Lindstrom, 1976). Stress theory predicts that monotonous jobs should increase physiological arousal, but this does not occur. Physiological arousal depends on other factors, such as the complexity or risks, or both, involved in the job itself. Boredom in itself does not appear to produce stress.

Richard Thackray (1981) strongly disputed the idea that boredom is a stressor. He based his argument on a review of laboratory and field studies. Thackray defined boredom and monotony as highly repetitive and unchanging job conditions. Lack of change normally produces a desire for change or variety. Yet laboratory studies of repetitive work show lowered levels of physiological arousal, not heightened arousal.

In a field study of highly mechanized logging work in Sweden, Johansson's team showed that certain groups of employees were more vulnerable to disturbances such as sleep disorders, gastrointestinal disorders, headaches, and nervous tension. Following these observations, another team examined physiological and psychological differences between a high-risk group and a low-risk control group (Johansson et al., 1976). They found higher levels of urinary adrenalin in the high-risk group. The high-risk group also reported stronger feelings of subjective tension and negative mood when compared with the control group. Physical symptoms of illness were higher in the high-risk group, although this difference was not statistically significant.

In looking at the jobs in the high-risk group, the research team noted several important characteristics that might account for the results. The high-risk workers were in positions that required complex judgments and continuous attention. Most importantly, they worked under a forced tempo. Their production rate was a bottleneck in the plant's flow of production. All employees worked on a piece-rate system. What these men produced determined how much all the men earned. The high-risk group thus bore a great responsibility. The objective features of the job, that it was mechanized and repetitive, made no difference. The group worked with a psychosocial pressure that radically changed the meaning of the job from "monotonous" to the "livelihood" of their fellow workers.

TECHNOSTRESS: THE CHANGING FACES OF JOBS

Job obsolescence is a major problem confronting workers in technological societies. Changing technology often forces workers to find new work, perhaps several times during their careers. Estimates now indicate that the average skill turnover for many jobs is around 10 to 15 years. In other words, many jobs that existed 10 years ago may have changed to such a degree that they now require substantially different skills. Because an average career now lasts about 40 to 45 years, many workers may need to retrain or find a new job three to four times during their career. Nowhere is this more evident than in technologically intensive industries.

Craig Brod (1982, 1988) defined **technostress** as "a condition resulting from the inability of an individual or organization to adapt to the introduction and operation of new technology" (1982, p. 754). Thus, technostress refers to the strain felt by workers who must change their skills to keep up with changing jobs or whose jobs may no longer exist because of new technology. As one example, in 1982, Gavriel Salvendy wrote that almost 10 million people were using computers in jobs which did not exist a few years before. According to his estimate, this number may now be closer to 25 million. By the year 2000, jobs in computer-related fields will have expanded at a rate faster than that of any other job area. By that time, blue-collar workers will account for only a small fraction of the total work force.

Technostress often intensifies because employees prefer to stay as comfortable as possible and usually resist change that requires adaptive effort. In addition, employees may view new skills as a threat to their self-esteem instead of as a positive road to personal growth and advancement. They may only come to accept technological change when management clearly and convincingly communicates the potential benefits and defuses the threats of new technology. As Naisbitt (1982) suggested, high tech must be balanced by high touch, the human side of innovation.

Brod (1982) suggested that technostress can be managed first through education aimed at understanding technostress and the human response to it. Second, the employee may apply several stress management techniques to technostress, such as cognitive reappraisal and stress inoculation. Finally, self-assessments may help the employee detect negative thoughts and attitudes that stand in the way of change.

JOB BURNOUT: THE END OF WORK STRESS

If the buzzword of the stress-prone personality is "Type A," the buzzword of work stress is **job burnout.** *Job burnout is not a symptom of work stress, it is the result of unmanaged work stress.* Robert Veniga and James Spradley (1981) conducted a detailed study of job burnout. They defined burnout as "a debilitating psychological condition brought about by unrelieved work stress, which results in:

1. Depleted energy reserves
2. Lowered resistance to illness
3. Increased dissatisfaction and pessimism
4. Increased absenteeism and inefficiency at work" (pp. 6–7)

When the symptoms appear in severe form, management or the employee or both must act quickly before stress turns into burnout.

According to the analysis of Veniga and Spradley, five stages lead to burnout. In the *honeymoon stage,* youthful ideals motivate the novice, who feels an abundance of energy, enthusiasm, and job satisfaction. The person may continue with energy and satisfaction if early problems are constructively managed. In the second, *fuel shortage* stage, the actual signs of burnout begin to appear and intensify as time goes on. In the third, *chronic* stage, symptoms of exhaustion, illness, anger, and depression are continuously evident. In the *crisis* stage, symptoms are so severe the person may feel as though life is falling apart. In the final stage, *hitting the wall,* the person can no longer function and shows signs of serious deterioration.

There is a tendency to equate **workaholism** with job burnout. While the association is not perfect, evidence shows that the more hours you work per week, the more likely you are to burn out. Industry now considers the workaholic a liability, not an asset. Many workaholics work 80 hours or more per week. Some have physical systems that allow them to work longer and run on less sleep than others. For most people, such long hours severely strain the physical system, even though the costs may not appear until later. Workaholics may be driven by a fear of failure. This is a negative, stifling motivation rather than a positive, enhancing one. While they work hard, workaholics are not necessarily productive and creative. In fact, the opposite may be closer to the truth. That is, workaholics may work long hours because they are unable to concentrate on one thing at a time and thus need more time to complete a task.

WORK STRESS IN SPECIAL GROUPS

Certain occupational groups apparently experience more stress than others. Space does not permit a lengthy discussion, but some groups merit comment.

Working Women and Job Stress

Women still face blatant discriminatory practices that add stress to their working conditions. Women still are locked into a variety of dead-end, lower paying, and lower prestige jobs compared with men. No more than 2% of senior managers in the private sector, and only 8.6% in government, are women (Morrison & von Glinow, 1990). Although federal and state legislation was designed to protect against discriminatory practices, recent evidence reveals that the earning gap between women and men is growing wider. For example, in 1965, white women earned about 60% of the salary of white men. In 1975, after ten years of effort and legislative work, women's economic value declined to 58% of what white males earn. Barbara Pletcher (1978) noted that any woman earning above $15,000 a year is earning more than about 99% of working women.

A study published by the U.S. Census Bureau (1983) reported that a bachelor's degree is worth $329,000 to a male worker compared with a high school–educated male. The same bachelor's degree provides the woman with $142,000 advantage compared with a high school–educated female. The man would earn $1,190,000 in his career, but the woman would earn only $523,000.

Employed women often live in a dual-career home that is not yet egalitarian. The woman then works two jobs, one on the outside, the other as a homemaker. Numerous social and economic values continue to support this practice. Women's position in the work force and the stress they bear are not likely to change dramatically unless social attitudes change. Macewen and Barling (1988) showed that conflict between the roles of mother and career woman has a negative effect on marital adjustment. Their research did not indicate support for the reverse notion, that marital adjustment influences interrole conflict. Sadly, there is still little research available to help couples deal with dual-career stress (Higgins, 1986; Kater, 1985).

Sexual Harassment: Women's Hazardous Work Conditions

Perhaps the most oppressive form of stress comes from **sexual harassment** on the job. Sexual harassment may be part of some misguided male's gamesmanship to prop up his ego. It may be a pervasive power game designed to keep women in their place, as Barbara Pletcher (1978) suggested. Still, the effect is the same: exploitation and oppression combined with personal conflict and higher levels of stress.

More active efforts may be needed to weed out those who harass. Women can use legal remedies, but these are still difficult to implement. Nonetheless, filing a legal suit against a supervisor or colleague may be an act of courage necessary to protect both a highly valued professional career and to advance the position of women.

Pletcher recommended that women keep a detailed diary of contacts, dates, times, incidents, words, and so forth. This may include instances of sexual innuendo, offensive jokes, and, of course, instances of pressure, coercion, or job blackmail. Periodically, the woman should send notes from this diary by registered mail to herself or a trusted friend. The envelope should remain sealed for use in future legal action. Courts generally admit such documents as evidence, and they can prevent a defense attorney's attacks on memory.

Although many would argue that this battle must be waged by women, there may be times when men are valuable, even necessary, allies. More men now recognize that men who engage in harassment are an embarrassment. More men are ready and willing now to help impose sanctions or rid the company of offenders. Finally, involving men may increase pressure for change of socio-cultural conditions that reinforce a dual standard of sexuality.

Stress in Air Traffic Controllers

Tragic air accidents often serve to focus attention on air traffic controllers (ATCs). The collision on February 1, 1991, of a USAir liner and a commuter plane at Los Angeles, probably the result of confusion in the control tower, reminds us again of this problem. In the world's most congested airports, airplanes take off or land every 30 to 45 seconds. ATCs are responsibile for the safety of thousands of people each day and for protection of the airlines' multimillion-dollar investments. Maintaining strained attention, as is necessary during long hours of radar monitoring, places extreme pressure on ATCs. Early studies of ATCs showed stress effects that included hypertension, peptic ulcers, diabetes, headaches, indigestion, chest pain, and burnout.

Subsequent studies began to question the generality of these early findings. A study of ATCs in low-density airports found none of the stress effects observed earlier (Melton et al., 1977). Another study revealed the mediating effect of air traffic density. Stress effects did not occur away from the most densely populated airports. Further, physical symptoms do not appear until after three years of service. This led John Crump (1979) to conclude that "the stress of ATC work is no greater than could be expected in 'normal' populations" (p. 244). In Europe's largest airport, in Frankfurt, Germany, ATCs indicated they were primarily dissatisfied with the administration, pay, and working conditions, not the stress of managing the airplanes (Singer & Rutenfranz, 1971). Thus, the potential dangers of this job must be considered on a site-by-site basis.

TELECOMMUTING OR THE ELECTRONIC SWEATSHOP?

An interesting, though controversial, development resulted from the personal-computer revolution. About 15 years ago, University of Southern California futurist Jack Nilles coined the term **telecommuting.** It refers to people who work at home on jobs that depend on the computer or who transfer the results of their work to their employer via computers (Nilles, Carlson, Gray, & Honneman, 1976).

The first signs of telecommuting or teleworkers appeared several years ago, primarily in large and specialized industries (Turnage, 1990). In the early 1980s, IBM, with a dozen other Fortune 500 companies, sponsored a study of telecommuting. They found about 100,000 people telecommuting. Recent estimates suggest that as many as 15 million teleworkers may exist in the United States (Turnage, 1990).

The hope for telecommuting is that it will reduce pressures experienced in the traditional workplace. In contrast to a centralized shop and direct supervision, telecommuting may offer solutions to several management/employee problems. Telecommuting removes the worker from office politics and assembly-line conflicts. It decentralizes work (flexplace) and reduces energy waste from commuting. Further, it offers flex scheduling and job sharing (between spouses or friends) with personal control over the flow of production, release time for personal business, and reduced difficulties in child care (Keita & Jones, 1990; Zedeck & Mosier, 1990). Business may benefit from lower overhead and higher productivity. Research shows that flextime increases productivity when resources have to be shared (Ralston, Anthony, & Gustafson, 1985). Whether this holds true of teleworkers remains to be seen, though anecdotal evidence suggests it does.

Some people believe that the promises of telecommuting are only hype that will ultimately lure workers into "electronic sweatshops." Union leaders are among the most vocal opponents of telecommuting. They see their control and influence in the work force eroding. They also see telecommuting as a computer-age excuse for exploitation. It is too early to say which view is more accurate. Still, we should carefully examine teleworking's potential for reducing job stress before we summarily dismiss it.

COPING WITH JOB STRESS AND BURNOUT

As noted earlier, dealing with job stress requires intervention at both the organizational and personal levels. Unfortunately, much of the emphasis in organizations has been solely on teaching workers how to manage or reduce stress. Very little emphasis has been placed on the sources of stress within the organization (Ivancevich et al., 1990; Murphy, 1984). In the next few pages, I will summarize several approaches that have proven helpful in dealing with job stress.

Personal Strategies for Relieving Job Stress

Managing work stress may operate on several levels. It may involve interventions to change perceptions and permit emotional catharsis. Educational and counseling interventions may target problem-solving skills to change negative aspects of the work environment, including organizational features. Finally, tension-reduction strategies can be used to reduce physical arousal.

Cognitive methods usually focus on the distorting perceptions and irrational thought patterns that contribute to stress. Veniga and Spradley (1981) suggested that the employee faced with burnout must give up the myth that something external is always responsible. While it may seem reasonable, blaming does nothing to correct the situation. Blaming also abandons personal control instead of encouraging belief in self-efficacy.

Many techniques reported in the literature depend on experimental models of stress management. Others are active employee assistance programs in major businesses. As an example, one program used cognitive reappraisal techniques to deal with thoughts and emotions associated with job stress (Ganster, Mayes, Sime, & Tharp, 1982). The program also used relaxation training to reduce tension and excess physiological arousal. The interventions helped employees reduce feelings of depression and lower physiological arousal as measured by epinephrine levels. Unfortunately, most of this research is still largely pragmatic and atheoretical (Ivancevich et al., 1990), which makes it difficult to know what elements are effective in producing change.

Jere Yates (1979) listed eight general rules for dealing with job stress, which can be paraphrased as follows:

1. Maintain good physical health.
2. Accept yourself as you are with all your strengths, weaknesses, successes, and failures.

3. Keep a confidante, a close friend you can talk to with complete candor.
4. Take positive, constructive action to deal with the sources of stress in your job.
5. Maintain a social life apart from the people with whom you work.
6. Engage in creative activities outside the workplace.
7. Engage in meaningful work.
8. Apply an analytic (scientific) method to personal stress problems.

Physical exercise is often ignored as a coping strategy for job stress. Physical exercise is an excellent change of pace from the job, especially for desk-bound workers. It provides release for emotional and mental tension. It reduces frustration and allows displacement of anger or aggression that might be self-destructive. Finally, it reduces risk of coronary disease and lowers absenteeism, job injuries, and health-care costs (Gebhardt & Crump, 1990).

Another effective coping technique is to *change gears* through some interesting hobby or creative activity. A hobby that keeps you active physically, mentally, and spiritually is important to maintaining a sense of perspective. Social activities can also provide a way of changing pace. However, people often socialize with people from work. This may transport job problems to the home and remove opportunities for relaxation.

Accuracy in self-assessment is also important in minimizing job stress. A mismatch between job requirements and job skills may occur because employees do not accurately evaluate their skills for the job demands. It is true that management makes promotion decisions based on assessments of performance in lower-level jobs that are not directly comparable to higher-level jobs. We often forget, though, that when the mismatch occurred there was also a person with an inaccurate self-assessment waiting to be promoted. After the promotion, when the employee is unable to keep up with the job, a cycle of frustration and recrimination may take place. The job that looked attractive in prospect may now threaten the employee's future with the company. Peter (1969) described this situation in *The Peter Principle,* which is promoting a person to their highest level of incompetency.

Using the scientific or analytic method in managing stress means forming hypotheses about what may be the source of the problem. Using the scientific method means that a person collects data from relevant sources, including friends and colleagues, then evaluates a hypothesis in light of the data. The person may use the information to intervene or plan some constructive course of action that will prevent the problem from recurring. In this sense, the scientific method is not for theory building but for application to the real world.

Perhaps the most important way a person can cope with job stress is to work on becoming more aware of the stressors that are unique to his or her position. A person can use a personal inventory or diary, use an objective resource person, or cultivate the art of listening to his or her own body. The body can sound the alarm in early stages of stress and enable a person to prevent the appearance of stress.

Coping by Taking Legal Action

Employees should be aware of the legal remedies at their disposal. These may be used to settle personal grievances or effect organizational reform. For example, employees have the right to file a complaint with the Occupational Safety and Health Administration (OSHA) regarding unsafe and hazardous work conditions. Federal agencies must then conduct site inspections and evaluations. The agencies may levy fines or recommend other sanctions against companies that do not correct the conditions.

Organizational Strategies for Relieving Job Stress

As noted earlier, participation in decisions that affect job conditions eliminates many employee complaints. For example, Veniga and Spradley (1981) reported on a group of computer keypunchers who redesigned their jobs. Absenteeism dropped by 24%, mistakes on the job dropped by 35%, and productivity increased 40%. The company eliminated supervisory positions, thus saving $64,305 per year.

Employee Assistance Programs

Many companies now have employee assistance programs. Ten years ago, fewer than 300 firms offered such programs. Today, over 2400 firms, including several prestigious Fortune 500 companies, provide employee assistance programs.

An employee assistance program offers a variety of services to deal with different facets of employee adjustments to work. Most programs extend to areas beyond the job and include assistance for problems that may have developed outside the job but that affect job performance. These services include personal counseling, classes on stress management and coping (Ivancevich et al., 1990), job retraining, career-change counseling, and support for families of employees in stressful occupations (Hildebrand, 1986). Some programs include a professional staff retained by the company solely to assist its employees. Beyond this, corporations are developing a broad range of services to help employees retain the enthusiasm and freshness of a new employee. Child-care programs, complete health gyms, spas, and exercise and nutrition programs are becoming more common (Gebhardt & Crump, 1990; Ilgen, 1990). These programs address some important needs but do not always directly deal with the issue of reform of the organization itself.

SUMMARY

This chapter has provided an overview of job stress and burnout. We have seen that job stress costs employers and employees millions of dollars each year. The symptoms of job stress include physical, psychological, and behavioral disturbances. Areas of stress include physical conditions of the job, role ambiguity, interpersonal relationships on the job, career development, organizational structure, and the home-work connection. Certain occupational groups, such as women and emergency service providers, are more subject to stress because of job discrimination or because of the dangerous nature of their jobs.

With early recognition of the onset of stress, effective interventions, including cognitive appraisal, relaxation training, and physical exercise may be applied to reduce, if not eliminate, the effects of stress. Personal coping skills must be combined with corporate interventions to reduce long-term stress.

KEY TERMS

assembly-line hysteria	job stress	technostress
boredom	Peter Principle	telecommuting
circadian rhythm	role ambiguity	workaholism
deprivational stress	sexual harassment	qualitative overload
dual-career stress	shift work	quantitative overload
job burnout	spillover	

REFERENCES

Adams, J. D. (1981). Health, stress, and the manager's life style. *Group and Organization Studies, 6,* 291–301.

American Psychiatric Association. (1987). *Diagnostic and statistical manual of mental disorders* (3rd ed., rev.). Washington, DC: Author.

Beehr, T. A., & Newman, J. E. (1978). Job stress, employee health, and organizational effectiveness: A facet analysis, model, and literature review. *Personnel Psychology, 31,* 655–699.

Brod, C. (1982). Managing technostress: Optimizing the use of computer technology. *Personnel Journal, 61,* 753–757.

Brod, C. (1988). *Technostress: Human cost of the computer revolution.* Reading, MA: Addison-Wesley.

Burke, R. J. (1986). Occupational and life stress and the family: Conceptual frameworks and research findings. *International Review of Applied Psychology, 35,* 347–368.

Caplan, R. D., Cobb, S., French, J. R. P., Jr., Van Harrison, R., & Pinneau, S. R. (1975). *Job demands and worker health: Main effects and occupational differences.* Washington, DC: U.S. Government Printing Office.

Cobb, S. (1976). Social support as a moderator of life stress. *Psychosomatic Medicine, 38,* 300–314.

Cooper, C. L. (1983). Identifying stressors at work: Recent research developments. *Journal of Psychosomatic Research, 27,* 369–376.

Cramer, S. H., Keitel, M. A., & Rossberg, R. H. (1986). The family and employed mothers. *International Journal of Family Psychiatry, 7,* 17–34.

Crump, J. H. (1979). Review of stress in air traffic control: Its measurement and effects. *Aviation, Space, and Environmental Medicine, 50,* 243–248.

Cullen, M. R., Cherniack, M. G., & Rosenstock, L. (1990). Occupational medicine [First of two parts]. *The New England Journal of Medicine, 322,* 594–601.

Czeisler, C. A., Johnson, M. P., Duffy, J. F., Brown, E. N., Ronda, J. M., & Kronauer, R. E. (1990). Exposure to bright light and darkness to treat physiologic maladaptation to night work. *The New England Journal of Medicine, 322,* 1253–1259.

Diamond, S. (1985, May 19). Warren Anderson: A public crisis, a personal ordeal. *The New York Times,* Section 3, pp. 1F, 8F.

Everly, G. S., Jr., & Girdano, D. A. (1980). *The stress mess solution.* Bowie, MD: Robert J. Brady.

Farrell, D., & Stamm, C. L. (1988). Meta–analysis of the correlates of employee absence. *Human Relations, 41,* 211–227.

Fisher, C. D. (1985). Social support and adjustment to work: A longitudinal study. *Journal of Management, 11,* 39–53.

French, J. R. P., Caplan, R. D., & Van Harrison, R. (1982). *The mechanisms of job stress and strain.* New York: Wiley.

Ganster, D. C., Mayes, B. T., Sime, W. E., & Tharp, G. D. (1982). Managing organizational stress: A field experiment. *Journal of Applied Psychology, 67,* 533–542.

Gebhardt, D. L., & Crump, C. E. (1990). Employee fitness and wellness programs in the workplace. *American Psychologist, 45,* 262–272.

Green, R. G. (1985). Stress and accidents. *Aviation, Space, and Environmental Medicine, 56,* 638–641.

Higgins, N. C. (1986). Occupational stress and working women: The effectiveness of two stress reduction programs. *Journal of Vocational Behavior, 29,* 66–78.

Hildebrand, J. F. (1986). Mutual help for spouses whose partners are employed in stressful occupations. *Journal for Specialists in Group Work, 11*(1), 80–84.

Hopkins, B. L., Conard, R. J., Dangel, R. F., Fitch, H. G., Smith, M. J., & Anger, W. K. (1986). Behavioral technology for reducing occupational exposures to styrene. *Journal of Applied Behavior Analysis, 19,* 3–11.

House, J. S. (1987). Chronic stress and chronic disease in life and work: Conceptual and methodological issues. *Work & Stress, 1,* 129–134.

Ilgen, D. R. (1990). Health issues at work: Opportunities for industrial/organizational psychology. *American Psychologist, 45,* 273–283.

Institute of Medicine (United States). (1979). *Healthy people : The Surgeon General's report on health promotion and disease prevention.* (Government Document No. HE20.2:H34/5). Rockville, MD: U.S. Government Printing Office.

Ivancevich, J. M., Matteson, M. T., Freedman, S. M., & Phillips, J. S. (1990). Worksite stress management interventions. *American Psychologist, 45,* 252–261.

Johansson, G., Aronsson, G., & Lindstrom, B. O. (1976). Social psychological and neuro-endocrine stress reactions in highly mechanized work (Report No. 488). Stockholm, Sweden: University of Stockholm, Department of Psychology.

Kater, D. (1985). Management strategies for dual-career couples. *Journal of Career Development, 12,* 75–80.

Katzell, R. A., & Thompson, D. E. (1990). Work motivation: Theory and practice. *American Psychologist, 45,* 144–153.

Keita, G. P., & Jones, J. M. (1990). Reducing adverse reaction to stress in the workplace. *American Psychologist, 45,* 1137–1141.

Levi, L. (1990). Occupational stress: Spice of life or kiss of death? *American Psychologist, 45,* 1142–1145.

Macewen, K. E., & Barling, J. (1988). Interrole conflict, family support and marital adjustment of employed mothers: A short term, longitudinal study. *Journal of Organizational Behavior, 9,* 241–250.

Martocchio, J. J., & O'Leary, A. M. (1989). Sex differences in occupational stress: A meta-analytic review. *Journal of Applied Psychology, 74,* 495–501.

McLaughlin, M., Cormier, L. S., & Cormier, W. H. (1988). Relation between coping strategies and distress, stress, and marital adjustment of multiple-role women. *Journal of Counseling Psychology, 35,* 187–193.

Melton, C. E., Smith, R. C., McKenzie, J. M., Wicks, S. M., & Saldivar, J. T. (1977). *Stress in air traffic personnel: Low-density towers and flight service stations* (FAA Office of Aviation Medicine Report No. AM-77-23). Washington, DC: U.S. Government Printing Office.

Moch, M. K., Bartunek, J., & Brass, D. J. (1979). Structure, task characteristics, and experienced role stress in organizations employing complex technology. *Organizational Behavior and Human Performance, 24,* 258–268.

Morrison, A. M., & von Glinow, M. A. (1990). Women and minorities in management. *American Psychologist, 45,* 200–208.

Murphy, L. R. (1984). Occupational stress management: A review and appraisal. *Journal of Occupational Psychology, 57,* 1–15.

Naisbitt, J. (1982). *Megatrends: Ten new directions transforming our lives.* New York: Warner Books.

Nilles, J. M., Carlson, F. R., Jr., Gray, P., & Honneman, G. J. (1976). *The telecommunications-transportation tradeoff.* New York: Wiley.

Pelletier, K. R. (1984). *Healthy people in unhealthy places.* New York: Delacorte Press.

Peter, L. J. (1969). *The Peter principle.* New York: Morrow.

Pletcher, B. A. (1978). *Saleswoman: A guide to career success.* Homewood, IL: Dow Jones–Irwin.

Quinn, R. P., & Staines, G. L. (1979). *The 1977 quality of employment survey.* Ann Arbor: Survey Research Center, University of Michigan.

Ralston, D. A., Anthony, W. P., & Gustafson, D. J. (1985). Employees may love flextime, but what does it do to the organization's productivity? *Journal of Applied Psychology, 70,* 272–279.

Rousseau, D. M. (1978). Relationship of work to nonwork. *Journal of Applied Psychology, 63,* 513–517.

Salvendy, G. (1982). Human-computer communications with special reference to technological developments, occupational stress and educational needs. *Ergonomics, 25,* 435–447.

Sauter, S. L., Murphy, L. R., & Hurrell, J. J. (1990). Prevention of work-related psychological disorders. *American Psychologist, 45,* 1146–1158.

Schuler, R. S. (1980). Definition and conceptualization of stress in organizations. *Organizational Behavior and Human Performance, 25,* 184–215.

Singer, R., & Rutenfranz, J. (1971). Attitudes of air traffic controllers at Frankfurt Airport towards work and the working environment. *Ergonomics, 14,* 633–639.

Spector, P. E. (1986). Perceived control by employees: A meta-analysis of studies concerning autonomy and participation at work. *Human Relations, 39,* 1005–1016.

Spector, P. E., Dwyer, D. J., & Jex, S. M. (1988). Relation of job stressors to affective, health, and performance outcomes: A comparison of multiple data sources. *Journal of Applied Psychology, 73,* 11–19.

Thackray, R. I. (1981). The stress of boredom and monotony: A consideration of the evidence. *Psychosomatic Medicine, 43,* 165–176.

Turnage, J. J. (1990). The challenge of new workplace technology for psychology. *American Psychologist, 45,* 171–178.

U.S. Bureau of the Census. (1983). *Lifetime earnings estimates for men and women in the United States: 1979* (Current Population Reports, Series P-60, No. 139).

Veniga, R. L., & Spradley, J. P. (1981). *The work/STRESS connection.* Boston: Little, Brown.

Yates, J. (1979). *Managing stress: A businessperson's guide.* AMACOM.

Zedeck, S., & Mosier, K. L. (1990). Work in the family and employing organization. *American Psychologist, 45,* 240–251.

CHAPTER 8

Social Sources of Stress: Social Changes, Technological Changes, and Life-Changes

OUR METHOD OF DEALING WITH [SOCIAL] DANGERS . . . IS LIKELY TO BE TOO SLOW AND DANGEROUS FOR THE RATE OF CHANGE THAT EXISTS TODAY.
AUBREY KAGAN

The years of 1968 through the early 1970s were exciting ones for America's space program. Americans saw the first of several lunar landings. Public interest and involvement through the mass media were at an all-time high. Still, there were those who would not or could not enter the space age no matter what kind of evidence they faced.

During an early lunar landing, an incident occurred that still stands out vividly. While the checkout of the lunar module progressed, the local station switched to a downtown shopping district for interviews with people on the street. The TV anchor asked several people, "What do you think of America's achievement in putting a man on the moon?" One person replied, "That's all a hoax. It's just the government tricking us. It can't be done. God didn't intend for us to be there and we'll never be there!"

In a lighter moment, one might suggest that this person proved the truth of the adage that ignorance is bliss. It is possible, of course, that the person firmly believed what he was saying. Perhaps he was ignorant of the technological power behind the space program. It is more likely that he was using a stress-reducing strategy to deal with a pace of change that was beyond him.

Coping strategies used in such situations include denial, defensive coping, and resistant coping or withdrawal. Oblivion and denial bestow a type of protection against stress for some people in some situations.[1] Still, when people react to change in a closed-in, defensive fashion, the result is usually unhealthy. To paraphrase a biblical maxim, they live in society but are not part of society. Change can exact heavy penalties from those unprepared or unwilling to meet the challenge.

---

[1]Research conducted on patients undergoing serious surgery suggests that they fare much better without knowledge of the seriousness of their situation. This is not directly comparable to the person who denied the reality of lunar landings.

STRESS AND ILLNESS:
THE ORIGINS OF SOCIAL THEORY

For many years, sociologists, psychologists, and politicians expended tremendous effort and enormous sums of money to identify pressures imposed by social conditions. Many studies suggested that crime, mental illness, and poor health increase in direct proportion to the degree of (1) financial stress, (2) urban crowding, and (3) lower socioeconomic status (Brenner, 1973; Faris & Dunham, 1939; Hollingshead & Redlich, 1958; Srole et al., 1962). Obviously, these three factors are closely related. The analyses often overlooked the effect of racism, which subjects certain groups to extreme stress. This stress is further intensified by lower socioeconomic status, crowded living conditions, and "programmed failure" in educational systems that do not readily accommodate to the psychosocial needs of culturally diverse students (Peters & Massey, 1983).

Economic stress is an issue that still sparks interest. Based on a survey of 8000 people, Dooley and Catalano (1984) concluded that economic factors have a small but direct effect on physical symptoms. Unemployment had an indirect effect on symptoms because it had the expected negative effect on economic stability.

Government agencies implemented many political action programs during this time, apparently motivated by the belief that social conditions provoke human misconduct. The logic was compelling: social pressures are the root of psychological stress and physical illness. Therefore, if we correct defects in the social environment, stress and illness will decline.

The Dodge-Martin Theory

Two social theorists, Dodge and Martin (1970), were among the first to state the relationship between social pressures and personal stress. Although they based their theory on statistics of *death rate* in the population (mortality), they believed that the theory applied to the *frequency of illness* (morbidity) as well. In brief, their theory states that social factors, including excessive stress, contribute to both chronic (long-term) and acute (short-term) illnesses. However, the specific social factors that contribute differ for each type of illness.

Preventive Action or Delayed Reaction

Other writers have noted similar connections between social upheaval, stress, and illness. One life-change researcher, Aubrey Kagan (1974), pointed to the dramatic increase in ill health associated with the Industrial Revolution. This era gained notoriety from the rapid expansion of technology and monstrous pressures on social structures. A similar analysis may be appropriate for the Great Depression. Still, Kagan saw a much greater danger:

Our method of dealing with the dangers was, and still is, to recognize them usually after a large measure of damage has been done and to apply rational corrections. This method—sometimes called "planning from crisis to crisis"—is likely to be too slow and dangerous for the rate of change that exists today. (p. 42)

Kagan's point makes plain the compelling motivation to understand the effects of social stressors in contemporary society.

Criticisms of Early Social Theory

Unfortunately, many early theories took a single-cause, single-effect approach. They looked for the cause of stress only in social structure (sociogenic) *or* only in the person (psychogenic). Social theories such as those just described focused solely on social structure, largely ignoring the person's contribution to stress reactions. *Relational analyses* were not yet considered.

These early theories also ignored contradictory data. For example, many people raised in poverty and ghetto conditions not only survived but seemed immune to stress (Werner, 1984). Hudgens (cited in Rabkin & Streuning, 1976a) observed that most people do not become disabled even when terrible things happen. A good stress theory should explain how people escape the effects of stress as readily as it explains why people succumb to stress. Suzanne Kobasa's (1979) work on hardiness is one example of a theory that tries to explain resistance.

This chapter and the next, then, will focus on society, life-changes, and environment. The separation of these topics from personality and attitudes is for organizational convenience and thematic coherence only. *The focus is still on the interaction between environment and personal appraisal.* From a systems perspective, a person is a complex, self-referenced, comparator system that is enmeshed in larger social-cybernetic systems.

A SEARCH FOR SOCIAL STRESSORS

A review of stress literature suggests that we can limit our focus to a few powerful sources of social stress. A major national study (Institute of Medicine, 1979) identified four sources contributing to stress and poor health: (1) uprooting stress, the effect of dislocation and frequent relocations; (2) dehumanizing societal institutions that deliver services mechanically and impersonally; (3) the existence of many obstacles to efficient and effective delivery of human services; and (4) the rapid spread of technology.

For our purposes, these may be condensed to three categories: (1) rapid sociological and technological change, (2) dehumanizing and victimizing forces, and (3) environmental stressors, including overcrowding, polluting, and so forth. The first two topics provide the major themes for this chapter. Environmental stress is discussed in Chapter 9.

STRESS AND SOCIAL CHANGE

Alvin Toffler presented two separate analyses of major contemporary stressors; both embraced the notion of rapid, continuous, and dramatic social change. In *Future Shock,* Toffler (1970) discussed the information overload that results from too much change in too short a time. Future shock is a disease characteristic of highly developed technological societies. It occurs when the pace of change is so rapid it exceeds our ability to integrate change. In short, future shock is the premature arrival of the future.

The pace of social and technological change is astounding. Technological changes dramatically alter the way people work, learn, and spend their leisure time. Technology changes the environment in which we live, and jobs change to keep pace with new technology. Education changes, and our children ask questions about problems that did not even exist 30 years ago. Science changes the amount and range of information available; *it will change even faster in the future.* Now scientists write nearly 6000 to 7000 articles each day. The amount of scientific and technical information published grows at the rate of 13% per year. At this rate, the volume doubles every 5.5 years. Current projections are that the growth rate will soon reach 40% (Naisbitt, 1982). Turnage (1990) notes that information technology has halved in cost and doubled in power every 2 to 4 years. Yet these technological changes only scratch the surface of what might lie ahead.

Lifestyle changes mirror social change. Changes in the family challenge old values and religious traditions. Common-law marriage, gay liberation, abortion, and lesbian adoption of orphans provoke heated exchanges among families, communities, cities, and governments. Use or misuse of environmental resources leads to competition, if not violent confrontation, between special-interest groups. Organized religion abandons traditions and revises once-unwavering positions, shaking the foundation of personal values in the process. The assumptive world, the world order constructed in our cognitive schema, has changed. For some, adjusting schemata to fit new realities may be easy. Others will simply endure with tension in a world they no longer know.

A Strange New Emerging World

Toffler's (1980) second work, *The Third Wave,* described the end of *second-wave* civilization. Industrialism, religious idealism, and a representative but centralized democracy formed the core of second-wave society. Second-wave civilization was the society of 300 years past, much of it the society of our immediate past, and it is still *part of a crumbling present.* Toffler suggested that current changes are not revolutionary in concept only, but also in pace and impact. The old society, with entrenched values and traditions, is being torn down to make way for a new society. The new society frames a new set of values and traditions on the rubble of the old. The transition will produce excitement for some but despair for others.

Confronted with technological developments such as surrogate mothers, test-tube babies, and organ transplants, choices are less certain. Family customs may not only leave many people unprepared, but also leave people antagonistic to change. Personal beliefs and ethical philosophies formed in the crucible of aging ideologies may be incompatible with the new order. For many, personal change may come only after fighting a private war in the human psyche as they struggle to extract personal meanings from change. Later, the conflict may be fought in open arenas such as marriage, the nuclear family, and the community.

Personal Stability and Social Change

The psychological impact of this revolution is highly visible. Confusion and anxiety tend to increase. Some authors have called this "the age of anxiety." Self-identity becomes less sure as relationships that provided personal security seem more tenuous. To use Durkheim's (1951) term, a feeling of **anomie** may increase. Anomie is a sense of being alone and lost in a huge, impersonal social structure that has no room for individual differences. This feeling may motivate a desperate, almost spiritual, quest for renewed stability. On one hand, a person may cling tenaciously to the structures of the past. On the other, he or she may be vulnerable to a variety of cults that seem to offer stability.

A rapidly fragmenting populace enthusiastically, and financially, supports new "cults" and "isms." Cultural diversity extends to religious pluralism. Each church has its own drive-up, tune-in, advice-column insights into human nature. Churches also have cash-and-carry solutions: buy a pamphlet, a book, an audio- or videotape and carry out the secret of happiness, marital bliss, or effective parenting. Each church captures some part of its followers' imagination by offering to restore sanity to a world that is no longer recognized.

Bernice Martin (1981) noted that myriad cults and religions exploded onto the American cultural scene in the 1960s and 1970s. She used a term from Berger and Luckmann, *plausibility structures,* to describe the attraction of these cults, which seem to "prop up the subjective self" in a time of extreme cultural fluidity. As Martin said of the cults,

> they claim to be liberating while much of their real appeal lies in the latent function of providing firm and definitive conceptions of private individual identity which can be strongly internalized and which are usually backed up by psycho-social support structures. (p. 222)

In a discussion of family structure, Robert Nisbet (1970) noted that social structure is typically stable and resistant to change, whereas people and processes may change rapidly, even explosively. People experience immense pressure when change cannot be personally controlled or is externally imposed. The mere perception of lack of control and lack of predictability of events may be enough to produce intense stress. Future shock is part and parcel of the unpredictable, uncontrollable, externally imposed change.

PERSONAL CONFRONTATIONS WITH RAPID CHANGE

Toffler confined his analysis to the shape of change itself. Recent research provided clues about the coping strategies people often choose in these circumstances (Gentry, Foster, & Harvey, 1972; Lazarus, 1966). Faced with rapid, incomprehensible change, people adopt a variety of defensive postures. Some strategies for coping with change are effective and promote personal growth. Other strategies are self-limiting, if not self-defeating. Forced to make too many choices without time to integrate old standards and values, many people will simply avoid making choices altogether. One major negative outcome of rapid change is **demoralization,** the psychological result that occurs when environmental demands exceed a person's capacity to meet them (Dohrenwend & Dohrenwend, 1982; Frank, 1973; Wills & Langner, 1980).

LIFE-CHANGE, STRESS, AND ILLNESS

Rapid social change appears to play a central role in the development of stress. Some outcomes of social change may exist as subtle, if not insidious, pressures on personal adaptive reserves. Other effects may be more direct, as well as much more serious. A 1949 Conference on Life Stress and Bodily Disease formally recognized the importance of life stress and illness (Rabkin & Streuning, 1976a). In the 1970s and 1980s, several investigators launched empirical research programs to discover the relationship, if any, between **life-change and illness.** The details and conclusions of this scientific pursuit will be the subject of the next few pages.

LIFE-CHANGE UNITS: THE EMPIRICAL STORY

Two separate teams of researchers began the most notable research on life-change and illness. The first team consisted of Thomas Holmes from the University of Washington and Richard Rahe of the U.S. Navy Medical Neuropsychiatric Research Unit. The second was the wife-and-husband team of Barbara and Bruce Dohrenwend (1982) at Columbia University. Because the Dohrenwends' work built on the legacy of Holmes and Rahe, we will treat the two lines of inquiry as a single program. Also, because this line of inquiry has been under attack recently for various reasons, I will summarize major criticisms later in this chapter.

Holmes and Rahe (1967) set out to answer two of the most important questions in stress research. First, they wanted to know what life-change situations are most stressful. Second, they wanted to know what physical problems, if any, may develop because of stressful life-changes. They reasoned that both constitutional variables and temporal factors in life govern risk for illness. In the words of Richard Rahe (1974):

Constitutional endowment helps to explain an individual's susceptibilities to particular types of illnesses but does little to explain why an individual develops an illness at a particular point in time. . . . Recent life changes appear to act as "stressors" partially accounting for illness onset. Conversely, when subjects' lives are in a relatively steady state of psychosocial adjustment with few ongoing life changes, little or no illness tends to be reported. (p. 58)

To answer the first question, Holmes and Rahe developed a scaling procedure to assess the degree of stress associated with commonly encountered life events. Taking a direct approach, they asked a large group of people to identify their most stressful events. Then Holmes and Rahe assigned weights to the events based on the group's ratings. They recognized that life events did not have to be extreme (such as war or pestilence) in order for stress to be present. Instead, they focused on naturally occurring stressors or life events such as marriage, divorce, childbirth, and death of a loved one (Dohrenwend & Dohrenwend, 1982).

In regard to the relationship between stress and illness, Holmes and Rahe followed an old trail. Early laboratory investigators had discovered that numerous physical ailments, including ulcers and death, may be related to severe stress. If this finding was also true of people in a natural environment, some important implications for detecting and preventing the sources of illness might emerge.

To begin this phase, Holmes and Rahe asked approximately 5000 clients to write down events they considered most stressful. From this pool of responses, they built a list of 43 life-change events that included positive (marriage), negative (going to jail), frequent (minor traffic violations), and rare (death of spouse or child) events. The common core is that these events require some adaptive struggle or **social readjustment** to manage them effectively. Social readjustment is "the intensity and length of time necessary to accommodate to a life event, *regardless of the desirability of this event*" (Holmes & Masuda, 1974, p. 49). Adaptive struggle may reveal itself in psychological conflict and anxiety for a time and may be the motivation for a lifestyle change.

In the next phase, Holmes and Rahe asked 394 people to rate the 43 events based on their experiences with the stressors. Further, they asked the clients to note the relative degree of disruption each event caused. Holmes and Rahe assigned marriage an arbitrary value of 500. Then each person judged whether the remaining events required more or less readjustment than marriage and assigned to each event a value proportionate to the value of 500. For example, if clients judged that the death of a spouse required twice as much readjustment effort as marriage, they assigned it a value of 1000. After collecting this information, Holmes and Rahe computed the average severity of life-change produced by each stressor. Finally, they ranked the events from most intense to least intense.

THE SOCIAL READJUSTMENT RATING SCALE

This resulted in the **Social Readjustment Rating Scale (SRRS)** shown in Table 8-1. Note that the first item, death of spouse, is assigned a value of 100.

TABLE 8-1
Rank of Life-Change Events with Associated LCUs

Rank	Life event	LCU
1	Death of spouse	100
2	Divorce	73
3	Marital separation	65
4	Jail term	63
5	Death of close family member	63
6	Personal injury or illness	53
7	Marriage	50
8	Fired at work	47
9	Marital reconciliation	45
10	Retirement	45
11	Change in health of family member	44
12	Pregnancy	40
13	Sexual difficulties	39
14	Gain of new family member	39
15	Business readjustment	39
16	Change in financial state	38
17	Death of close friend	37
18	Change to different lines of work	36
19	Change in number of arguments with spouse	35
20	Mortgage over $10,000	31
21	Foreclosure of mortgage or loan	30
22	Change in responsibilities at work	29
23	Son or daughter leaving home	29
24	Trouble with in-laws	29
25	Outstanding personal achievement	28
26	Wife begins or stops work	26
27	Begin or end school	26
28	Change in living conditions	25
29	Revision of personal habits	24
30	Trouble with boss	23
31	Change in work hours or conditions	20
32	Change in residence	20
33	Change in schools	20
34	Change in recreation	19
35	Change in church activities	19
36	Change in social activities	18
37	Mortgage or loan less than $10,000	17
38	Change in sleeping habits	16
39	Change in number of family get-togethers	15
40	Change in eating habits	13
41	Vacation	13
42	Christmas	12
43	Minor violations of the law	11

SOURCE: Holmes & Rahe (1967).

The original rating used an arbitrary maximum value of 500, but after computing the final mean ratings, the investigators assigned the most severe stressor a value of 100. They adjusted all the means to this standard so the relative intensity of each event is still reflected accurately. Holmes and Rahe called this adjusted event value a **Life Change Unit (LCU).** Now, presumably, the total amount of stress a person experienced in a given time could be measured by adding together all the LCUs for the items checked.

Note that the three items ranked most stressful by this sample (death of spouse, divorce, and separation) involve life-changes in marital status. In fact, eight of the top ten stressors are either family- or work-related. Also note that very few items are *high-severity* stressors, whereas a large number are *low-to-moderate-severity* stressors.

In addition, you can see that many events are pleasant events. Most people probably think that marriage, pregnancy, completion of school, change in line of work, outstanding personal achievement, vacation, and Christmas are positive events. Still, these events produce stress, some events more than others. As Selye's definition of stress suggests, the body does not distinguish between positive and negative stressors. The excitement of marriage is almost as taxing as the grief suffered with the loss of a close member of the family.

Take a moment to respond to the scale before reading further. Circle the number on the left for any events you have experienced in the past six months. After you have done this, locate the LCU score for the event in the right-hand column and circle it. Then sum the circled LCU scores. Information on interpreting the results will be provided in the following pages.

DO STRESSFUL LIFE EVENTS REALLY PRODUCE ILLNESS?

After they obtained these severity ratings, Holmes and Rahe wanted to know if life-changes affect personal adjustment and health, and if so, how. Previous research suggested that stressful life-changes could precipitate a variety of harmful effects, including psychological disturbances and physical illness. Three lines of evidence contributed to the belief that stressful life-changes produce some deterioration in health, if not outright illness. One line of evidence comes from laboratory and clinical research programs based on the work of Selye and others. Much of this research appeared in earlier chapters of this book.

The second line of evidence comes from observations of reactions to natural disasters, such as earthquakes and floods, and observations of individuals under conditions of abnormal stress, such as soldiers in combat. The term **post-traumatic stress syndrome** refers to the emotional-behavioral pattern that follows such extreme conditions. Information on stress reactions to catastrophic events will be presented in more detail in the next chapter.

The third line of evidence represents the concerted effort of many investigators working over nearly two decades. Most have used the scaling techniques of Holmes and Rahe; others have adapted their scaling procedure or developed similar techniques. In all cases, the efforts shared a common goal: to assess the relationship between the amount of stress and the amount of illness in populations in the natural environment.

Physicians and Life Crises

Holmes and Rahe asked a group of 200 resident physicians to list all the "major health changes" they had experienced in the previous ten years and to fill out the SRRS. Each responding physician (88 total) received a score based on the sum of LCU values. Of the 96 major health changes reported, 89 occurred with total LCU scores over 150. When the LCU score was under 150, the majority reported good health in the following year. When the LCU score was above 300, over 70% of the physicians reported illness in the following year (Rahe, 1974). Holmes and Rahe used 150 as a preliminary definition of *life crisis*.

Further analysis permitted Holmes and Rahe to establish more precise categories for life crises: 150 to 199 LCUs defined a *mild* life crisis, 200 to 299 LCUs defined a *moderate* life crisis, and anything over 300 LCUs defined a *major* life crisis (Holmes & Masuda, 1974). (If you have already responded to the scale, you can compare your score against this standard.) The working assumption is that the more life crises that accumulate, the more likely the person will incur some illness shortly afterward.

In an extensive review of studies aimed at testing this assumption, Holmes and Masuda found an impressive array of supporting evidence. Retrospective studies found increased life-change associated with myocardial infarction, fractures, diabetes, tuberculosis, pregnancy, and leukemia (Rabkin & Streuning, 1976a; Rahe & Arthur, 1978). Another study showed that as life-change increased among college freshmen, their grade point averages went down. Similar outcomes obtained in other cultures established the cross-cultural generality of this relationship.[2] Studies of children, of identical twins, and of college students provided similar results. Among adults, the findings appear to hold across various occupational groups.

Telephone Operators, Hungarian Refugees, and Carrier Pilots

Hinkle (1974) and his colleagues were among the first to provide evidence of this type. They began with a large group of female (1327) and male (1527) telephone company employees. Using a random sampling technique, they reduced this group to a smaller sample of 226 employees with 20 years or more of company service. A review of the medical histories of this group revealed phenomenal differences in sickness. One group took no sick leave at all during the 20 years. Members of another group each had less than five days' total absence due to sickness and only one or two episodes of illness-related leave each year. Company records on a third group of employees revealed some startling facts. Members

---

[2]The countries included in cross-cultural replications include England, Wales, Norway, Sweden, Denmark, France, Belgium, Switzerland, Japan, Malaysia, San Salvador, and Peru, and the state of Hawaii.

of this group missed up to 1000 workdays during the 20-year period. Some had nearly 100 episodes of disabling illness during the same 20-year period. All told, *that is equivalent to missing three years of work,* with roughly five illness disability episodes per year.

The next step in the investigative process was even more revealing. Hinkle wanted to confirm whether particular biological or psychosocial patterns might explain the major differences between the healthy and the sick group. While the researchers could not statistically rule out the possibility that these differences were due to chance, strong evidence existed of a differing psychosocial pattern for each group. In Hinkle's (1974) own words:

> the "healthy" telephone operators were women . . . who liked their work, found it easy and satisfying, liked their families and associates, and were generally content and comfortable with their lot in life. This was often not the case with the frequently ill telephone operators . . . many of them were working at this job not because they liked it but from necessity. They often described it as confining or boring. For various reasons these women were unhappy with their lot in life, with their families, their associates, and their communities. (p. 21)

Hinkle studied two other groups. One group consisted of Chinese-born graduate students, technicians, and professional people living in New York City. The second was a group of Hungarian refugees who escaped to America following the "Black October" Russian invasion of Hungary. Both groups had undergone severe dislocation, separation from families and stable social support groups, and extreme culture shock.

For the most part, the Chinese group showed little evidence of illness. At first this result seemed to contradict the pattern observed in previous studies. Information from the Hungarian group, though, provided a possible explanation for the paradox. Compared with the telephone operators, the Hungarian group showed the same distribution of illness *during the ten years preceding their flight.* They described their time leading up to the confrontation with the Hungarian regime as one of insecurity and frustration. During the revolution and escape, and in spite of severe disruption in their lives, they actually showed improved health. It appeared that the general excitement and the anticipation of making a fresh start in a new country served as a type of inoculation against sickness. Hinkle concluded that the effect of dramatic social change on a person's health could not be judged solely from the nature of the change itself. Other factors must be important, including a person's psychological characteristics.

Other investigations confirm this conclusion. For example, observations of enlisted sailors showed that only a few men accounted for most of the sick days taken. Sailors who worked in routine, menial jobs that required less skill were sick most frequently. Often their jobs were either hazardous or uncomfortable or both. Further, these sailors were less mature and less capable compared with those who did not report illness (Nelson, 1974).

Rubin (1974) conducted an interesting study in the real-world environment of aircraft carrier pilot trainees. The situation these trainees encountered appears similar in many respects to the one in the Brady "Executive monkey" study reviewed earlier. As we shall see shortly, the physical reactions observed were also similar. Here is how Rubin described the training situation and aircraft:

> The F-48 Phantom jet fighter-bomber is a two-man aircraft. The pilot, in the front cockpit, has complete flight control. The radar intercept officer (RIO), in the rear cockpit, monitors the radar and other instruments but has no flight control. He does have excellent visibility. In an emergency both the pilot and the RIO can eject themselves from the aircraft, a procedure not without hazard. The RIO is aware of these hazards and the aircraft's position during the landing attempt, but he must rely completely on the pilot's skill for his own personal safety. (p. 228)

In other words, the RIO is in exactly the same situation as the monkeys who could do nothing to control the shock. The RIOs could only put their safety in the hands of the pilot and hope.

Measurements of the physical responses of both the pilots and the RIOs showed an interesting pattern of reactivity. While the RIOs showed higher levels of subjective anxiety on all days tested, the pilots showed the type of stress reaction pattern observed in the laboratory animals. Again, in the words of Rubin (1974):

> These results indicate that aircraft carrier landing practice was considerably more stressful for the pilots than for their RIOs. In the context of the "executive" monkey paradigm, the "executive" naval aviator, who had to perform a highly complex task while avoiding serious potential harm to himself, his partner and his aircraft, showed an unequivocal adrenal cortical stress response. The passive partner, on the other hand, although completely aware of the risks involved, showed only a slight, statistically insignificant adrenal response. (pp. 231–232)

David Krantz and Shera Raisen (1988) reviewed a growing body of biobehavioral literature concerned with the effects of social stress on ischemic heart disease. They conclude from this review that three environmental variables contribute to increased coronary risk. These are low socioeconomic status, low social support, and occupational settings marked by low control and high demand. Krantz and Raisen point out that the effects are often small and the relationships complex. Thus, the notion of simple, one-way paths of causation does not fit the data.

THE CASE AGAINST LIFE-CHANGE AND ILLNESS

Research on life-change and illness has been criticized since it began. As Dohrenwend and Dohrenwend (1982) said, "at present the belief that life stress causes illness is based on faith bolstered by some scientific evidence" (p. 91). Lost in the shuffle is the counterargument that life stress may be growth promoting, a position that has drawn little empirical attention (Zautra & Sandler, 1983). The substance of life-change criticism will be examined briefly.

Most of the early studies on life stress and illness used retrospective designs, which contain several weaknesses. First, reliability of retrospective data is suspect because of errors in memory, subjective biases in reporting illness, overreporting, and intervening distortions that may affect subjects' perceptions of the events (Rabkin & Streuning, 1976a). Further, early prospective studies showed the expected relationship, but it was much weaker in the prospective studies than in retrospective studies. This led to a skeptical attitude in the scientific community.

More carefully designed prospective studies followed that caused even more skepticism. David Schroeder and Paul Costa (1984) reported on a prospective study that found no evidence for the connection. Subjects took a medical examination prior to a year designated as the target year. Later, the subjects reported on life-change using a "56-item Holmes-Rahe–style" checklist. Schroeder and Costa employed physicians' records of illness to assess the number of *new diseases not present at the pre-stress examination.* They found no correlation between the amount of life-change in the previous 12 months and the incidence of illness.

Still, disconfirming prospective studies such as Schroeder and Costa's must be weighed against positive prospective studies. It may be that moderator variables will be discovered that resolve the discrepancy between outcomes. Sarason, Levine, and Sarason (1982) point to three broad classes of moderator variables that may be closely related to the life-change and illness issue. These three variables include: relatively stable personal characteristics, such as locus of control and psychological hardiness; prior experiences that influence how a person responds to stress; and environmental factors, such as social support.

One argument against the life-stress–illness connection was both simple and powerful. This argument states that illness is often confounded with psychiatric and psychological problems. Psychiatric disability is stressful and causes disruptions in life. Evidence shows that illness occurs with greater prevalence in psychiatric populations. Thus, illness shows a correlation to life stress with no necessary causal connection. It may be also that psychiatric disability leads to distorted perceptions of life stress and biased reporting.[3] These important arguments cannot be easily discounted.

Another criticism focused on the biased content of life-change scales. Life-stress scales appear to be contaminated with items related to mood and disposition. New evidence reveals that ratings of life stress may reflect a pessimistic style and negative emotional set more than they reflect inherent properties of the event. Support for this argument comes from the work of Brett and her colleagues, who use the notion of negative affect (Brett, Brief, Burke, George, & Webster, 1990). Negative affect is a mood-dispositional dimension that reflects pervasive individual differences in negative emotionality and self-concept. When Brett's group used measures of life-change free of negative affect bias, the

---

[3]For a review of confounding variables, see Rabkin and Streuning (1976b).

relationship to physical symptoms mostly disappeared. When they constructed scales with extreme negative affect, the relationship to physical symptoms was even stronger than to total life-events scores. This provided even stronger evidence that the major contributing factor to the life-change–illness connection was negative affect. This finding is all the more interesting when we consider the role negative affect played in coronary risk research.

Finally, Brett's group showed that the negative affect scale correlated even more strongly with depression. Negative affect may be a general mood-dispositional tendency that carries with it the burden of depression and lower quality of health. The stress connection may be incidental or only a reflection of the person's dispositional tendencies. This would argue against life stress as a cause of illness.

COPING WITH SOCIAL CHANGE

The complexity of social change precludes giving specific recommendations, as we might with more specific stresses. Social change is global, pervasive, insidious, and constant. As several writers have suggested, change may be the most constant part of our environment. Accepting the fact of change may be an important first step in coping with it. Preparation and self-education are also vital. The well-read, socially alert, and culturally aware person may have the greatest likelihood of managing innovation, technology, and lifestyle choices with the least amount of stress. Ostrichlike responses to unwanted change do nothing. Naisbitt (1982) commented that the appropriate response to technology is to accommodate it, respond to it, and shape it.

Stress-inoculation methods may also help (Meichenbaum & Jaremko, 1983). This approach focuses on imagining worst-case scenarios that might induce a high degree of stress. The assumption is that once you have anticipated your worst fears and thought about strategies for managing them, you will manage the situation better when it happens. In addition, change will be easier to tolerate because you have already worked out the emotional side of it.

The report *Healthy People* presented several ways for people to cope with social stress (Institute of Medicine, 1979). These included belonging to a group, having acceptable substitute activities available, having ready access to advice, having someone to talk to about personal troubles, and having an education. Belonging to a group is important for social support (Cohen & Wills, 1985). Social support is helpful when one makes stressful decisions such as quitting smoking and going on a diet. Conversely, lack of social support may contribute to psychological disorders (Leavy, 1983).

COPING WITH VICTIMIZATION

Tuesday, November 20, 1984, should have been just another school day for 17-year-old Ben Wilson, student and all-star basketball player at Simeon Vocational

High School in Chicago. Instead, it would be the last day of his life. Two 16-year-old students shot Ben Wilson to death when they became angry after he "bumped" into them on the sidewalk near the high school (Berkow, 1984). Ben Wilson was just one victim that day. As in many cases like this, the effect of the crime reaches out to others and endures (Hepburn & Monti, 1979). Wilson's family and friends, also victims, must suffer the consequences of this senseless crime for years.

Crime creates nearly 15 million victims each year, while family violence and abuse occurs in nearly 1.5 million homes (Flanagan & Maguire, 1990). According to FBI statistics, nearly 952,000 aggravated assaults and 21,500 murders occurred in 1989 (Federal Bureau of Investigation, 1990). In the same year, nearly 95,000 women were forcibly raped.[4] Material loss from all types of robbery is approximately $9.5 billion annually. Corporate and white-collar crime bilks untold millions through coercion, extortion, and fraud (Meyer, 1981). Terrorism on an international scale has disrupted the lives of thousands (Fields, 1980; Ochberg, 1978).

Great as the immediate physical and material losses may be, the aftermath of crime produces even more sinister, pervasive, and debilitating effects. Call it "mind-rapes"— the unwanted, continued forced entry into one's consciousness of the memories, feelings, pain, and terror of the event. For many, this continued intrusion into the inner sanctum of the mind is the greater crime and the source of recurrent stress (Janoff-Bulman, 1988).

POSTTRAUMATIC STRESS DISORDER: A FIRST LOOK

Traumatic events may include natural disasters, murder, rape, combat, accidents, or terrorism. Still, there is a common behavioral pattern that typifies victims' reactions called *posttraumatic stress disorder* (American Psychiatric Association, 1987). Four signs lead to the diagnosis of posttraumatic stress disorder (PTSD). First, evidence must exist of a recent stressor such as those identified above. Second, the victim relives the event through dreams, intrusive thoughts, or feelings that the traumatic event is happening again. Third, the victim experiences numbing of responsiveness, which may appear as decreased interest in activities, detachment from others, or flattening of emotional affect. Finally, the person may show two or more symptoms, including startle responses, sleep disturbance, survival guilt, or cognitive impairment, among others. The symptoms of rape-trauma syndrome are the same as those of PTSD (Burgess, 1983).

---

[4]This figure is regarded as far too low because of the flawed methodology used by the FBI for collecting its data. Mary Koss (cited in Freiberg, 1990), in testimony before Congress, reported that 76 in 1000 college women were subjected to rape or attempted rape in a 12-month period. Further, in a sample of 2300 working women, 27.5% reported being victimized by rape or attempted rape since their 14th birthday.

FEAR—THE VICTIM'S JAILER

The most pervasive psychological effect is fear. An assault or robbery does not even have to take place for fear to weave its web. William Berg and Robert Johnson (1979) speak of the **"fear of crime" syndrome** (p. 58) and of "self-defined prisoners" (p. 59) who no longer have safe havens when crime follows them into their homes. Fear becomes their jailer and gatekeeper, shutting off free access to an outside world that still beckons but is too frightening to explore. Personal freedom seems limited because victims generally feel compelled to alter patterns of social, market, and work behavior (Brooks, 1981). They feel constant vigilance is necessary to ensure that personal injury or loss does not occur again. Disillusionment about society in general and justice in particular become enduring attitudes. Victims expend mental energy in conflict that could be used for creative pursuits. In effect, fear changes the victim's reality.

VICTIMOLOGY: INVESTIGATING CRIMINAL-VICTIM RELATIONSHIPS

Criminologists are specialists who investigate the relationships between social systems and criminal behavior. Another group of specialists, **victimologists,** try to discover the factors that contribute to becoming victims (Schafer, 1977).[5] Among many questions raised by these investigators, three are central. One issue is **risk**: What factors predispose some individuals to be targets of crime? A second question has to do with **prevention**: What can be done to educate people to reduce their risk? Another is *coping*: What can be done to help victims put their work, social, family, and personal lives back together?

The Question of Risk: Who Are the Victims?

Victims of crime exist in every segment of society, though some groups are more vulnerable than others. The term **vulnerable** refers to groups with shared demographic or personal characteristics who are susceptible to becoming victims through no fault of their own (Galaway & Hudson, 1981). One research team, headed by Michael J. Hindelang, began to piece together a picture that describes high-risk groups (Hindelang, Gottfredson, & Garofalo, 1978). The four demographic characteristics that seem most important are summarized as follows.

Age Younger persons have a higher likelihood of becoming victims, probably because of mobility and social behavior. The elderly experience more anticipatory fear and are more likely to feel the effects of victimization because of their relative lack of power (Berg & Johnson, 1979).

[5]Victimology is the science that explores the role of the victim in crime. Hans von Hentig and B. Mendelsohn developed the field in the 1940s.

Marital status   Unmarried people have a greater risk of becoming victims than married people, generally because of socializing activities. On the other hand, married people generally spend more time at home or work than on the move.[6]

Employment status   Unemployed people have a higher risk of becoming victims than employed people.

Sex   Men are at higher risk than women. This finding mirrors the patterns previously described: the most vulnerable people are young, unmarried, unemployed males who may be in the wrong place at the wrong time. Although young males may be at higher risk, females report more fear of victimization (Hindelang et al., 1978).

Prevention: How to Avoid Becoming a Victim

To be sure, modern living entails risks. Still, the likelihood of serious loss or injury from personal crime is less than that from driving a car. Further, a few simple steps can be taken to reduce the risks of becoming a victim. In other words, *reducing risk does not require monumental changes in lifestyle.* Hindelang's group concluded that "for most people, the behavioral effects of crime or the fear of crime appear more as subtle adjustments in behavior than as major shifts in what can be called behavioral policies" (Hindelang et al., 1978, p. 224). This notion, that reducing risk does not require major lifestyle changes, is *the single most important idea* in this entire discussion.

Lifestyle Assessment

Lifestyles are significant factors in personal crime because lifestyles relate to being in places and situations with high *opportunities* for criminal actions. *Lifestyle* refers to routine work or leisure activities (Hindelang et al., 1978). A lifestyle assessment may be helpful, then, to understand how personal behavior alters environmental risks.

The first step is to identify personal habits of shopping, socializing, and movement in your locale. Habits by definition are automatic and require little or no conscious attention. Keeping a diary for one or two weeks may bring unattended trouble spots into focus. By cross-checking habits against the risk information that follows, you may see that certain adjustments are desirable.

---

[6]Schafer (1977) presents information that disputes this general pattern. He suggests that both the number of criminals and the number of violent crimes is largest among married persons. The argument, though, uses frequency rather than proportional statistics; this casts doubt on the argument. Schafer qualified the argument as pertaining to violent crime and not to all instances of victimization.

Adjusting time   According to Hindelang, the time between midnight and 6 A.M. carries the highest risk for injury (Hindelang et al., 1978). There are several reasons for this. First, fewer bystanders are present to notice or intervene at night. Second, people consume more alcohol at night, and alcohol plays a significant role in criminal acts. Most importantly, *the contribution of alcohol to the risk of criminal assault comes as much from the victim as from the offender.* Alcohol affects decision-making processes and lowers important protective social inhibitions. Steele and Josephs (1990) call this an "alcohol-induced myopia." It appears to contribute to provoking criminal attacks or increasing the likelihood of injury or both.

Avoiding high-risk places   Two places are notably high-risk places: home and the street. However, crimes occurring in these two arenas are dramatically different. Assaults in the home are most often crimes of passion, committed by a spouse, lover, or friend after some serious domestic strife. These crimes have a high injury rate because the partner tends to react with physical aggression.

Criminal assaults on the street are often crimes of profit or power (territorial imperatives) precipitated by strangers experiencing personal frustrations (Schafer, 1977). Street assaults can be avoided largely through adjusting time schedules, using modes of transportation that avoid prolonged contact on the street, and traveling in groups.

Taking self-protection measures   After a crime has occurred, victims frequently replay the episode and second-guess their reactions to the event. They wonder what they could have done differently. The basic principles of self-protection can be summarized briefly. Where profit seems to be the motive, it is less risky to let the thief carry on without resisting. When engaging in self-protection, physical counterattack more than doubles the risk. The most successful means of warding off attacks include verbal resistance through threats of detection, persuasion, or talking the offender out of committing the crime (20% injury rate, 80% injury free); evasive action (16% injury rate, 84% injury free); and simply yelling or screaming (36% injury rate, 64% injury free) (Hindelang et al., 1978).

Adjusting daily activities   As noted earlier, only minor behavior adjustments are necessary to reduce risk. For example, you should vary routine market behaviors (shopping for food, clothing) instead of maintaining a rigid schedule. Also, shop during the day or early evening hours. Adjust job-related behaviors so hours of transit and mode of transit are optimal. Leave the office early to take a crowded metro, not late when you will be traveling alone. Attend social activities (such as movies and dining out) in small groups. On university campuses, late-night escort services are becoming more common to enable people to move about with safety. If one exists, consider making use of it when appropriate.

BARRIERS TO EFFECTIVE PREVENTION

Three psychological processes seem to influence both the risks we take and the stress reactions we experience from victimization. These are cognitive appraisals, beliefs, and emotional reactions. Cognitive appraisals include evaluating the risk of becoming a victim and making causal attributions about crime. Beliefs refer to our readiness to act based on the perceptions that our behavior will be beneficial in some respect. Fear is the emotional reaction of primary concern, as noted earlier.

Misattributions about Crime

Three attribution errors play a crucial role in adaptive behaviors to avoid becoming a victim. These include attributions about *local versus distant distribution* of crime, *local versus outside involvement,* and **self-blame** for cause of the crime.

Misattribution 1: Crime is worse elsewhere   On average, people think crime is a big problem elsewhere, but not in their community. This is true even where crime rates are high, such as in urban inner-city districts (Hindelang et al., 1978). People are more likely to evaluate threat in their community as less than that in other communities even within their city. This misattribution may enable people to diffuse threat so it will not be a constant burden. It may also contribute to reduced vigilance, which increases the risk for subsequent victimization.

Misattribution 2: Outsiders are doing it   People tend to attribute crime in their area to outsiders. Using data from a Florida sample, Schafer (1977) showed that the majority of offenders (61.5%) lived only a few miles and a few minutes from their victims.

Misattribution 3: I am to blame   The process of self-blame has been the subject of much research over the past two decades. At least two motives affect the way people cope with serious accidents, injuries, or illness. The first, described in the work of Lerner, suggests that people need to maintain their belief in a just world (Lerner & Matthews, 1967; Lerner & Simmons, 1966). That is, people get what they deserve and deserve what they get. Misfortune cannot be just random. Therefore, if something bad happens, the victim must have done something to deserve it.

The second motive, described in the work of Elaine Walster, concerns the perception of control over the environment. Walster (1966) suggests that most people attribute blame to a victim to reassure themselves that they will not be likely to suffer the same misfortune. The basis of the reasoning is, again, that if the event is unpredictable or uncontrollable, it could happen to anyone, including themselves, at any time. Therefore, the victim must have had something to do with the accident.

Whether an individual *personally accepts blame* for a misfortune depends on the person's perception of control. If the victim perceives that he or she had control over circumstances leading up to an incident, they are more likely to engage in *behavioral self-blame* (Janoff-Bulman, 1988). This usually allows the victim to retain credible belief in the utility of preventive behaviors. *Characterological self-blame* occurs when the victim believes some enduring trait contributed to the incident. This usually involves self-esteem deficits and consequent depression. Bulman and Wortman (1977) also observed cognitive reappraisal. Some people evaluate the outcome as desirable. They may believe that "God is testing me," or "It really is a blessing in disguise," or "I know I will grow a lot because of this."

Attributing personal blame adds a significant load to the coping process and may interfere with recovery from life-threatening assaults and illness. Denial of blame may be a necessary short-term defense after a traumatic event. Continued denial, on the other hand, may interfere with assessment and implementation of adaptive changes in the lifestyle that contributed to the risk in the first place. Denial may also impair the healthy sense of caution needed to live safely and securely.

Beliefs about Personal Vulnerability

Beliefs we hold about crime are also important. Beliefs are predispositions to act in certain ways based on positive and negative evaluations of people, places, and things. One belief system, beliefs about vulnerability, is paramount in this regard. Beliefs about vulnerability may change behavior in one of two ways. First, belief in continuous vulnerability may heighten fear and thus become disabling. Taken to the extreme, it approaches a paranoid-like state that may produce undesirable side effects, such as depression and disorientation, while placing unnecessary limits on personal freedom. On the other hand, people who believe that they are invincible tend to take unnecessary risks. Such people are likely to scorn suggestions to assess their lifestyle and to ignore most of the preventive actions suggested earlier. Beliefs, then, can increase or decrease the likelihood of engaging in suitable preventive behaviors. They can help or hinder coping efforts in the aftermath of crime.

COPING WITH THE AFTERMATH OF CRIMINAL ASSAULT

As noted earlier, the effects of a criminal attack can be revealed in several physical and psychological disturbances (American Psychiatric Association, 1987). Sleep disorders, anxiety attacks, and changes in appetite may all occur (Silver &

Wortman, 1980). Compulsive lock checking, becoming housebound, and experiencing feelings of extreme terror may go on for weeks or months.[7] John Hepburn and Daniel Monti (1979) studied adaptive responses among a population of high school victims. They found that fear of crime was the most significant variable explaining why the subjects avoided groups and social places.

Reconstructing Assumptive Worlds

Another significant change occurs in the aftermath of traumatic events. Schemata constructed through experience are damaged, if not destroyed (Janoff-Bulman, 1988). Victims lose their sense of control and invulnerability. They feel their world is no longer safe and benevolent. The most important assault, the most hurtful injury, is to their schema of self-worth and self-acceptance. As Janoff-Bulman (1988) notes,

> the key to the victim's recovery process is the reestablishment of an integrated, organized set of basic assumptions or schemas. The traumatic event must be assimilated into the victim's assumptive world, or the assumptive world must accommodate to the new data. . . . (p. 107)

Managing Fear from Victimization

The most powerful emotion victims feel is fear. Fear is a complex response that includes thoughts, feelings, and bodily reactions. It generalizes to encompass people who look similar to the offender and places that remind the victim of the original situation. Eliminating fear thus requires methods that will deal with these three channels of involvement and that can help the victim deal with generalized fears.

The most successful method for treating specific fears over the past few years has been systematic desensitization, which will be discussed in detail in Chapter 12. Another technique that may help combat fear is rational-emotive therapy (RET). Rational-emotive therapy assumes that irrational thoughts bolster the fear and underlie self-limiting behavior. As practiced by Ellis (1962), the therapist attempts to point out the link between the person's emotions and thought processes. The goal is to replace irrational constructs, which stand in the way of healthy behavior, with rational assessments.

Another technique is stress inoculation, a multimodal method that combines several specific techniques. Stress inoculation attempts to get the individual to deal with small fears one at a time. A program can be structured so that success in dealing with little fears is almost a sure thing. As successes build, the person builds resistance so that larger fears do not seem as overwhelming as

---

[7]Studies of victims reveal that the mental maelstrom following a personal assault or loss may last up to 3 years. Severity of the crime and personal characteristics of the victim influence duration.

before. As the process continues, larger fears become more manageable until the person can deal successfully with the normal range of activities and people. This technique will be discussed in more detail in Chapter 12.

One behavioral manifestation of fear is avoidance of people, places, and things that remind the victim of the original event. This is anticipatory fear. Any behavior that leads to fear reduction is more likely to be repeated. Thus, avoidance behaviors are likely to increase after the assault. This is generally unnecessary, but it constitutes a restriction on personal freedom that needs to be considered. Positive assertion to gradually increase the frequency and range of encounters with people and social situations is one approach that can be used.

Active Mastery: Keys to Coping with Victimization

In the preceding sections, we reviewed positive steps to reduce stress and develop active coping skills. These steps were lifestyle assessment based on knowledge of personal and environmental risks; inspection of cognitive misattributions; evaluation of potentially misleading beliefs; and coping with fear. In addition, we may consider environmental design (or lack thereof, such as poor street lighting) that contributes to increased risk. Another strategy is to seek restitution through a state victim assistance program. Finally, many local organizations provide educational and counseling programs that speed recovery and help reduce future risks. It appears that people who ignore or avoid such assistance may continue to be at risk compared with those who use these services. For example, one group of victims decided not to participate in a prevention education–counseling program. Three years later, this same group had burglary rates almost three times greater than normal (Schneider & Schneider, 1981).

SUMMARY

In this chapter, we have traced briefly the concern for social stress and social stability in early research and theory. This work identified several primary conditions (such as poverty, overcrowding, and unemployment) thought to be the origins of frustration and stress in modern society. We also examined the idea that social stress is linked to both mental and physical illness. The most important source of stress is social change.

Change confronts us with many personal and social dilemmas. We must cope with new decisions, technologies, jobs, environments, and lifestyles. Many of these changes are not under our personal control and they confront us with a range of value conflicts that present difficulty, especially for the unprepared. Preparation through self-education, stress inoculation, and value clarification may be the best way to deal with social change.

A major source of stress in urban areas is victimization. We discussed identification of risk factors, prevention of risk, and use of coping strategies to deal with the aftermath of crime. Information on risk factors shows that the young, unmarried, and unemployed male has the highest risk, although the impact of victimization is probably most keenly felt by women and the aged.

Prevention involves lifestyle assessment to identify habitual behaviors that may place the person at risk. Both misattributions and faulty beliefs tend to prevent effective coping behaviors. We reviewed guidelines to help examine problematic causal attributions and beliefs.

Finally, we suggested coping strategies that may be appropriate for dealing with fear. Fear can be reduced through desensitization and rational-emotive therapy. Stress inoculation may be used to reduce the potential for overwhelming stress. Positive assertion and social action are also helpful in removing the restrictive effects of fear. The key idea is to obtain active mastery of one's environment through personal and social actions designed to reduce risk.

KEY TERMS

anomie
criminologist
demoralization
Dodge-Martin theory
fear-of-crime
   syndrome
life-change and
   illness

Life Change Unit
   (LCU)
lifestyle
posttraumatic stress
   syndrome
preventing
   victimization
risk of victimization

self-blame
social readjustment
Social Readjustment
   Rating Scale (SRRS)
stress inoculation
victimologists
vulnerability

REFERENCES

American Psychiatric Association. (1987). *Diagnostic and statistical manual of mental disorders* (3rd ed., rev.). Washington, DC: Author.

Berg, W. E., & Johnson, R. (1979). Assessing the impact of victimization: Acquisition of the victim role among elderly and female victims. In W. H. Parsonage (Ed.), *Perspectives on victimology* (pp. 58–71). Newbury Park, CA: Sage.

Berkow, I. (1984, November 25). The shooting of Ben Wilson. *The New York Times*, p. S-7.

Brenner, M. H. (1973). *Mental illness and the economy.* Cambridge, MA: Harvard University Press.

Brett, J. F., Brief, A. P., Burke, M. J., George, J. M., & Webster, J. (1990). Negative affectivity and the reporting of stressful life events. *Health Psychology, 9,* 57–68.

Brooks, J. (1981). The fear of crime in the United States. In B. Galaway & J. Hudson (Eds.), *Perspectives on crime victims* (pp. 90–92). St. Louis, MO: C.V. Mosby.

Bulman, R. J., & Wortman, C. B. (1977). Attribution of blame and coping in the "real world": Severe accident victims react to their lot. *Journal of Personality and Social Psychology, 35,* 351–363.

Burgess, A. W. (1983). Rape trauma syndrome. *Behavioral Sciences and the Law, 1,* 97–113.

Cohen, S., & Wills, T. A. (1985). Stress, social support, and the buffering hypothesis. *Psychological Bulletin, 98,* 310–357.

Dodge, D. L., & Martin, W. T. (1970). *Social stress and chronic illness.* Notre Dame, IN: University of Notre Dame Press.

Dohrenwend, B. S., & Dohrenwend, B. P. (1982). Some issues in research on stressful life events. In T. Millon, C. Green, & R. Meagher (Eds.), *Handbook of clinical health psychology* (pp. 91–102). New York: Plenum.

Dooley, D., & Catalano, R. (1984). The epidemiology of economic stress. *American Journal of Community Psychology, 12,* 387–409.

Durkheim, E. (1951). *Suicide: A study in sociology.* New York: Free Press.

Ellis, A. (1962). *Reason and emotion in psychotherapy.* New York: Stuart.

Faris, R., & Dunham, H. W. (1939). *Mental disorders in urban areas.* Chicago: University of Chicago Press.

Federal Bureau of Investigation. (1990). *Uniform crime reports for the United States.* Federal Bureau of Investigation, U.S. Department of Justice. Washington, DC: U.S. Government Printing Office.

Fields, R. (1980). Victims of terrorism: The effects of prolonged stress. *Evaluation and Change, 8,* 76–83.

Flanagan, T. J., & Maguire, K. (Eds.). (1990). *Sourcebook of criminal justice statistics— 1989.* U.S. Department of Justice, Bureau of Justice Statistics. Washington, DC: U.S. Government Printing Office.

Frank, J. D. (1973). *Persuasion and healing.* Baltimore, MD: Johns Hopkins University Press.

Freiberg, P. (1990, Nov.). APA testifies: Rape estimates far too low. *APA Monitor, 21,* p. 25.

Galaway, B., & Hudson, J. (Eds.). (1981). *Perspectives on crime victims.* St. Louis, MO: C.V. Mosby.

Gentry, W. D., Foster, S., & Harvey, T. (1972). Denial as a determinant of anxiety and perceived health status in the coronary care unit. *Psychosomatic Medicine, 34,* 39–44.

Hepburn, J. R., & Monti, D. J. (1979). Victimization, fear of crime, and adaptive responses among high school students. In W. H. Parsonage, *Perspectives on victimology* (pp. 121–132). Newbury Park, CA: Sage.

Hindelang, M. J., Gottfredson, M. R., & Garofalo, J. (1978). *Victims of personal crime: An empirical foundation for a theory of personal victimization.* Cambridge, MA: Ballinger.

Hinkle, L. E. (1974). The effect of exposure to culture change, social change, and changes in interpersonal relationships on health. In B. S. Dohrenwend & B. P. Dohrenwend (Eds.), *Stressful life events: Their nature and effect* (pp. 9–44). New York: Wiley.

Hollingshead, A. B., & Redlich, F. C. (1958). *Social class and mental illness: A community study.* New York: Wiley.

Holmes, T. H., & Masuda, M. (1974). Life change and illness susceptibility. In B. S. Dohrenwend & B. P. Dohrenwend (Eds.), *Stressful life events: Their nature and effect* (pp. 45–72). New York: Wiley.

Holmes, T. H., & Rahe, R. H. (1967). The social readjustment rating scale. *Psychosomatic Medicine, 11,* 213–218.

Institute of Medicine (United States). (1979). *Healthy people: The Surgeon General's report on health promotion and disease prevention.* (Government Document No. HE20.2:H34/5). Rockville, MD: U.S. Government Printing Office.

Janoff-Bulman, R. (1988). Victims of violence. In S. Fisher & J. Reason (Eds.), *Handbook of life stress, cognition and health* (pp. 101–113). New York: Wiley.

Kagan, A. (1974). Psychosocial factors in disease: Hypotheses and future research. In E. K. E. Gunderson & R. H. Rahe (Eds.), *Life stress and illness* (pp. 41–57). Springfield, IL: Charles C Thomas.

Kobasa, S. C. (1979). Personality and resistance to illness. *American Journal of Community Psychology, 7,* 413–423.

Krantz, D. S., & Raisen, S. E. (1988). Environmental stress, reactivity and ischaemic heart disease. *British Journal of Medical Psychology, 61,* 3–16.

Lazarus, R. S. (1966). *Psychological stress and the coping process.* New York: McGraw-Hill.

Leavy, R. L. (1983). Social support and psychological disorder: A review. *Journal of Community Psychology, 11,* 3–21.

Lerner, M. J., & Matthews, G. (1967). Reactions to suffering of others under conditions of indirect responsibility. *Journal of Personality and Social Psychology, 5,* 319–325.

Lerner, M. J., & Simmons, C. (1966). Observer's reaction to the "innocent victim": Compassion or rejection? *Journal of Personality and Social Psychology, 4,* 203–210.

Martin, B. (1981). *A sociology of contemporary cultural change.* New York: St. Martin's Press.

Meichenbaum, D., & Jaremko, M. E. (1983). *Stress reduction and prevention.* New York: Plenum.

Meyer, P. B. (1981). Communities as victims of corporate crimes. In B. Galaway & J. Hudson (Eds.), *Perspectives on crime victims* (pp. 33–44). St. Louis, MO: C.V. Mosby.

Naisbitt, J. (1982). *Megatrends: Ten new directions transforming our lives.* New York: Warner Books.

Nelson, P. D. (1974). Comment. In E. K. E. Gunderson & R. H. Rahe (Eds.), *Life stress and illness* (pp. 79–89). Springfield, IL: Charles C Thomas.

Nisbet, R. A. (1970). *The social bond.* New York: Knopf.

Ochberg, F. (1978). The victim of terrorism: Psychiatric considerations. *TERRORISM: An International Journal, 1,* 147–167.

Peters, M. F., & Massey, G. (1983). Mundane extreme environmental stress in family stress theories: The case of black families in white America. In H. I. McCubbin, M. B. Sussman, & J. M. Patterson (Eds.), *Social stress and the family* (pp. 193–218). New York: Haworth Press.

Rabkin, J. G., & Struening, E. L. (1976a). Life events, stress, and illness. *Science, 194,* 1013–1020.

Rabkin, J. G., & Struening, E. L. (1976b). Social change, stress, and illness: A selective literature review. *Psychoanalysis and Contemporary Science, 5,* 573–624.

Rahe, R. (1974). Life change and subsequent illness reports. In E. K. E. Gunderson & R. Rahe (Eds.), *Life stress and illness* (pp. 58–78). Springfield, IL: Charles C Thomas.

Rahe, R. H., & Arthur, R. J. (1978). Life change and illness studies: Past history and future directions. *Journal of Human Stress, 4,* 3–15.

Rubin, R. T. (1974). Biochemical and neuroendocrine responses to severe psychological stress. In E. K. E. Gunderson & R. H. Rahe (Eds.), *Life stress and illness* (pp. 227–241). Springfield, IL: Charles C Thomas.

Sarason, I. G., Levine, H. M., & Sarason, B. R. (1982). Assessing the impact of life changes. In T. Millon, C. Green, & R. Meagher (Eds.), *Handbook of clinical health psychology* (pp. 377–400). New York: Plenum.

Schafer, S. (1977). *Victimology: The victim and his criminal.* Reston, VA: Reston.

Schneider, A. L., & Schneider, P. R. (1981). Victim assistance programs: An overview. In B. Galaway & J. Hudson (Eds.), *Perspectives on crime victims* (pp. 364–373). St. Louis, MO: C.V. Mosby.

Schroeder, D. H., & Costa, P. T. (1984, May). *Do stressful life events influence objectively-measured health? A prospective evaluation.* Paper presented at the Midwestern Psychological Association Annual Conference, Chicago.

Silver, R. L., & Wortman, C. B. (1980). Coping with undesirable life events. In J. Garber & M. E. P. Seligman (Eds.), *Human helplessness* (pp. 279–375). New York: Academic Press.

Srole, L., Langner, T. S., Michael, S. T., Opler, M. K., & Rennie, T. A. C. (1962). *Mental health in the metropolis*. New York: McGraw-Hill.

Steele, C. M., & Josephs, R. A. (1990). Alcohol myopia: Its prized and dangerous effects. *American Psychologist, 45,* 921–933.

Toffler, A. (1970). *Future shock*. New York: Bantam Books.

Toffler, A. (1980). *The third wave*. New York: Bantam Books.

Turnage, J. J. (1990). The challenge of new workplace technology for psychology. *American Psychologist, 45,* 171–178.

Walster, E. (1966). Assignment of responsibility for an accident. *Journal of Personality and Social Psychology, 3,* 73–79.

Werner, E. E. (1984). Resilient children. *Young Children, 40,* 68–72.

Wills, T. A., & Langner, T. S. (1980). Socioeconomic status and stress. In I. L. Kutash, L. B. Schlesinger, and Associates (Eds.), *Handbook on stress and anxiety* (pp. 159–173). San Francisco: Jossey-Bass.

Zautra, A., & Sandler, I. (1983). Life event needs assessments: Two models for measuring preventable mental health problems. *Prevention in Human Services, 2,* 35–58.

CHAPTER 9

Environmental Stress: Disasters, Pollution, and Overcrowding

MAN'S ATTITUDE TOWARD NATURE IS TODAY CRITICALLY IMPORTANT SIMPLY BECAUSE WE HAVE NOW ACQUIRED A FATEFUL POWER TO ALTER AND DESTROY NATURE.
RACHEL CARSON

The night of December 2, 1984, was much like any other night in Bhopal, India. Before the dawn would break, though, a nightmare would leave over 2500 of Bhopal's citizens dead and as many as 250,000 more scarred, blinded, disfigured, or disabled permanently. A combination of technical problems, mechanical failures, and human error led to the leakage of deadly methyl isocyanate fumes from the Union Carbide plant in Bhopal. Until that night, the plant had offered the hope of improved agricultural productivity to help feed India's 700 million people.

Natural catastrophes and technological disasters produce intense suffering for living victims, survivors who must rebuild shattered lives and reconstruct dreams around a new reality. Less intense, though no less real, is the stress endured by the worried well. They wait and wonder when and where the next disaster will occur. Schemata that once were organized around the notion of a safe, supportive habitat may be reorganized around imminent danger and the awesome power of natural or technological forces. The more ruinous outcome, then, may be the effect such disasters have on perceptions.

In recent years, we have identified several stressors that occur because humans have altered, exploited, or dumped on their environment. It is small consolation that alterations of the environment were designed to benefit humankind. The truth is that human tinkering often brings disaster and destruction instead of safety and support. We now combat air and noise pollution in crowded urban areas. Chemical wastes dumped into streams and on once-virgin soil endanger the earth's species. Toxins created to control pests infiltrate the food chain.

The study of environmental stress deals with natural, technological, and social disasters. The results of this study should provide answers to pressing questions. What differences in individual perceptions and thoughts turn disaster into defeat for one but challenge for another? What environment-behavior interactions are most likely to increase physical illness, emotional distress, and mental disturbance? What promising applications emerge from the study of environmental stress? Can we learn how to design self-control procedures so people will

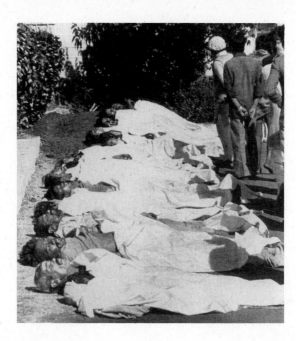

Bhopal, India, viewing the bodies of victims of a lethal gas that seeped into the city
SOURCE: UPI/Bettmann Newsphotos.

be less wasteful of natural resources? Can we discover ways to intervene in the environment without disrupting habitats and destroying nature's balance? Answers to these questions could reduce both strain on the environment and the psychological impact of environmental stressors.

The purpose of this chapter, then, is to provide a perspective on environmental stress by focusing on the most commonly encountered environmental stressors. Along the way, prominent theories of environmental stress will be presented. To begin, a few definitions are in order.

ENVIRONMENT AND ECOLOGY

Some terms commonly encountered in environmental stress literature are **environment, habitat,** and **ecology.** Environment refers to surroundings, the physical space that we perceive and in which we behave. Habitat is where a particular animal resides. The natural habitat for a trout is the lake; for deer, the forest. Humans are gregarious creatures. We are fond of living together, sharing companionship and trading services. The town is our natural habitat. Still, humans are endlessly adaptable. We can survive over a much wider range of climates and conditions than any other animal (Moran, 1981). Thus the notion of habitat may be less useful in the study of human-environment relations than in that of animal-environment relations.

The term *ecology* refers to a distinct branch of biology that studies relationships between living organisms and their environment. The relationship between an organism and the environment is reciprocal, an exchange that goes on over several cycles. For example, at one time hunters in the Southwest received bounties for killing pests. As a result, coyotes and wildcats became rare in and around the Kaibab forest of Arizona. This produced a rapid increase in the deer population. Deer overgrazed the land, which destroyed ground cover and increased erosion. Tragically, thousands of deer died for lack of food.

Mounting concern for ecology may be due in part to our harmful environmental manipulations. We are not content to build shelters to protect us from the elements; we believe we can and should harness and control the elements as well. To exercise control, we seed clouds, drill wells, drain swamps, build dams, design earthquake-proof buildings, and harness nuclear energy. As we change the environment, though, we change relationships between animals, humans, and their environmental niches. Some of these changes are beneficial, but some are not. Examples of injurious influences on the ecology of an area are abundant. The Aswan Dam—built to control floods along the Nile and provide hydroelectric power—had a devastating effect on fish and fishing all along the river's course. The same thing happened with other dams, including the Tennessee Valley Authority project. Acid rain, extinction of several species caused by civilization's encroachments on natural habitats, and pollution of Love Canal furnish other examples. Viewed in this light, disturbing the ecological balance can produce powerful sources of stress for many organisms.

THEORIES OF ENVIRONMENTAL STRESS

Numerous theories seek to explain environmental stress. These include **arousal theories,** learning theory, **behavior constraint theory, ecological theory,** and **environmental stress theory.** As will become apparent, environmental stress theory integrates Hans Selye's general adaptation syndrome theory and Richard Lazarus's cognitive-transactional theory. These theories are summarized in Table 9-1.

Arousal and Stimulation Theories of Stress

One way to view the relationship between the environment and human behavior is in terms of the amount of stimulation the environment provides. These arousal theories are more simplistic and restrictive than other environmental stress theories. Still, some support exists for the notion that stress varies with level of arousal. Albert Mehrabian and James Russell (1974) tried to identify the dimensions that best describe *any* environment. They found this could be done with just three dimensions: pleasure, dominance, and arousal.

The major idea common to arousal theories is that different degrees of stimulation produce varying degrees of arousal. Very intense stimulation, such as a rock band rehearsing in the upstairs apartment, probably will lead to too much arousal and feelings of distress. On the other hand, very low levels of stimulation, such as stimulus deprivation, can result in too little arousal and feelings of boredom. This is a **stimulus load theory.**

Cohen (1978) proposed an overload theory. This model assumes that stimulation is a type of information, and human behavior is the outcome of information processing. When too much information bombards a person, overload occurs. Attention is divided as we try to carry out two or more cognitive tasks at the same time, and strain results. When too little information exists, the person may not be able to make wise, appropriate decisions.

Another stimulation approach is Wohlwill's (1974) **adaptation level theory.** Wohlwill assumed that each person has a preferred and optimal level of stimulation. This optimal level varies between people; some people prefer more stimulation than others. Optimal levels also vary within people over time; we prefer more stimulation at some times than at others. Finally, the current level of preferred stimulation is a result of adaptation; we adjust the value we place on stimulation because of continued exposure. Whether something is understimulating or overstimulating depends on the current level of adaptation. For example, after spending an intense day at an amusement park, you might consider a comedy movie boring. Conversely, after being confined in a hospital for an extended time, you might think that same movie very entertaining.

Conditioning and Environmental Stress

Learning models have been widely used to explain adaptive behaviors, including adaptation to the effects of stress. Byrne and Clore (1970) extended the classical conditioning model to environmental stress. Their **classical conditioning theory** includes a role for the conditioning of attitudes, something that was not part of the original theory. Specifically, Byrne and Clore propose that attitudes are conditioned to distinctive environmental stimuli and carry positive and negative valences. Attitudes are predispositions to act in certain ways. When an attitude is associated with an event, the recurrence of the event may evoke a stress reaction through the associated attitude.

For example, a child goes to a doctor's office and receives a painful injection. The office and other related stimuli (doctors, nurses, uniforms, odors) become signals for pain. Later, when the child expects to return to the office, a strong negative emotional response occurs. Based on this emotional response, a negative attitude forms: "I don't like that place."

In the Byrne and Clore model, pain from the injection is an unconditional stimulus, while fear and avoidance are part of the unconditional response. The office is the conditional stimulus, which was neutral before the injection. Afterward, it takes on the power of the unconditional stimulus and produces fear and avoidance, the conditional or learned response. Fear and avoidance may occur even when the doctor's office is only symbolically represented in conversation. Figure 9-1 shows the relationships suggested by Byrne and Clore with added examples.

TABLE 9-1
Comparison of Key Features of Environmental Stress Models

Stress model	Definition of stress	Source(s) of stress	Model's strengths	Model's weaknesses
Arousal theories	No specific definitions provided but suggests stress is negative reaction to variations in stimulation	Overarousal Underarousal Mismatch between preferred arousal and current level of stimulation	Main constructs are easy to grasp Seems easy to operationalize and test empirically	Extremely simplistic view of stress Places major emphasis on stimulaion Ignores biological factors Largely ignores cognitive-appraisal factors Little extensive or intensive testing to verify theories
Conditioning theory	Faulty conditioning arousing negative attitudes and/or conditional emotional response	Presence of any conditional stimuli that evoke negative attitudes or emotions	Empirically based Clear operational definitions for basic terms and procedures Extends classical model to arena of cognitions	Mostly indirect testing rather than direct testing Limited in scope Does not provide integrated view of biological or social variables

Theory	Definition	Focus	Strengths	Weaknesses
Behavior constraint model	No specific definition provided	Real or perceived limits on behavior	Incorporates three well-defined and tested constructs in coherent theory Empirically based	Indirect evidence rather than direct tests Limited in scope Seldom used
Ecological theory	No specific definition provided	Behavior settings or factors such as undermanning	Incorporates social/normative notions of relations between settings and behavior Has led to variety of applications for environmental design	Limited in scope Little or no consideration of biological factors Little interest in individual or cognitive variables Difficult to test
Environmental stress theory	Combination of the biological and cognitive models of Selye and Lazarus	Real or perceived psychosocial pressures	Incompasses a broad range of variables from biological to psychological and social	An eclectic approach to theory, taking the best of current theories Not directly tested but logically synthesized

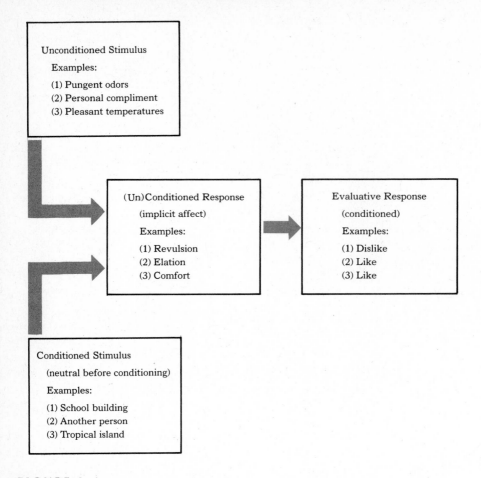

FIGURE 9-1
The Byrne-Clore Reinforcement-Affect Model, a conditioning model of environmental perceptions
SOURCE: Byrne and Clore (1970).

The Behavior Constraint Model

On occasion, the environment can produce effects over which we have little or no control. Severe storms, hurricanes, and blizzards are forces that usually require a "ride it out" response. We may minimize the likelihood of personal damage by taking certain precautions, but no effort will alter or stop the forces in motion.

Work situations may take on similar uncontrollable features. Job security for many workers depends on their company's ability to compete in a volatile market. Over the past few years, the computer industry has provided numerous examples of uncontrollable situations. Some companies offered excellent, even superior, products. Still, the companies folded either because they lacked market clout or advertising budgets or because they were competing against "name" companies. For the employees, it made no difference how hard they worked or controlled quality.

Under such conditions, behavior is constrained, or limited. We cannot do all the things we would like to do. We may feel we cannot control our destiny. However, according to the behavior constraint model, the limits imposed on behavior need not be real limits; they can be imaginary as well. If we merely *believe* the situation is out of control, our behavior will be as limited as if we really do lack control. Several authors have discussed environmental stress in these terms.

The work of Judith Rodin and Andrew Baum (1978) provides a noteworthy example. According to their analysis, three steps lead to behavior constraint: perceived loss of control, as described in the preceding paragraph; psychological reactance; and a feeling of learned helplessness.

Brehm and Brehm (1981) used the notion of *reactance* to explain some consumer behaviors. As an example, a salesperson comes to your door with a product you need and the product is a good one. But the salesperson makes you feel manipulated, or "sold." According to reactance theory, people do not like feeling out of control, so they take steps to regain control. You might even refuse to purchase the product solely to avoid being manipulated; this is reactance.

When people try to regain control but repeatedly fail to do so, they may develop learned helplessness (Seligman, 1975). Learned helplessness is a condition in which the person could exert control but does not because of previous failures. In emergency situations, such as natural and technological disasters, people may give up because they feel there is nothing they can do. While the behavior constraint model contains some interesting elements, it is seldom used in environmental psychology.

Behavior Settings and Ecological Psychology

Roger Barker (1968) advocated an ecological view of environmental stress. The key concept in his theory was **behavior settings.** A behavior setting is a culturally determined physical milieu that calls for certain fixed patterns of behavior. These include group behaviors as well as individual behaviors. For example, a church is a behavior setting that has several predictable behavior patterns. Classrooms and restaurants are other examples, as are business and faculty meetings. Knowing the setting enables one to predict with some certainty what behavior should occur. Change the setting, and the behavior also changes.

Related ideas in Barker's theory include undermanning and overmanning. For example, amusement parks can be "overmanned" when large crowds exceed the park's capacity. In such circumstances, people may feel frustrated and stressed. In large universities and large classes, students may feel left out, uninvolved, and anonymous. On the other hand, in smaller universities and smaller classrooms, students may feel involved and worthwhile. Barker's model has proven useful in studying stress in business, mental institutions, schools, and churches. It has also been helpful in suggesting ways to engineer the environment to eliminate or reduce stressors.

Environmental Stress Theory

Environmental stress theory combines the best of both Hans Selye's general adaptation syndrome and Richard Lazarus's cognitive-transactional theory. Andrew Baum's research group analyzed environmental stressors, such as the Three Mile Island incident, in terms of these two theories (Baum, 1990; Baum, Singer, & Baum, 1981). They concluded that the cognitive processes suggested by Lazarus and the physiological arousal proposed by Selye occur consistently in several environmental stress situations, including catastrophic events, noise, and crowding. This suggests that a specialized theory of environmental stress does not add much explanatory power, if any, to that provided by these two well-known, well-researched models. Figure 9-2 shows the two theories in integrated form (Fisher, Bell, & Baum, 1984).

CATEGORIES OF ENVIRONMENTAL STRESS

Work on environmental stress has focused on several major stressors. There is, first, the short-term catastrophic disaster, which affects few people. Its effect on the environment and people is usually severe, but such events tend to happen infrequently. Natural, technological, and social disasters[1] fit this category. Second, ongoing, chronic stressors affect many more people daily but in less severe ways. Their effects may not appear for years. Fisher and his colleagues labeled these **background stressors** (Fisher et al., 1984), whereas Holahan (1986) labeled them **ambient stressors. Noise pollution, air pollution,** chemical pollution, **crowding,** and commuting are examples of this type of environmental stress. The remainder of this chapter focuses on the most important environmental stressors.

NATURAL DISASTERS

For those people unfortunate enough to be in harm's way, natural disasters threaten physical destruction, psychological trauma, and family disorganization on a scale not encountered with most other stressors. Hurricanes and tornadoes, floods and blizzards, volcanic eruptions and earthquakes are among the most catastrophic natural disasters. For some, the immediate impact may be no more

---

[1]The term *social disaster* is my own. It refers to those events that do not readily fit the natural and technological categories but nonetheless share the elements of unpredictability and lack of control and produce a powerful impact on people's lives. The 1984 McDonald's massacre and the Jonestown suicides belong in this category.

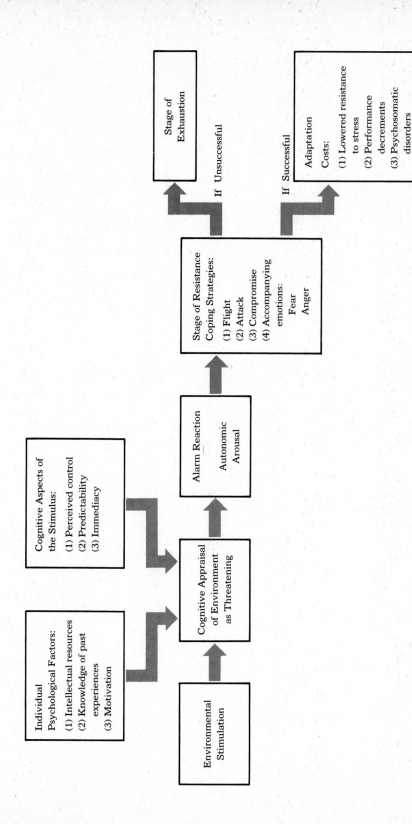

FIGURE 9-2

The environmental stress model proposed by Fisher, Bell, and Baum

SOURCE: Fisher, Bell, and Baum (1984).

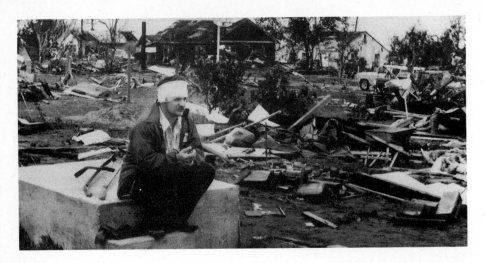

Destruction and despair in the wake of tornadoes at Sweetwater, Texas, April 20, 1986
SOURCE: AP/Wide World Photo.

than a fleeting panic. Later, when the family finds that its members are unharmed, the response is probably relief and joy coupled with renewed respect for nature's fury.

At the other extreme is the wholesale disruption of lifestyle. In such cases, a comfortable existence is temporarily replaced by discomfort, severe deprivation, and physical fatigue. Lengthy periods of cleanup, recovering personal effects from the devastation where possible, rebuilding, caring for sick or injured family members, and arranging for the burial of deceased family members are some of the activities that consume enormous amounts of physical and psychological energy. States of anxiety may overwhelm victims who perceive an uncertain future. Fear of a recurrence of the dread event may erode decision-making ability and interfere with appropriate problem-solving behavior. Television replay of scenes from Mexico City and Armenia following devastating earthquakes vividly illustrated some of these reactions.

Natural disasters share several common characteristics. They are mostly unpredictable. Consider, for example, nature's lottery, the tornado. No matter how sophisticated modern weather reporting may be, warning of an approaching tornado is all that can be done. Where and when a tornado will touch down is anyone's guess. Natural disasters are also largely uncontrollable. Consequently, people may feel they are temporarily at the mercy of forces much more powerful than anything they could have imagined. Finally, natural catastrophes require short-term and long-term coping responses from both victims and the community.

Studies of natural disasters have noted a typical pattern of responding, which seems to occur in three stages. There is first a *shock stage* in which victims appear to be stunned, dazed, and apathetic. Second, a *suggestible stage* occurs in which victims tend to be passive, suggestible, and willing to take directions from others. Finally, in the *recovery stage,* individuals are tense and apprehensive. They often show a frequent need to recount details of the catastrophic event at this time (Coleman, Butcher, & Carson, 1980).

Effects of Natural Disasters

Many psychological and physical symptoms appear after a natural calamity. Psychological symptoms include initial panic, anxiety, phobic fear, vulnerability, guilt, isolation, withdrawal, depression (including some suicide attempts), anger and frustration, as well as interpersonal and marital problems (McLeod, 1984). Disorientation, lack of attachment, and loss of a sense of security may occur for a time. Sleep and eating disturbances are common. Some people report that they continuously relive the agony in their dreams, as though they cannot escape from the horror. The severity and duration of these effects seem to depend on the magnitude of the loss.

These psychological symptoms can be described as posttraumatic stress disorder (PTSD), a syndrome discussed previously. While most clinicians accept PTSD as a reliable description, McFarlane (1988) warns against its uncritical acceptance. He points to the lack of research supporting the contention that different types of traumatic events produce the same outcome. McFarlane studied a group of Australian fire fighters who fought a disastrous bush fire. Core signs of PTSD, intrusive thoughts and recurrent intense images, appeared in one group not diagnosed with PTSD. In spite of the cognitive disruption, they showed no significant long-term disability. Further, survival guilt and detachment were not observed. McFarlane observed the opposite, namely that many fire fighters became more socially involved following the disaster. Finally, a comparison of fire fighters diagnosed with PTSD with fire fighters without PTSD showed little difference in morbidity. McFarlane questioned whether these core symptoms are sufficiently specific to be helpful diagnostic criteria.

Physical symptoms following a natural disaster include increased fatigue, headaches, colds and other illnesses, and weight loss from both sleep and eating disturbances. The amount of physical illness, though, is much less than what might be expected. One possible explanation for this is that the short-term, acute nature of disaster stress triggers the body's natural self-defense mechanisms. Because the stress is over quickly, lowered resistance and exhaustion do not occur (Baum, 1990). This is also consistent with the observation that the severity and duration of both psychological and physical effects depend on the significance of the loss produced by the disaster.

The symptoms reported here appear to be nearly universal. The Sri Lanka cyclone of 1978, for example, provides one well-documented, confirming case study (Patrick & Patrick, 1981).

THE AFTERMATH OF MOUNT SAINT HELENS

One of the most widely publicized natural disasters of the recent past was the eruption of Mount Saint Helens on May 18, 1980. The 9600-foot mountain, located in the southwestern part of the state of Washington, exploded with a force that lifted a cubic mile of debris from its peak.[2] The force of the eruption hurled ash as high as 50,000 feet into the atmosphere and covered several thousand square miles with volcanic ash. Nearly 300 people were working, camping, or sightseeing near the volcano. More than 200 escaped or were rescued, although 2 of these died later. Another 60 persons died or disappeared and are presumed dead (Murphy, 1984).

Shortly after the eruption, a team of investigators collected data from cities and towns in the impact area (Pennebaker & Newtson, 1983). What they found confirmed earlier findings. The data showed a pattern of initial short-term panic with little or no long-term effect. Within the first 24 hours, outgoing telephone calls ran a full 100% above normal levels, jamming phone lines in the process. This level of activity subsided quickly, however.

Both physical symptoms and negative emotional moods occurred at a higher rate than in a normal population, but the frequency of symptoms varied with both proximity and temporal factors. People living in a dangerous area while trying to deal with the day-to-day necessities of living reported *fewer* physical and emotional symptoms. They were also less willing to provide information to interviewers, which suggests that their anxiety levels were still high. The investigators concluded that these people had not allowed themselves time to work through their feelings about the disaster. As time went on, people in the dangerous areas became more willing to talk. Most residents showed few effects of the eruption in a follow-up survey about a year later.

Shirley Murphy (1984) studied victims of the Mount Saint Helens eruption to assess how quickly and completely people recover from the effects of a natural catastrophe. Dr. Murphy classified victims into four categories. One group consisted of victims who had suffered the *presumed* loss of a relative or close friend. The second group had suffered the *confirmed* loss of a relative or close friend. The third and fourth groups had lost, respectively, permanent or vacation homes. A fifth group, which served as a control group, suffered no loss at all.

Dr. Murphy found that bereaved victims reported higher levels of emotional stress and poorer mental health status compared with other victims. But they did not seem to suffer any poorer physical health than the group that had experienced no loss. Those who had relatives or friends *presumed* dead appeared to show the most distress when interviewed. They talked about how "waiting was agony," how they went on "hoping, yet knowing they were dead," and that "it's hard to come to terms with no body" (Murphy, 1984, p. 212). People who lost permanent homes reported levels of stress similar to those of the bereaved group, but they reported no greater physical or emotional difficulties than the control group. These people also experienced greater amounts of anger, blame,

---

[2]To appreciate the volume of a cubic mile of earth, consider this. A cubic mile of earth is equal to 5.5 billion cubic yards. Most standard gravel trucks carry approximately 14 cubic yards of dirt. If you could line up enough trucks to haul away all the debris from Mount Saint Helens, it would take a string of 390,741,623 trucks. If you could fill one truck every ten minutes working 24 hours a day, it would take 7434 years to do what Mount Saint Helens did in a matter of minutes!

and dissatisfaction with financial aid for rebuilding than any other group. Those who lost vacation homes did not show differences from the control group on any of the measures. Most victims reported that they felt only partially recovered even 11 months after the disaster.

TECHNOLOGICAL DISASTERS

Technological disasters share several characteristics with natural disasters. They tend to be unpredictable and uncontrollable and can produce intense physical suffering, psychological stress, and social disruption. In fact, one must look to the very worst of the natural disasters to find destruction on a par with the disasters of Hiroshima and Nagasaki, the Vietnam War, or the Bhopal tragedy. Most technological disasters subject people to acute stress because they last only a short time. Still, certain types of technological disasters can produce stress effects over long time frames. Love Canal, for example, was a hazard for several years. The incident at Three Mile Island probably has passed into memory for those living outside the region. For those living in the immediate vicinity, however, it continues to be a source of fear.

In other ways, technological disasters are very different from natural disasters. Technological disasters usually result from human miscalculation, carelessness, and greed. Sometimes they result from flagrant disregard for the value of human life compared to the corporate balance sheet. They are, in a word, preventable. From the vantage point of hindsight, at least, it seems that someone could have done something to prevent these disasters from happening. To the victim, someone is to blame, and that someone must pay. The gas in Bhopal had not even settled when residents began to blame Union Carbide and others for the accident. It is difficult to accuse a Supreme Being of malice when a tornado strikes, but sins of human error are not so easily forgiven. It is hardly surprising, then, that more anger and resentment follow technological disasters than natural disasters (Lystad, 1985). Our sense of control is also threatened. We think that what we create, we also control. After a technological disaster, it is indisputable that what we created, we could not and did not control.

BUFFALO CREEK AND THREE MILE ISLAND

Few technological disasters have been more extensively studied than the Buffalo Creek flood of 1976 and the nuclear accident at Three Mile Island in 1979. These studies reveal patterns of physical and psychological symptoms similar to those found following natural disasters. They also suggest that the effects of technological disasters are more long-term than those of natural disasters.

The Buffalo Creek Flood

The Buffalo Mining Company built a dam of coal slag to control flooding in towns along the Buffalo Creek Valley in West Virginia. In February 1976, after rains had swollen the creek behind the dam, the dam collapsed. In 15 minutes of unbridled fury, the wall of water destroyed the town of Saunders and several other valley settlements. Over 5000 people were left homeless, while 125 would never come home again. The physical and psychological effects of the flood were still evident two to four years later. The physical and psychological scars discovered by researchers were as follows:

1. anxiety, grief, and despair
2. apathy and withdrawal
3. depression
4. stomach problems
5. anger and rage
6. regression in children
7. nightmares and sleep disturbances
8. survival guilt

Some combination of these symptoms occurred in roughly 80% of the adults and 90% of the children.

Many of these symptoms also occurred in the aftermath of Bhopal, although these observations were not made in a systematic fashion. Citizens of Bhopal reportedly suffered from a generalized fear of additional gas leaks. This led to a mass exodus from the city in the days following the accident. Other symptoms reported included nightmares, sleeplessness, depression, and anxiety (Bales, 1985).

The Three Mile Island Nuclear Accident

Among the most frightening of disasters is a nuclear plant explosion or meltdown. Many movies have exploited the theme and graphically depicted a vision of wholesale destruction that might transpire. In spite of assurances of safety from various sources, many people remain unconvinced. Until the meltdown at the Chernobyl nuclear power plant in 1986, the world had witnessed only limited danger from nuclear accidents. The immediate reaction to the Chernobyl meltdown was largely restricted to medical and technical aid. It did not include studies of the psychosocial impact, as has occurred in other nuclear accidents. As a result, Chernobyl can only stand as a grim reminder of the horrendous forces and frightful damage that could engulf the world with a full-scale meltdown. Unlike Chernobyl, Three Mile Island was extensively studied from a psychosocial view.

The incident began when the reactor dubbed Unit 2 malfunctioned and radioactive gases escaped into the atmosphere. The crisis lasted several days, with evacuations and disruption of life in the immediate region. Plant personnel quickly brought the reactor under control and reduced the potential for serious danger. Still, the threat of radioactive leaks continued for some time. It was more than a year before workers could clear contaminated water and gases from the building and erase the threat entirely. Even today, the plant remains a focal point of contention.

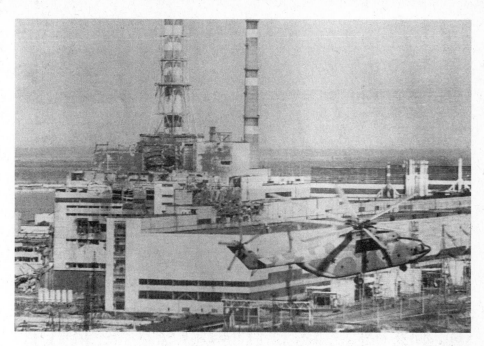

Chernobyl nuclear power plant in the Ukraine. Technological disasters are often more difficult to deal with because human error is usually involved.
SOURCE: Reuters/Bettmann Newsphotos.

Several studies in the first two years following the accident reported that psychological distress increased. There were more physical complaints and increased physiological arousal as indicated by levels of adrenaline in urine samples. Residents who had little or no social support showed more evidence of stress than those who had strong support (Baum, 1990; Fleming, Baum, Gisriel, & Gatchel, 1982). This finding confirms the notion advanced by Cobb (1976) that social support operates as a buffer against the effects of stress.

Love Canal: The Silent Killer

In contrast to these dramatic disasters, Love Canal was a silent killer. Its onset was slow and insidious, and most people were unaware that anything was wrong. Although people are once again settling in Love Canal, the total cost may still not be known.

Love Canal was a 16-acre chemical dump site for the Hooker Chemical Company of Niagara Falls, New York. The company used the abandoned canal to dispose of nearly 20,000 tons of chemical wastes over a period of roughly ten years, ending in 1953. Hooker Chemical then covered the canal and sold it to the local school district for $1. Families built homes on the site over the next 20 years. But no one told them the open field in their midst contained the seeds of deadly destruction; it was to be a park for the children (Gibbs, 1983). Officials did not begin to seriously investigate the problem until 1976, and they did not take any substantive action until 1978, when they developed a relocation plan that allowed 237 families at the center of Love Canal left to seek homes elsewhere. Unfortunately, 700 families on nearby streets were not included in the relocation plans. They were left alone to worry about their safety and their fate.

Residents were frightened, frustrated with the lack of action by government offices, and angry at the coverup that had occurred in years past. The most extreme frustration and anger arose when residents felt they had no control and when no progress was evident. Many residents reported feeling helpless and trapped.

Perhaps the most difficult problems were due to uncertainty and lack of information. Residents feared for their own safety and that of their young children. They also feared that pregnant women would bear deformed children. Pregnant women and children under 2 were the only residents "officially" declared at risk in the area. Officials knew that chromosome damage and ovum damage could result. Yet no one had any concrete answers to the residents' questions.

As Lois Gibbs reports, many people threatened to take their lives because of inability to deal with the constant stress. Several people tried and succeeded. Gibbs (1983) also said that "it [was not] uncommon to watch my neighbors, who before Love Canal were calm easygoing people, throw books at officials, use profanity in public, or threaten officials with physical harm at heated public meetings" (pp. 123–124). The litany of problems confronted by Love Canal residents included disruption for children, who had to relocate in different homes and schools as often as four times.

COPING WITH THE EFFECTS OF DISASTER

While it is one thing to identify the problems resulting from natural and technological disasters, it is another to provide information on how to cope with disasters. At least one team of investigators attempted to address this issue. Another team found that survivors of a natural disaster may come out of the experience with much better coping skills than they had before the disaster (Quarantelli & Dynes, 1977). The following information is based on one such analysis plus a composite of findings from the studies reported in the preceding sections.

Following the Three Mile Island incident, an investigative team headed by Andrew Baum studied the coping strategies used by residents in the vicinity (Baum, Fleming, & Singer, 1983). Baum's team asked a small sample of people to describe the coping strategies they used over the months following the accident. The research team used a scale that measured the extent to which each person used an emotion control coping style as opposed to a problem control coping style (Folkman & Lazarus, 1980). They defined emotionally focused coping as a strategy in which a person tries to control and release negative feelings (such as anger, frustration, and fear) provoked by the incident. Problem-focused coping was defined as a strategy in which a person tries to develop concrete plans of action and exerts as much direct control as possible.

Based on this initial assessment, Baum's group classified each person as high or low for emotionally focused coping and high or low for problem-focused coping. Then the group counted the number of symptoms reported for each coping style. The results were revealing. People who were *low* on emotionally focused coping reported nearly three times the number of symptoms compared with those who were high on this dimension. People who were *high* on problem-focused coping reported nearly three times the number of symptoms compared with those who were low on this dimension.

This suggests that, in disaster situations, the most effective strategy is to focus first on ridding oneself of the negative emotions. Victims should seek ways of bringing emotions out in the open and avoid locking them up inside. In addition, victims probably should not be concerned about trying to control through direct problem confrontation. This advice does not apply to all stress situations, though, for a specific reason.

The investigative team reasoned that a disaster such as Three Mile Island confronts people with a situation that is inherently uncontrollable for anyone without technical training. Attempts to assert direct control, then, seem to add stress by increasing personal feelings of frustration at not being able to do anything about the disaster. In other stressful situations, such as interpersonal conflict, a problem-solving approach may be the most effective means of managing the stress. Personal control may be both possible and effective for resolving interpersonal conflict.

Information seeking is also a highly visable coping strategy in disaster situations. Uncertainty is a major cause of stress; obtaining relevant and concrete information can help reduce uncertainty. The problem is that information provided during and after disasters may be inaccurate, unclear, and confusing. This was the case with much of the information supplied during the Love Canal controversy. People often received mixed messages on health problems, relocation efforts, economic support, and so forth. In this situation, people who sat back and waited were often better off than those who actively pressed for information. Thus, officials charged with the responsibility of providing information should be careful to provide only information that is accurate and clear.

The Crash of Flight 232

A clinical intervention study following the July 19, 1989 crash of United Airlines Flight 232 at Sioux City, Iowa, confirmed several of these issues (Jacobs, Quevillon, & Stricherz, 1990). News coverage of this crash was extensive, due in part to the time that elapsed between the first warnings that the plane had lost hydraulic power and the actual crash. The pilot displayed courage and calmness through the ordeal, and his heroic efforts enabled 184 passengers to survive.

Jacobs, Quevillon, and Stricherz (1990) were part of the mental health disaster team whose responsibility was to provide crisis counseling for the families and friends of passengers on Flight 232. Their article provides insights

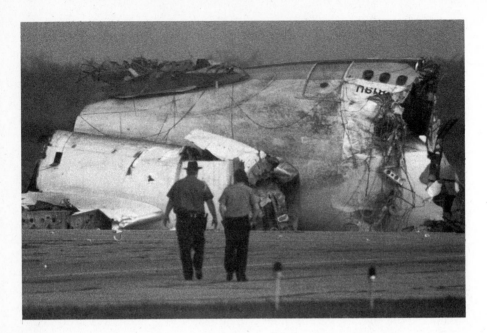

Sioux City police stand guard over the fuselage of United Airlines Flight 232. The pilot's courage in crisis is credited with saving nearly 200 of the 300 passengers.
SOURCE: UPI/Bettmann.

into the difficulties of critical-incident stress debriefing and makes suggestions for mental health disaster planning in the future. Medical response to the disaster was superbly handled, but provision of emotional support to the families was hindered by diffusion of responsibility and official misinformation.

During the chaotic morning following the crash, the team received four different reports on the imminent arrival of family members. First, it was reported that 100 family members would arrive, and the team called in the 80 mental health counselors needed to deal with that number. Then the airline reported that only 7 family members were arriving; as a result, half the counselors were sent home. Shortly afterward, 100 family members were expected again, and the counselors were called back. Less than 10 minutes later, the 7 family members arrived.

The press, however unwittingly, also contributed by publishing inaccurate information. Incorrect lists of passengers led to confusion, with alternating hope and grief. One man noted that his loved one's name did not appear on the list, and his hope for her safety was reborn. Only 30 minutes later, he had to be told of her death.

NOISE POLLUTION

Urban residents often seek the silence of forest and field as a vacation from the din of traffic, the clatter of jackhammers, and the roar of airplanes. The fact that people try to escape noise, reduce noise, or engage in political battles to control noise suggests that the properties of noise are unpleasant. In extreme cases, people even kill because of noise. Such was the case one warm summer night.

A normally quiet and responsible young man, Mike came home from his night-shift job tired and looking for a peaceful night's sleep. He awakened to the sounds of loud music, laughter, and talking at a nearby party, a party to celebrate Kelly's 21st birthday. Mike asked the partygoers to quiet down, and heated words passed between Mike and Kelly. Some shoving occurred, and Mike ran across the street, with Kelly and his friends in hot pursuit. After an altercation at Mike's apartment, Mike shot Kelly to death. Noise does not usually produce such extreme outcomes. Nonetheless, it is a source of stress for millions of people each day.

As the case of Mike and Kelly illustrates, noise is a relative matter. One person's noise is another person's music. There may be individual differences in sensitivity to noise that also influence response (Topf, 1989). We usually define noise in terms of the effect it has on people. More formally, *noise* is unwanted sound. We perceive noise as an unwarranted, offensive, and mostly uncontrollable intrusion on our peace.

The three dimensions of sound most closely related to whether we perceive it as noise are intensity, predictability, and controllability. The measure of intensity is the decibel (dB), a standard that provides a physical reference for measuring and comparing sounds. Normal conversation is about 60 dB. Street noise is about 80 dB. Rock bands often play at 120 dB to 140 dB. Auditory pain begins to occur around 100 dB. Permanent damage can occur with sustained exposure to sounds above 100 dB such as encountered in foundries. The U.S. Occupational Safety and Health Administration (OSHA) has set a 90-dB ceiling for business and industry, but more than half the production workers in America are exposed to sound levels that can produce hearing loss. Table 9-2 lists decibel levels for sounds people commonly hear at home and at work.

Generally, predictable noise is less disturbing than unpredictable noise. People can adapt readily to the effects of consistent, predictable noise. For example, most people who have grown up in Chicago around the elevated trains can sleep through the night without great difficulty because they have adapted to the noise. A person moving to Chicago from a rural area might have great difficulty sleeping at first.

An isolated event dramatically illustrated the importance of predictability and adaptation. One night, police stations along one train route in Chicago were inundated with calls from curious residents. "What happened?" "I know something is wrong, but I don't know what it is. Can you help?" The explanation turned out to be very simple: A power outage had shut down the trains! People awoke because of the silence. The more unpredictable and inconsistent the noise is, the more stressful it is. When it is predictable, we can adapt to it, anticipate it, and thus minimize its impact.

Finally, when we can control noise, it is less aversive than when we cannot control it. Consider this example: Your radio is playing loudly when someone suggests looking for a different station. If someone else dials in a new station,

TABLE 9-2
Decibel Levels for Common Sounds at Home and Work

Source	Decibel level	Effect
Rocket engine	180	
	160	
Aircraft carrier deck	140	Intense pain
Emergency sirens at 100 feet		
Rock concert/discotheque	120	Moderate auditory pain
Automobile horn at 3 feet	110	
Off-road motorcycle		
Garbage truck	100	Beginning of pain
Subway station	90	Maximum OSHA level
Lawn mower/outboard motor		Hearing damage begins
Noisy restaurant	80	
Freeway at 50 feet	70	Interference with use of phone
Washing machine		
Normal conversation	60	
Residential street noise	50	Quiet
Living room with TV on		
Refrigerator	40	
Library		
Whisper at 15 feet	30	Very quiet
	20	
Broadcasting studio	10	Barely audible
	0	Threshold of hearing

you probably will react more negatively to the white noise between stations than if you do it yourself. Muting switches are built into some stereo receivers to avoid this very problem, an example of engineering to control the aversive properties of noise.

Research shows that noise impairs performance in schoolchildren (Bronzaft & McCarthy, 1975). It reduces the production efficiency of factory and clerical workers. Noise also increases certain types of illnesses, although the evidence for this is often weak. Nonetheless, gastrointestinal disturbances such as ulcers, vaso-constriction, higher blood pressure, and increased secretions of catecholamines (adrenaline and noradrenaline) occur consistently in association with high levels of noise (Cohen, Evans, Krantz, & Stokols, 1980). After a review of literature on noise exposure and subjective reactions, Job (1988) concluded that the findings are similar across different nationalities using different measuring techniques.

Even if noise is not strongly linked to health problems, it may have severe disruptive effects on social behavior. Noise apparently causes distortions in our perceptions of other people. It may affect our liking or disliking another person (Siegel & Steele, 1980). In addition, research confirms that noise tends to increase the likelihood of aggression, but this may only occur when a person is already angry. Thus, noise may facilitate, but not instigate, aggression (Konecni, Libuser, Morton, & Ebbesen, 1975). When Mike shot Kelly, something that happened earlier that day might have annoyed Mike; the noise of the party may only have provided the excuse for ventilating anger. By the way, a jury later found Mike innocent.

COPING WITH NOISE POLLUTION

Numerous techniques are available to deal with noise. In ecological terms, we call these *noise abatement procedures.* Noise control techniques can be divided into two broad categories: one approach is to control noise at the source. This would involve stricter laws and enforcement for mufflers on trucks, automobiles, and motorcycles. Quiet airplanes would have to be designed, and quiet office equipment, typewriters, and printers would have to be built. Even then, we could not effectively eliminate all unpleasant sounds that are part of modern industrial society.

The second general approach is to engage in better environmental design for work and living space that minimizes the potential for intrusion of unwanted sounds. Increased thickness of walls, with attention to economically feasible soundproofing, may go a long way to reducing the side effects of noise. Thicker carpets, acoustic dampening on ceilings, sound-absorbing wall surfaces, curtains, and plants may reduce the spread or influx of sound. Masking, which uses a desirable sound to drown out an undesirable sound, is sometimes effective. Some masking may occur without design, such as the masking that occurs from heating and ventilating fans. Masking also may be by design. Offices use music to reduce background noise, and you might use the stereo to mask street sounds at home.

The Walkman Environment

An interesting recent phenomenon is the Walkman environment. It is common to see people running, driving, biking, or "malling," living in a world created by their portable stereos. Entire city populations seem to be plugged in, turned on but tuned out to whatever is going on outside those two cushioned pads on their ears. The popularity of portable stereos may be due more to the control it gives people over noise than to the convenience of having portable music. In addition to providing a portable means for masking noise, Walkmans give people great control over the type and volume of music they hear. This also makes the sound environment predictable. The Walkman may be an effective remedy for noise pollution while on the move.

AIR POLLUTION

The Taj Mahal is one of the world's great architectural achievements. Design of the building took 7 years, and construction took nearly 22 years. More than 20,000 workers labored year-round to complete the project. It was finished in exquisite detail with precious and semiprecious stones inlaid in marble. Now, a massive effort is under way to restore, preserve, and save the Taj Mahal from destruction. It is slowly being eaten away by corrosive air pollutants from a nearby power plant.

Although air pollution does not seem to cause the psychological distress that disasters, crowding, or noise do, it is nonetheless important. At least three harmful effects are related to air pollution. First, it directly threatens human and animal health. Second, air pollution can have sweeping effects on the environment through a variety of atmospheric and climatic changes, including ozone depletion, smog, and acid rain. Third, air pollution has the potential to harm and destroy buildings through corrosive effects, as illustrated by the Taj Mahal.

One problem with air pollution is that it is not always detectable to the senses. The most apparent sign of air pollution is smog, the haze we can see on the horizon. We can smell air pollutants, such as gases from automobiles, smoke from processing plants, and odors from smoking tobacco. Other pollutants, such as carbon monoxide and radon gas, are undetectable to either the eye or the nose. Airtight homes illustrate this problem. Such homes can be more polluted inside than outside, yet the owners are not aware of it (Guenther, 1982).

The Air Pollution Syndrome

The health hazards of air pollution are well known. At the extreme end of the spectrum, 50 to 90% of cancer cases may result from air pollution. In the United States alone, health officials estimate that 140,000 deaths result from air pollution each year. In Mexico City, with a population of 18 million people and dense industrialization, 100,000 people die each year from air pollution, 30,000 of whom are children. Fisher's group reported that one breath of air in an average city contains 70,000 dust and dirt particles; just living in New York City is equivalent to smoking 38 cigarettes a day (Fisher et al., 1984).

Doctors have identified an **air pollution syndrome (APS)** (Hart, 1970). The syndrome includes headaches, fatigue, insomnia, depression, irritability, eye irritation, and stomach problems. Fisher's team also provided a short but detailed summary of additional health hazards from air pollution (Fisher et al., 1984). Long-term exposure to carbon monoxide, for example, can result in headaches, epilepsy, memory disturbances, visual and auditory impairments, Parkinsonism, and physical fatigue. In addition, carbon monoxide deprives body tissue of oxygen, a condition known as hypoxia. Particulates, such as those emitted from smokestacks, exhausts, and other sources, include lead, mercury, and asbestos. These pollutants can cause cancer, anemia, and respiratory and neural problems. Psychiatric problems are also aggravated by air pollution, as indicated by increased hospital admissions.

Air pollution has other effects as well. Human performance suffers as pollutants increase. Reaction time, attention, and perceptual motor deficits occur. It is possible that such effects contribute to the frequency of automobile accidents in heavily congested cities. Air pollution also may change social behaviors, including increasing aggression.

Involuntary (Passive) Smoking

Among the most divisive issues in recent years is the rights of nonsmokers and smokers and the issue of **passive smoking.** Several studies have shown that inhaling the smoke from someone else's cigarette can have detrimental health effects. Breathing rate, heart rate, and blood pressure increase. The Surgeon General and the National Academy of Science both published reports in 1986 stating for the first time that passive smoke inhalation causes disease (Fielding & Phenow, 1988). They singled out the increase in risk for lung cancer as the most notable.

In their review of this issue, Fielding and Phenow (1988) compared mainstream smoke, inhaled by smokers, with sidestream smoke, the aerosol given off by the end of smoldering tobacco. They noted that sidestream smoke "has a higher pH, smaller particles, and higher concentrations of carbon monoxide, as well as many toxic and carcinogenic compounds" (p. 1452). Among the strongest evidence suggesting a direct association between passive smoke inhalation and disease is the dose-response relationship. Risk increases (response) with increased exposure (dose) on a continuum that includes low-dose smokers (one or few cigarettes per day). One widely used short-term urinary marker, cotinine, correlates positively with increased exposure to tobacco smoke. In addition, evidence exists of respiratory disorder as measured by reduced expiratory volume and flow and of upper-respiratory problems in both adult and child nonsmokers living with smokers.

Combining the results of several studies, the best estimate of the relative risk for lung cancer is 1.34.[3] Compared to unexposed persons, then, exposed individuals are at increased risk for lung cancer. This estimate may seem small, but the cost in human lives is not, as Fielding and Phenow point out. Of the 12,200 annual deaths from lung cancer, 2500 to 8400 deaths may be attributable to involuntary smoke inhalation.

---

[3]Recall that relative risk as defined in Chapter 2 is the ratio of disease in the exposed group to disease in the nonexposed group. Thus, if 500 nonexposed people showed clinical signs of lung cancer, 670 exposed people would show signs of lung cancer.

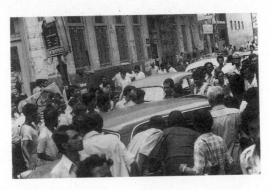

Calcutta, India—Crowding may influence social behavior, but people can adapt to crowding.
SOURCE: Photo by author.

STRESS AND OVERCROWDING

The management, or mismanagement, of space frequently contributes to stress. Perhaps the most important issue in this context is that of overcrowding. Researchers use two terms, **density** and *crowding,* when discussing overcrowding (Baron & Needel, 1980). Density is the physical condition of overpopulation. Crowding, on the other hand, is "a psychological state characterized by stress and having motivational properties (e.g., it elicits attempts to reduce discomfort)" (Fisher et al., 1984, p. 216).

To illustrate density, consider that in a city the size of San Francisco one can encounter 300,000 people in a 15-minute walk. Calcutta, India, has inner districts that are among the most densely populated in the world, with nearly 35,000 people per square kilometer. That is equivalent to 35,000 people in the space of five square blocks! That is density. However, even where the population is very dense, some people may not feel crowded. Without doubt, a complex web of psychosocial factors combines to produce the subjective feeling.

The effects of overcrowding on human behavior can be summarized as follows

1. High density frequently produces negative moods. This is true only for men, as women appear to have negative moods more frequently in low-density conditions. This suggests a *socialization* process that differs for males and females (Freedman, 1975).

2. Physiological arousal—as measured by higher blood pressure, skin conductance, sweating, and increased cortisol and epinephrine output—occurs in a variety of laboratory and natural settings under conditions of crowding. One study of commuters noted that the intensity of arousal, however, depended on the degree of control that commuters had in choosing their space on the train

(Lundberg, 1976). This suggests that the effect of crowding is dependent on how the person appraises the *controllability* of the situation.

3. Illness increases as density increases, as studies of prison inmates, college students, and naval crews show. The types of illnesses reported are not serious, but the frequency increases.

4. Overcrowding also may increase withdrawal and aggression. Withdrawal responses include lower levels of eye contact and maintenance of greater interpersonal distance (Baum & Koman, 1976). If aggression increases at all, it does so only in males. The findings are somewhat weak and inconsistent on the latter issue.

Most negative outcomes of overcrowding are consistent with the cognitive-transactional model and the idea of loss of control. As Baum and Valins (1979) noted, overcrowding generally leads to an increase in unwanted interactions, which itself is a basic loss in controlling the range and quality of interactions. Fisher and his colleagues also saw stimulus overload and behavior constraint as potentially contributing factors, but these are still consistent with the cognitive model (Fisher et al., 1984). Loss of control could mediate physiological arousal, leading to increased sympathetic arousal and illness.

Coping with Crowding

At least two different means of coping with overcrowding have been suggested. The first focuses on environmental design aimed at reducing the feeling of crowding. Bright colors, wall decorations, higher ceilings, and rectangular rooms can increase the perception of space and reduce the feeling of crowding. Design of space to stir symbolic and affective qualities can also be helpful, especially in major metropolitan areas (Stokols, 1980).

The second approach focuses on the feelings of anxiety or apprehension felt by people in situations of crowding. One study used three different techniques to reduce anxiety in commuters (Karlin, Katz, Epstein, & Woolfolk, 1979). The three techniques included relaxation training (discussed in Chapter 11), cognitive reappraisal, and imagery (both discussed in Chapter 12). The results suggest that each technique provided some help, but cognitive reappraisal produced the most positive results.

Commuting in Urban Environments

Commuting may be one of the more stressful experiences for urban workers living in the suburbs. Above and beyond the time and expense of commuting, commuters face the daily hassle of traffic jams; accidents; rude, if not hostile, drivers; and competition for right-of-way, position at stoplights, access to freeway ramps, and parking. Research shows that commuting stress increases with the volume of traffic, changes in the weather, and two-lane or curving roads (Stokols & Novaco, 1981). Several factors affect commuting stress, including personality and the degree of control the person can exert in crowded conditions.

SUMMARY

This chapter has reviewed the status of research on stress and health related to environmental factors such as disasters, pollution, and crowding. While disasters produce more intense but acute stress, pollution and crowding produce less intense but chronic stress. Negative health effects of environmental stress are generally mild, including short-term disturbances in eating, sleeping, and physical fatigue, with some increase in the frequency of normal illnesses. Severe effects, short of death, occur primarily with long-term environmental hazards.

Explanations of these effects can be encompassed in a cognitive-transactional model through mediators such as perception of loss of control and predictability. The effects of these stressors can be reduced through environmental design and personal interventions aimed at reducing anxiety, ventilating negative emotions, and increasing the perception of personal control. Stress management techniques may be useful in this regard.

KEY TERMS

adaptation level
  theory
air pollution
air pollution syn-
  drome (APS)
ambient stressors
arousal theory
background stressors
behavior constraint
  theory

behavior setting
classical conditioning
  theory
crowding
density
ecological theory
ecology
emotionally focused
  coping
environment

environmental stress
  theory
habitat
noise pollution
passive smoking
problem-focused
  coping
reactance
stimulus load
  theory

REFERENCES

Bales, J. (1985, July). Fear is residue of Bhopal tragedy. *APA Monitor, 16,* p. 15.
Barker, R. G. (1968). *Ecological psychology: Concepts and methods for studying the environment of human behavior.* Stanford, CA: Stanford University Press.
Baron, R. M., & Needel, S. P. (1980). Toward an understanding of the differences in the responses of humans and other animals to density. *Psychological Review, 87,* 320–326.

Baum, A. (1990). Stress, intrusive imagery, and chronic stress. *Health Psychology, 9,* 653–675.

Baum, A., Fleming, R., & Singer, J. (1983). Coping with victimization by technological disaster. *Journal of Social Issues, 39,* 117–138.

Baum, A., & Koman, S. (1976). Differential response to anticipated crowding: Psychological effects of social and spatial density. *Journal of Personality and Social Psychology, 34,* 526–536.

Baum, A., Singer, J. E., & Baum, C. S. (1981). Stress and the environment. *Journal of Social Issues, 37,* 4–35.

Baum, A., & Valins, S. (1979). Architectural mediation of residential density and control: Crowding and the regulation of social contact. In L. Berkowitz (Ed.), *Advances in experimental social psychology* (Vol. 12, pp. 131–175). New York: Academic Press.

Brehm, S. S., & Brehm, J. W. (1981). *Psychological reactance: A theory of freedom and control.* New York: Academic Press.

Bronzaft, A. L., & McCarthy, D. P. (1975). The effects of elevated train noise on reading ability. *Environment and Behavior, 7,* 517–527.

Byrne, D., & Clore, G. L. (1970). A reinforcement model of evaluative responses. *Personality: An International Journal, 1,* 103–128.

Cobb, S. (1976). Social support as a moderator of life stress. *Psychosomatic Medicine, 38,* 300–314.

Cohen, S. (1978). Environmental load and the allocation of attention. In A. Baum, J. E. Singer, & S. Valins (Eds.), *Advances in environmental psychology* (Vol. 1, pp. 1–29). Hillsdale, NJ: Lawrence Erlbaum Associates.

Cohen, S., Evans, G. W., Krantz, D. S., & Stokols, D. (1980). Physiological, motivational, and cognitive effects of aircraft noise on children: Moving from the laboratory to the field. *American Psychologist, 35,* 231–243.

Coleman, J. C., Butcher, J. N., & Carson, R. C. (1980). *Abnormal psychology and modern life* (6th ed.). Glenview, IL: Scott, Foresman.

Fielding, J. E., & Phenow, K. J. (1988). Health effects of involuntary smoking. *The New England Journal of Medicine, 319,* 1452–1460.

Fisher, J. D., Bell, P. A., & Baum, A. (1984). *Environmental psychology* (2nd ed.). New York: Holt, Rinehart & Winston.

Fleming, R., Baum, A., Gisriel, M. M., & Gatchel, R. J. (1982). Mediating influences of social support on stress at Three Mile Island. *Journal of Human Stress, 8,* 14–22.

Folkman, S., & Lazarus, R. S. (1980). An analysis of coping in a middle-aged community sample. *Journal of Health and Social Behavior, 21,* 219–239.

Freedman, J. L. (1975). *Crowding and behavior.* San Francisco: W. H. Freeman.

Gibbs, L. M. (1983). Community response to an emergency situation: Psychological destruction and the Love Canal. *American Journal of Community Psychology, 11,* 116–125.

Guenther, R. (1982, August 4). Ways are found to minimize pollutants in airtight houses. *Wall Street Journal,* p. 25.

Hart, R. H. (1970). The concept of APS: Air Pollution Syndrome(s). *Journal of the South Carolina Medical Association, 66,* 71–73.

Holahan, C. J. (1986). Environmental psychology. *Annual Review of Psychology, 37,* 381–407.

Jacobs, G. A., Quevillon, R. P., & Stricherz, M. (1990). Lessons from the aftermath of Flight 232: Practical considerations for the mental health profession's response to air disasters. *American Psychologist, 45,* 1329–1335.

Job, R. F. S. (1988). Community response to noise: A review of factors influencing the relationship between noise exposure and reaction. *Journal of the Acoustical Society of America, 83,* 991–1001.

Karlin, R. A., Katz, S., Epstein, Y., & Woolfolk, R. (1979). The use of therapeutic interventions to reduce crowding-related arousal: A preliminary investigation. *Environmental Psychology and Nonverbal Behavior, 3,* 219–227.

Konecni, V. J., Libuser, L., Morton, H., & Ebbesen, E. B. (1975). Effects of a violation of personal space on escape and helping responses. *Journal of Experimental Social Psychology, 11,* 288–299.

Lundberg, U. (1976). Urban commuting: Crowdedness and catecholamine excretion. *Journal of Human Stress, 2,* 26–32.

Lystad, M. H. (1985). Human response to mass emergencies: A review of mental health research. *Emotional First Aid, 2,* 5–18.

McFarlane, A. C. (1988). The phenomenology of posttraumatic stress disorders following natural disaster. *The Journal of Nervous and Mental Disease, 176,* 22–29.

McLeod, B. (1984, October). In the wake of disaster. *Psychology Today,* pp. 54–57.

Mehrabian, A., & Russell, J. A. (1974). *An approach to environmental psychology.* Cambridge, MA: MIT Press.

Moran, E. F. (1981). Human adaptation to arctic zones. *Annual Review of Anthropology, 10,* 1–25.

Murphy, S. A. (1984). Stress levels and health status of victims of a natural disaster. *Research in Nursing and Health, 7,* 205–215.

Patrick, V., & Patrick, W. K. (1981). Cyclone '78 in Sri Lanka—The mental health trail. *British Journal of Psychiatry, 138,* 210–216.

Pennebaker, J. W., & Newtson, D. (1983). Observation of a unique event: The psychological impact of the Mount Saint Helens volcano. *New Directions for Methodology of Social and Behavioral Sciences, 15,* 93–109.

Quarantelli, E. L., & Dynes, R. R. (1977). Response to social crisis and disaster. *Annual Review of Sociology, 3,* 23–49.

Rodin, J., & Baum, A. (1978). Crowding and helplessness: Potential consequences of density and loss of control. In A. Baum & Y. Epstein (Eds.), *Human response to crowding* (pp. 390–401). Hillsdale, NJ: Lawrence Erlbaum Associates.

Seligman, M. E. P. (1975). *Helplessness.* San Francisco: W. H. Freeman.

Siegel, J. M., & Steele, C. M. (1980). Environmental distraction and interpersonal judgments. *British Journal of Social and Clinical Psychology, 19,* 23–32.

Stokols, D. (1980). Instrumental and spiritual views of people–environment relations. *American Psychologist, 45,* 641–646.

Stokols, D., & Novaco, R. (1981). Transportation and well-being: An ecological perspective. In I. Altman, J. F. Wohlwill, & P. B. Evertt (Eds.), *Transportation and behavior* (pp. 85–130). New York: Plenum.

Topf, M. (1989). Sensitivity to noise, personality hardiness, and noise-induced stress in critical care nurses. *Environment and Behavior, 21,* 717–733.

Wohlwill, J. F. (1974). Human adaptation to levels of environmental stimulation. *Human Ecology, 2,* 127–147.

PART FOUR

COPING, RELAXATION, AND IMAGERY

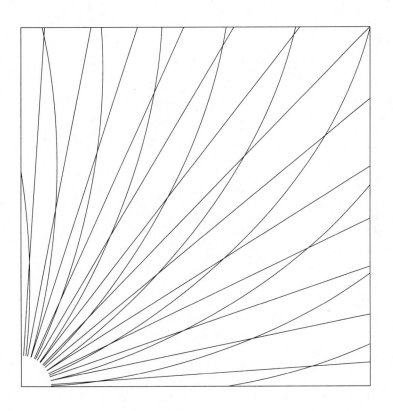

CHAPTER 10

Coping Strategies: Controlling Stress

In this chapter, we begin to focus on coping skills, the means we use to combat or prevent stress. We will discuss problematic issues in coping, including how to define the term and how to classify **coping strategies.** We will discuss one classification scheme that will provide the organizing structure for the rest of the chapter. We will also examine **coping resources,** coping behaviors, and **coping styles** that help or hurt coping efforts. As a beginning, consider the coping cameos in the following section as illustrations of how people managed to cope with a variety of problems.

COPING CAMEOS: STRUGGLES AND STRATEGIES

For Todd and Ann Marie, life had been every couple's dream. Their parents managed a successful business. School had been a breeze, and both had been popular members of their class. They expected marriage to be the beginning of a life distinguished by adult career successes, punctuated by fun and romantic interludes. The birth of their first child burst the bubble, leaving them shocked and dismayed for a time. Their child, far from being perfect, was mentally handicapped and would require substantial care throughout life. Todd and Ann Marie drew strength from their religion and support from their friends in the church. Before long, they felt their child was a gift to be nourished and cherished.

Brian was successful throughout high school, earning satisfactory, though not stellar, grades. He planned to follow the family tradition by pursuing a medical career. Nothing and no one ever suggested he might not succeed. Then he met disaster in a major laboratory sequence in the university pre-med program. All his life, he had focused on this one ambition only to be frustrated now by failure. Because he had no forewarning, Brian felt the blow more keenly. After little more than a week, Brian suddenly announced to his family that he was leaving school to pursue a business venture with a high school friend. The reasons for this sudden change were not clear, and the plans for the business were vague. He rejected all the family's attempts to give advice.

A modestly successful farmer became involved in a tax protest group. The federal government charged him with issuing illegal sight drafts and income tax evasion. He lost his farm, and, after a short flight to avoid prosecution, his freedom. When it came time to appear in court, the farmer refused to walk, talk, or cooperate with authorities. Officers rolled him into court on a hand-cart. Still, he refused to open his eyes or talk to the judge. He seemed to think that he could avoid reality by simply shutting it out.

Jan Kemp blew the whistle on preferential treatment of athletes at the University of Georgia. At the outset, it was a case of a teacher's conscience asking for academic honesty and integrity. Kemp could not have anticipated the shock waves that would reverberate through the academic and athletic communities. Along the way, she decided to take on the Cyclops of big-time college athletics through legal means. It cost Jan her job, placed her career in jeopardy, nearly destroyed her family, and led to two suicide attempts. During the trial against the university, Jan described herself as shy but courageous. A journalist called her another "Iron Magnolia," which was Rosalyn Carter's nickname. *Sports Illustrated* described Jan as tough and resilient (Nack, 1986). In the end, Jan Kemp won a moral and legal victory with reinstatement to her job and a major damage award. Her methods of coping with this threat were not always positive. Still, she met the challenge and won the battle.

These coping cameos were real dilemmas faced by real people. Each was trying in some fashion to offset stress that accompanied the situation. These people used an assortment of coping strategies, both positive and negative, to manage pressures. We may not agree with the way they met their personal threats, but each was successful to some degree.

These cameos also highlight several problems in the literature on coping skills. What does it mean to say that we "cope" with stress? Should we evaluate coping solely in terms of outcome? In other words, should we make no distinction between positive and negative strategies and judge only whether the strategy led to success? Do certain coping strategies work best in specific situations, or are they general methods? We turn our attention now to these issues.

COPING SKILLS: ISSUES AND DEFINITIONS

In an early attempt to define **coping,** Haan (1977) stated that coping is any effort that seeks to preserve reality. There are two problems with this view. First, it is much too vague to direct research. Second, it omits non–reality-oriented strategies. Non–reality-oriented coping may be evaluated negatively by others but still be successful for the person suffering from overwhelming stress. We might regard the farmer's refusal to walk, talk, or open his eyes as negative coping and non–reality-oriented. His behavior would not qualify as coping in Haan's definition. Still, the behavior apparently allowed the protester to maintain a private sense of control and success in defiance of authority.

Stone and Neale (1984) suggested that coping involves only conscious efforts to deal with stressful demands. This makes no allowance for unconscious or subconscious coping processes. Yet abundant evidence exists that psycho-dynamic defense mechanisms, some of which are presumably unconscious, are important for coping with emotional conflict and ego injury.

Folkman and Lazarus (1980) offered a very inclusive definition as part of the cognitive-transactional theory of stress. They defined coping as all cognitive and behavioral efforts to master, reduce, or tolerate demands. These demands could be external or internal. Internal demands may reflect the outcome of cognitive appraisals or emotional conflict. Further, coping usually aims at one of two outcomes: It seeks to alter the relationship between self and environment, or it seeks to reduce emotional pain and distress. A cognitive reappraisal that alters the meaning of an event is one way to change the relationship between self and environment. **Instrumental coping,** such as problem solving directed toward the source of the threat, is also a way to change this relationship. Coping must also deal with emotions aroused by stress. Emotional regulation is **palliative coping** in the Lazarus model. This model seems comprehensive on the surface.

After Kenneth Matheny and his associates conducted an extensive review of coping literature, they apparently could add little to Lazarus's definition (Matheny et al., 1986). They defined coping as "any effort, healthy or unhealthy, conscious or unconscious, to prevent, eliminate, or weaken stressors, or to tolerate their effects in the least hurtful manner" (p. 509). This will be the working definition for this chapter.

TAXONOMIES OF COPING

As we have seen, stress is a complex concept. To make sense of it, we broke it down into smaller units such as different sources of stress, different regulatory systems, and different responses. This was a way of classifying stress to better study and understand it. Classifying is typical of any scientific enterprise. We call formal classifying and naming schemes *taxonomies.*

Just as stress is a complex notion, so is the idea of coping. A taxonomy of coping should help impose order and enable us to study and understand it better. Billings and Moos (1981) provided an early taxonomy of coping responses. They suggested that coping behaviors could be categorized first in terms of the method of coping: active or avoidant. Further, the focus of the response could be categorized as problem oriented or emotion oriented. This dichotomy, problem versus emotion oriented, parallels the one used by Baum, Fleming, and Singer (1983) in their study of coping with nuclear disaster at Three Mile Island. It also appears similar to Folkman and Lazarus's instrumental versus palliative model. In the Billings and Moos scheme, we probably would view Brian's leaving school as an emotional, avoidant strategy. Billings and Moos used these two dimensions—active versus avoidant and problem versus emotion oriented—to construct a two-way table of coping, shown in Table 10-1.

Reliance on simple dichotomies has seldom been useful, especially when dealing with something as complex as stress or coping strategies. Thus,

TABLE 10-1
A Classification of Coping Methods Related to the Focus of Coping

	Active method	*Passive method*
Problem-oriented focus	Cognitive-behavioral	Cognitive-behavioral
Emotion-oriented focus	Cognitive-behavioral	Cognitive-behavioral

SOURCE: Billings and Moos (1981).

Elizabeth Menaghan (1983) proposed that coping could be broken down into coping resources, coping efforts and strategies,[1] and coping styles. Each category has traits or events that can be defined (operationalized) more precisely. To date, the most comprehensive attempt to classify coping strategies comes from the work of Matheny and his colleagues. Before turning to specific coping skills, therefore, I will describe Matheny's model in more detail.

A COPING MODEL: COMBATIVE VERSUS PREVENTIVE COPING

After a lengthy review of the coping literature and a meta-analysis, Matheny's group proposed that coping can be viewed first in terms of its combative or preventive nature (Matheny et al., 1986). **Combative coping** occurs when a stressor triggers a reaction. It is an attempt to subdue or defeat a stressor that is present and needs to be eliminated. **Preventive coping,** on the other hand, attempts to prevent stressors from appearing either through cognitive structuring that buffers the perception of demand or through increasing resistance to the effects of stress. Building resources increases resistance to stress. In this model, combative coping is escape learning, whereas preventive coping is avoidance learning. Matheny's model appears in Table 10-2.

According to Matheny's analysis, preventive coping involves four strategies: "(1) avoiding stressors through life adjustments, (2) adjusting demand levels, (3) altering stress-inducing behavior patterns, and (4) developing coping resources" (Matheny et al., 1986, p. 531). Avoiding stressors may entail leaving a dead-end job or a dead-end, unrewarding relationship.

Adjusting demand levels means that demands must match the limits of one's resources. Tackling jobs beyond one's competency may induce stress. Buying expensive gifts for family members beyond one's financial means may lead to combative coping, as when the bill collector shows up at the door. Adjusting demands to meet resources prevents that from happening.

Examples of altering stress-inducing behavior patterns include modifying the Type A behavior pattern, reducing impulsive traits, or tempering hyperreactivity such as that of anxiety-prone individuals. Developing coping resources includes building self-efficacy and a sense of control, developing time manage-

---

[1]*Coping strategies* and *coping efforts* are interchangeable terms. Both refer to direct plans and actions used to reduce or eliminate stress.

TABLE 10-2
Preventive and Combative Coping Methods

Preventive strategies	*Combative strategies*
1. Avoiding stressors through life adjustments	1. Monitoring stressors and symptoms
2. Adjusting demand levels	2. Marshaling resources
3. Altering stress-inducing behavior patterns	3. Attacking stressors a. problem solving b. assertiveness c. desensitization

4. Developing coping resources
 a. physiological assets
 b. psychological assets
   confidence
   sense of control
   self-esteem
 c. cognitive assets
   functional beliefs
   time management skills
   academic competence
 d. social assets
   social support
   friendship skills
 e. financial assets
	4. Tolerating stressors
	 a. cognitive restructuring
	 b. denial
	 c. sensation focusing
	5. Lowering arousal
	 a. relaxation
	 b. disclosure
	 c. catharsis
	 d. self-medication

SOURCE: Adapted from Matheny et al. (1986).

ment skills, and cultivating social networks. Although time management may not seem as crucial as some other coping skills, King, Winett, and Lovett (1986) showed that time management can serve as an effective coping strategy leading to reduced stress. McLaughlin, Cormier, and Cormier (1988) also showed that dual-career women frequently use time management and that it is positively related to better marital adjustment and lower levels of stress.

In the combative coping group, Matheny's team suggested five general classes of behaviors. **Stress monitoring** is necessary to initiate use of other strategies. *Marshaling resources* includes organizing and structuring for an effective coping effort.

The third combative strategy, *attacking stressors,* seeks to eliminate stressors directly. This may involve the use of problem-solving skills, information seeking, social skills, assertive responses, and altering patterns of hyper-reactivity. The person may need to alter cognitive structures to prevent intrusive self-limiting assumptions, to remove self-defeating thoughts, and to remain open to suitable options. Matheny's group strongly emphasizes this strategy because they believe it is desirable to eliminate stressors instead of just tolerating them.

Tolerating stressors is the fourth combative strategy. **Cognitive restructuring** may be essential when a stressor cannot be eliminated by direct action. "Cognitive restructuring aims to jettison . . . neurotic programming through reframing the perceived seriousness of demands and the limitations of one's resources" (Matheny et al., 1986, p. 535). Finally, *lowering arousal* involves reducing tension through a variety of means, as described earlier.

To discuss coping skills, we will use the three categories suggested by Menaghan in combination with Matheny's work. We will also examine evidence relevant to each skill as we progress.

COPING RESOURCES: WHAT IS AVAILABLE FOR COPING EFFORTS?

Resources are the basic supplies of coping strategies. They can be personal, social, or physical. Personal resources include traits or attitudes that are helpful in many situations. The most important personal resources appear to be **self-esteem,** self-denigration, perception of control, and self-efficacy. Jan Kemp held to a basic virtue of honesty and integrity both for herself and for her students. She also had a quiet courage that saw her through the toughest time of her life. Social resources include intimate relationships and extended networks. Todd and Ann Marie used an important social resource, their church support group, to help them cope with the demands of their handicapped child. Physical resources include satisfactory health and adequate physical energy to meet demands. They also involve practical resources, such as safe and functional housing and money for basic needs.

Social Support as a Coping Resource

Matheny's group found five coping resources in their literature review (Matheny et al., 1986). These were **social support,** beliefs and values, self-esteem, confidence control, and wellness. Social support was a central coping strategy in 54% of the studies reviewed. There are at least two possible views of how social support may operate. It may provide a buffering effect, protecting the person from the adverse effects of stress, or it may operate through a direct effect; that is, social support may be valuable and beneficial in its own right. Cohen and Wills (1985) argue that each model is correct and reflects multiple paths through which social support may influence stress and health outcomes. Further, it may be better to think of social support in a systems context. That is, the relationship between the individual and any support network is an ongoing transaction that involves two-way feedback of both positive and negative information. Each party may exercise regulatory or disregulatory effects on the other as interactions proceed (Leavy, 1983).

The effect of social support on coping is small when assessed by itself but large when combined with other treatments. Schultz and Saklofske (1983) argue that quality of social support is important, not quantity. Even if support is extensive, a person receiving low-quality support is more likely to report feeling lonely than one who receives less support, but of a higher quality.

Social support may be more important for certain types of stressors. Families with handicapped children face numerous stressors that never occur in other families (Yablin, 1986). They apparently benefit from social support networks (Kirkham, Schilling, Norelius, & Schinke, 1986). In addition, families coping with illness seem to fare better when strong social support networks are in place compared with those who do not have such support (Shapiro, 1983). Men with AIDS and AIDS-related complex (ARC) report increased distress when they perceive less support available (Zich & Temoshok, 1987). Social support also seems to be a buffer against severe coronary artery disease in Type A people (Blumenthal et al., 1987).

Beliefs and Values as Coping Resources

Beliefs and values are important because certain beliefs and values may lead one to appraise events as less stressful. Witmer (1986) noted that use of religious practices and spiritual beliefs is an overlooked element of coping strategies. We should also note that religious groups are strong social support systems whose influence has not been systematically assessed. Another general value scheme, optimism, may prove important. Optimism is the expectation that good things will happen. Michael Scheier and Charles Carver (1987), who wrote extensively on a systems view of stress, believe that optimism is an intriguing personality trait with important implications for coping and health. Optimism is a type of perceptual filter that colors a wide range of situations. Unfortunately, little research exists to suggest whether it can be treated as an enduring characteristic and, if so, how it may serve to offset the effects of stress.

Coping efficacy and control is a self-referent belief. It is the confidence that one can control events or cope with stressful demands. Bandura (1977) called this *self-efficacy.* Self-efficacy is part of secondary appraisal, the perceptual match we make between demands and the ability to cope with stress. Those who have a high degree of confidence in their own ability experience lower levels of stress. Matheny's team used the analogy of a magnifying glass to suggest how distorted appraisals can produce difficulty for some people. Think of times when you played with a magnifying lens or telescope. If you look through one end, everything suddenly looms larger. From the other end, though, everything appears much smaller or distant. In Matheny's analogy, some people seem to see demands through the magnifying end and their resources through the dwarfing end (Matheny et al., 1986).

The perception of coping efficacy appears to act as a cognitive mediator of anxiety. Bandura's research group noted several adverse outcomes that occur when people perceive coping inefficacy. These adverse outcomes include high levels of subjective distress, increased autonomic arousal, and elevated plasma catecholamine secretions (Bandura, Reese, & Adams, 1982). It is important to note that the perception of coping inefficacy does not have to be accurate to produce this outcome. Bandura also noted that faulty appraisal of coping efficacy can lead to anxiety and behavioral dysfunction just as readily as accurate appraisals can lead to distress.

Self-efficacy may foster positive health outcomes. The success of several intervention strategies appears to depend on changes in perceived self-efficacy

(O'Leary, 1985). These include smoking cessation and pain management programs. Diet and exercise regimens following heart attacks may also depend on changes in self-efficacy. As Ann O'Leary points out, the actual competence is not as important as the perception of efficacy. Self-efficacy also appears to enhance immune system function (Wiedenfeld et al., 1990). Before leaving the topic of self-efficacy, one last note is in order. *Self-esteem* means to accept and have high regard for oneself. It is not synonymous with self-efficacy, but theoretically self-esteem should increase with increases in perceived self-efficacy. Indirect support for the latter notion comes from research that shows good copers have a higher sense of self-worth than poor copers (Witmer, Rich, Barcikowski, & Mague, 1983).

Finally, *wellness* is the quality of health one enjoys, including physical fitness, energy level, weight control, and avoidance of high-risk behaviors. Of the studies that Matheny's group reviewed, 37% considered wellness a resource. In spite of the interest in wellness as a coping technique, Matheny's meta-analysis found that wellness was least effective in altering coping outcomes to the positive side (Matheny et al., 1986). We should be cautious about this interpretation, however, because very few studies assessed wellness interventions as coping methods. Further, many of the studies that considered wellness contained methodological weaknesses, including failure to control for differences in fitness before the study.

COPING EFFORTS:
WHAT CAN YOU DO TO COPE WITH STRESS?

Coping behavior may be positive or negative, active or avoidant, direct or indirect (Suls & Fletcher, 1985). It may include seeking help, seeking information, or diverting attention. Whatever their nature, coping efforts have just one function: to prevent, eliminate, or reduce stress. The extensive literature on coping reveals no less than a dozen behaviors that may be used for this purpose. The discussion in this section follows the summary of Matheny's group, with examples, supporting evidence, and types of training procedures added (Matheny et al., 1986). The first four coping efforts—**tension reduction,** cognitive restructuring, problem solving, and social skills—showed the strongest effect on coping outcome.

Tension Reduction: The Aspirin for Distress

The most commonly used coping skill is tension reduction. Tension is a physical warning that something is wrong. It usually means that an event in the environment or an unresolved internal conflict has increased physiological arousal to uncomfortable, if not harmful, levels. Tension can perpetuate stress even after removal of the stressor, so reducing tension can have positive outcomes. We may attain tension reduction through such methods as progressive relaxation,

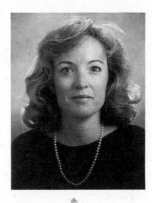

Shelley Taylor, prominent health psychologist
SOURCE: Courtesy of Dr. Shelley E. Taylor.

meditation, or autogenics. Matheny's group found that relaxation was the most widely used single treatment procedure and had the greatest positive effect on coping outcome. Many clinicians recommend relaxation for a wide range of stress-related conditions, including migraine headache (Sorbi & Tellegen, 1988).

Cognitive Restructuring: Changing Perceptions

Cognitive restructuring changes the meaning of an event or changes perceptions of personal adequacy to handle the situation. Coping is often an anticipatory process that begins before meeting threat or stress such as impending surgery. For example, ruminations are the Achilles's heel of coping efforts. Children waiting for dental work report many "catastrophizing" thoughts that increase their anxiety and make the dentist's work more difficult. Still, some children apparently use positive coping strategies spontaneously (Branson & Craig, 1988). Their cognitive efforts include positive self-talk ("I tried to think good thoughts"), thought stopping (eliminating bad thoughts), and emotional control cognitions ("Try not to worry"). They also seek information and support from the dentist, engage in attention diversion, and practice relaxation or deep breathing to reduce tension.

Fernandez and Turk (1989) showed that cognitive coping strategies are effective in alleviating pain.[2] Klingman (1985) provided training in cognitive-behavioral coping to girls preparing for inoculation against rubella. The girls showed lower levels of anxiety and were more cooperative compared with a control group that received only technical information.

Shelley Taylor's (1983) theory of cognitive adaptation integrates many important components of coping with threatening events. Taylor argues that readjustment to threat involves three general themes. First, we look for meaning

[2]This study was discussed at length in Chapter 2.

in the experience. We may even change the meaning of an event after reflection or after obtaining a different perspective from a friend or confidante. Next, threat often makes us feel insecure about our control or efficacy. So we try to regain mastery over the event and over life in general. Finally, because threat often attacks self-esteem, we may try to enhance self-esteem through positive self-evaluations.

Clinical interventions commonly use rational-emotive therapy and stress inoculation to bring about cognitive restructuring. In Matheny's meta-analysis, cognitive restructuring was second only to relaxation training in frequency of use. It also had the highest positive effect on coping outcome, matching the strength of relaxation training as an intervention procedure.

Humor may be a means of restructuring perceptions of stressful events. Gordon Allport (1937) discussed the role of **humor** in personality. He considered humor a prime correlate of insight. People can reformulate ordinary problems and misfortunes through humor. They gain a new perspective, a novel frame of reference induced by humor. Rod Martin and Herbert Lefcourt (1983) discovered that humor moderates the relation between negative life events and mood disturbance. Individual differences exist, though, in preference for humor, as do gender differences in the type of humor used to cope with stress (Schill & O'Laughlin, 1984).

Problem Solving: Rational Steps to Stress Reduction

Many events are stressful because they involve elements of problem solving that we are ill-prepared to handle. When we can solve a problem readily, we experience little stress or only challenging stress. When the solution to the problem eludes us or involves competencies beyond what we possess, stress is likely to occur. Brian might have engaged in some problem solving to evaluate other career options before leaving school. Jan Kemp, on the other hand, employed extensive problem solving by retaining a lawyer and following a legal process to reach a solution. Bandura (1989) suggested that people who believe in their problem-solving ability remain more effective analytic thinkers in difficult situations. Success in problem solving, then, may feed back to increase self-efficacy.

One might learn problem solving as a general strategy. On the other hand, one might learn specific problem-solving strategies for specific issues or situations. Maura Kirkham and her colleagues adapted a general problem-solving model called SODAS to help mothers of handicapped children (Kirkham, Schilling, Norelius, & Schinke, 1986). SODAS is an acronym for Stop, Options, Decide, Act, and Self-praise. It means to *S*top and identify the problem. Then, list all the solution *O*ptions. Next, *D*ecide which option is probably best. Outline a step-by-step plan to implement the decision and then *A*ct. Finally, reinforce yourself for solving the problem with *S*elf-praise. Most often, problem-solving classes focus on specific issues, such as study skills, weight control, escaping cycles of abuse, single parenting, effective parenting, and so forth.

Social Skills: Communication and Assertion

Problems with interpersonal relationships create many stressors. We may read signals of friendliness as overtures for intimacy and get hurt. We may talk too much, listen too little, and hear even less. We may seek positive evaluations to bolster our self-esteem, then fail to respond positively to the efforts of someone trying desperately to please us. Each of these situations involves social skills, the ability to navigate the troubled waters of interpersonal exchange in a mutually satisfying way (Marsh, 1988; Richmond, McCroskey, & Payne, 1987). Practicing social skills should enable us to achieve needs and goals in a way that does not harm others in the process. Social skills training includes interpersonal communication (Hargie, 1986; Mader & Mader, 1990), intimacy and **self-disclosure,** and **assertiveness,** among others (Cotler & Guerra, 1980; Zuker, 1983). As a group, social skills may positively influence coping outcomes, but they do not contribute greatly to coping success when learned as simple separate interventions (Matheny et al., 1986).

Positive Diversions: Filling Time Constructively

Positive diversions, also called **attention diversion,** use constructive activities to divert attention from painful or distressing thoughts. For example, a widow who takes on volunteer service may find that the new involvement reduces the frequency of memories of the spouse who died recently. Hobbies such as music, reading, acting, and exercise can also serve this purpose. Diversions may be useful in situations of uncertainty. For example, waiting for a call that means getting a special job can be difficult, especially if one conjures up scripts that anticipate a negative outcome. A similar situation exists when waiting for results from medical tests or when dealing with a family member with long-term illness.

Open and Closed Systems: Letting Out or Holding In

Another coping effort is **self-disclosure** and **catharsis.** *Self-disclosure* refers to being open as a person, being able to share thoughts and feelings with others. *Catharsis* means release of or purification of emotions. In clinical practice, it means bringing unexpressed, repressed emotions into the open so they can be dealt with directly. Closed-in people often suffer because they distance themselves from social support by their behavior. Also, they are like a dam stopping up a huge reservoir of emotionality. When emotion finally breaks out, it does so in a torrent instead of a controlled release. Irving Janis (1983a) provides some perspective, however, in noting that high disclosure can be harmful if it leads to demoralization.

The ideal is to maintain a balance between control and expression of emotions. Extreme or inappropriate emotions need to be controlled to some extent, whereas less extreme and appropriate emotions can be expressed more openly. The process of **ventilating emotions** can have a therapeutic effect and reduce stress. Similarly, self-disclosure can be beneficial if it is not too rapidly paced or done under duress.

Seeking Information: Ignorance Is Not Bliss

Information seeking is a very important cognitive skill when dealing with uncertainty. People using this skill aim to obtain information that will reduce uncertainty and the stress that goes with it. Patients considering a doctor's advice for elaborate tests may ask friends for information about the doctor, about the tests, or even about where to get more information. They may go to the library to read about symptoms, treatments, and prognosis before undergoing the lab tests. This can be beneficial and reduce stress in certain situations. In other situations, it may increase stress.

Doleys, Meredith, and Ciminero (1982) reported an early, successful cognitive intervention that depended on giving information to peptic ulcer patients. In this 1936 study by Chappell and Sevenson, patients received information on the relationship between emotions and gastric physiology. Then they learned how to change habitual patterns of thinking that increase gastric hyperactivity. The authors called their method *directive therapy,* but it was similar to cognitive restructuring therapy.

Stress Monitoring: Keeping an Eye on Distress

One train of logic suggests that being oblivious to stress is desirable. Another suggests that being aware of stress is of importance to survival. The argument for stress monitoring depends on the notion that awareness of stress is necessary to identify sources of stress in events and people. This view is consistent with a control theory of stress management (Suls & Fletcher, 1985). If we can identify stress-inducing events and people, then presumably we can engage in problem-solving behavior that will reduce, if not eliminate, stress from these sources. If we cannot, then disregulation may occur, leading to even more stress.

Stress monitoring includes awareness of increasing tension in muscles. This signal should enable us to take steps to halt or reduce the tension (Suls & Fletcher, 1985). The exercises used in progressive relaxation focus attention on tension and develop awareness of the contrast to relaxation. Stress monitoring also involves awareness of one's optimal range of stimulation.

Matheny's group found that stress monitoring could sensitize people to the existence of stress. In this case, the effects on coping efforts was negative. Suls and Fletcher (1985) studied coping with painful medical procedures, and their analysis provided some insights into this phenomenon. They showed that when monitoring focuses on threat, it increases distress. On the other hand, when monitoring focuses on sensory information, it does not. Further, if stress monitoring includes constructive efforts, such as identifying problem spots and engaging in problem solving, then stress monitoring can have a positive effect on coping outcome.

Assertive Behavior: Standing Firm, Not Angry

Many people encounter stress in normal transactions because they lack assertion skills. When someone cuts in line at the theater ahead of a nonassertive person, instead of gently but firmly asserting the social norm of turn taking, the nonassertive person says nothing. The event, though, may fester inside the person, welling up as a seething anger directed toward others. This cycle may also lead to lowered self-esteem. Learning appropriate assertion can help remove this source of distress (Cotler & Guerra, 1980; Zuker, 1983).

Negative Coping: Avoidance and Withdrawal

Avoidance or withdrawal is another coping strategy commonly used to protect against unwanted emotions. A person using avoidance usually seeks to eliminate stress by physically or mentally leaving the scene. People may avoid seeing a doctor for fear of hearing bad news. They may avoid the banker for fear of being pressured about a loan or an overdrawn account. Students may skip class for fear of bad news on a test. Avoidance is not reality oriented and, when used to the extreme, it can interfere with effective stress management. This happens when excessive avoidance feeds back negatively to self-esteem and self-efficacy. Then the behavior adds distress to the system instead of removing it.

Suls and Fletcher (1985) provided evidence from a meta-analysis of coping literature that avoidant strategies show their strength compared to other coping strategies only in the short run. That is, immediately after the appearance of a stressor, avoidance is superior to attention strategies. Yet, within two to six weeks, the pattern reverses when attention strategies become superior. They suggest that this may be due to a time lag required for the person to marshal resources to begin a more direct attack on the stressor.

Denial and Suppression: Intrapsychic Defenses

A person may escape mentally through **denial** or suppression. These control procedures usually seek to eliminate unpleasant emotions. In Freud's popular theory of personality, denial and suppression had a special name—*defense mechanisms*. Denial ignores a stressor, and suppression pushes the event deeper into the morass of the unconscious. These defenses constitute a refusal to accept objective reality for what it is. This cognitive escape route can be helpful when life-threatening illnesses first appear (Druss & Douglas, 1988). It is also a major, possibly necessary, stage in grieving.

TABLE 10-3
Signs and Symptoms of Denial Phase of Stress Response Syndromes

Signs	Symptoms
Perception and attention	Daze
	Selective inattention
	Inability to appreciate significance of stimuli
Consciousness	Amnesia (complete or partial)
	Non-experience
Ideational processing	Disavowal of meanings of stimuli
	Loss of reality appropriacy
	Constriction of associational width
	Inflexibility of organization of thought
	[F]antasies to counteract reality
Emotional	Numbness
Somatic	Tension–inhibition-type symptoms
Actions	Frantic overactivity to withdrawal

SOURCE: Horowitz (1979).

Mardi Horowitz (1979) wrote extensively about the psychological responses to serious life events. He outlined the signs and symptoms of denial that occur in stress reactions; these appear in Table 10-3. Despite its helpfulness in some situations, denial may be self-defeating. Extreme denial may prevent healthy coping and slow down progression to other stages of adjustment to and recovery from emergency situations. The more denial or suppression distort reality, the more likely the outcome will be negative.

Another intrapsychic defense is **intellectualization,** a process of translating feelings into a thought process. It blocks out feelings we do not want to deal with immediately. Clinical theory treats denial as a primitive defense and intellectualization as a more mature means of defending against unwanted emotions (Vaillant, 1977). A major problem exists when people intellectualize to such an extent that they filter all feelings through the rational net and thus can never express their emotions.

Negative Coping: Escape through Self-Medicating

Finally, some people cope through **addictions** or *self-medication* behaviors. Using tranquilizers, alcohol, and other drugs to reduce arousal or blunt the effect of stress falls in this category. Excessive use of medications for pain relief is also negative coping. Even children dealing with dental or arthritic pain reported taking medicine as a likely means of coping with pain (Branson & Craig, 1988).

These behaviors are negative diversions, although they may be successful from a personal point of view. The long-term effects are generally self-defeating, and the behaviors themselves entail risks and health hazards. Sorbi and Tellegen

(1988) showed that migraine patients reduced their use of medications following either cognitive stress-coping training or relaxation training. They also increased assertive and problem-solving behaviors and reduced depressive reactions.

Structuring: Putting It All Together

Structuring refers to ways in which we assemble or organize coping resources, then use these resources in anticipation of a stressful event. Stress inoculation is a technique that serves this purpose.

COPING STYLES: HOW DO YOU TYPICALLY MANAGE STRESS?

Coping styles are stereotypic reactions to stress. They are habitual or preferred ways to approach a problem or crisis (Menaghan, 1983). Some people tend to be aggressive and combative in the face of threat, whereas others are submissive and reticent. Cohen and Roth (1984) used the labels of "approachers" and "avoiders" to capture this distinction in their study of women coping with the stress of abortion. In common parlance, the approacher feels that doing something is better than doing nothing. The avoider feels that you can wait it out before you can beat it out. Some may blame others and thus blunt potential stress, whereas others perpetually blame themselves and add to their stress.

One research group distinguished between *proactive* and *reactive* styles (Adams, Hayes, & Hopson, 1976). The proactive person tries to act early to prevent stress from developing. The reactive person takes few preventive measures and reacts impulsively whenever stress occurs. Another difference in coping concerns cognitive styles. Some people are more reflective, whereas others are more impulsive, which also may influence the course of coping efforts.

Irving Janis (1983b) described the following five patterns of coping strategies associated with specific prior conditions and levels of stress:

1. *Unconflicted adherence.* This can also be called the bulldozer or submarine strategy. The strategy is to put the blade to the wall and keep pushing, or damn the torpedoes, full speed ahead. The person continues past action patterns, displaying little interest in outside information and slight regard for risks.

2. *Unconflicted change.* Here, the person would rather switch than fight. It makes little difference what friends or professionals recommend as long as the recommendation carries strong conviction. The person immediately and uncritically follows the recommended new course of action.

3. *Defensive avoidance.* In this type of coping strategy, the person uses cognitive and behavioral schemes to avoid confronting the situation. This avoidance may involve denial, procrastination, blaming someone else, rationalization, and selective inattention.

4. *Hypervigilance.* More commonly called panic, hypervigilance is evident when the person engages in frantic searches for solutions. The person makes impulsive decisions that only compound the problem, then regrets making the decision. Hypervigilant people show evidence of deterioration in cognitive skills, probably a result of extreme emotional arousal. Deterioration occurs in repetitive thinking, reduction in the pool of available ideas, and appearance of simplistic ideas.

5. *Vigilance.* Vigilance is the most mature form of coping with stress. The person uses rational problem-solving skills and engages in systematic information searches. Vigilant people consider alternative hypotheses about the source of the difficulty and evaluate solutions in a flexible, unbiased fashion.

BUILDING COPING SKILLS

Stevens and Pfost (1984) identified eight components of typical stress management programs. These include stress information, assessment, relaxation training, cognitive restructuring, problem solving, time management, nutritional counseling, and exercise planning.

The preceding chapters provided essential principles and theories about stress and health. This information should enable you to identify sources of stress in family, school, social, and work environments. You should recognize the attitudes, beliefs, behavioral patterns, and high-risk behaviors that can add to stress. You should also understand how these sources of stress alter internal functions and thus can damage the body. These ideas form the foundation of any informed, focused stress management program. They also provide a sound base for implementing a personal health program.

Although space does not permit thorough discussion of stress assessments, your instructor may include stress assessments as class activities. In this chapter, we identified coping resources and behaviors to manage stress and reduce risks. Subsequent chapters will show how specific techniques work, including the rationale, theory, and supporting research. The first set of techniques presented will be *stress management skills.* The second set deals with *personal health programming skills.*

One widely used and generally applicable stress management technique, progressive muscle relaxation, is presented in Chapter 11. Relaxation is a tension-reduction skill. Several methods build on relaxation training, including cue-controlled relaxation, differential relaxation, and desensitization. In Chapter 12, we will discuss imagery procedures, including autogenics, desensitization, cognitive restructuring, and stress inoculation. We will review meditation and biofeedback in Chapter 13. Chapter 14 describes time management techniques, and Chapter 15 discusses nutrition, diet, and exercise.

SUMMARY

In this chapter, we have discussed various models of coping and several coping skills. The first models of coping were simple two-category models that were replaced by more sophisticated models such as Matheny's. Now, we consider several dimensions of coping efforts. Combative coping is reactive coping, putting out fires after they start. Preventive coping seeks to keep stressors from appearing.

Another important part of coping is the personal resources we bring to stressful situations. Resources include personal traits and cognitive abilities. Problem-solving ability is an important cognitive skill that usually requires high-quality information, and seeking information in general appears to be an effective coping strategy. Belief in self-efficacy is also important to effective coping efforts. One cognitive coping strategy involves restructuring. With this method, we change the meaning of stressors so they become less threatening, or possibly even challenges. Finally, social support appears to help ward off stressors, but its absence appears to be more important than its presence.

Social skills may be important as a group, but individual social skills (such as assertiveness) do not seem to enhance coping significantly. The practical implication is that one should work on a range of social skills instead of depending on only one. Negative coping strategies, such as withdrawal or denial, may be helpful in short-term coping, but long-term coping depends on more mature coping strategies.

KEY TERMS

addiction	coping strategies	positive (attention)
assertion skills	coping styles	diversion
avoidance	denial	preventive coping
catharsis	humor as coping	self-disclosure
cognitive restructuring	behavior	self-esteem
combative coping	information seeking	social support
coping (defined)	instrumental coping	stress monitoring
coping efficacy	intellectualization	tension reduction
coping resources	palliative coping	ventilating emotions

REFERENCES

Adams, J. H., Hayes, J., & Hopson, B. (1976). *Transition: Understanding and managing personal change.* London: Martin Robertson.

Allport, G. (1937). *Personality: A psychological interpretation.* New York: Henry Holt.

Bandura, A. (1977). Self-efficacy: Toward a unifying theory of behavioral change. *Psychological Review, 84,* 191–215.

Bandura, A. (1989). Human agency in social cognitive theory. *American Psychologist, 44,* 1175–1184.

Bandura, A., Reese, L., & Adams, N. E. (1982). Microanalysis of action and fear arousal as a function of differential levels of perceived self-efficacy. *Journal of Personality and Social Psychology, 43,* 5–21.

Baum, A., Fleming, R., & Singer, J. (1983). Coping with victimization by technological disaster. *Journal of Social Issues, 39,* 117–138.

Billings, A. G., & Moos, R. H. (1981). The role of coping responses and social resources in attenuating the stress of life events. *Journal of Behavioral Medicine, 4,* 139–157.

Blumenthal, J. A., Burg, M. M., Barefoot, J., Williams, R. B., Haney, T., & Zimet, G. (1987). Social support, Type A behavior, and coronary artery disease. *Psychosomatic Medicine, 49,* 331–340.

Branson, S. M., & Craig, K. D. (1988). Children's spontaneous strategies for coping with pain: A review of the literature. *Canadian Journal of Behavioural Science, 20,* 402–412.

Cohen, L., & Roth, S. (1984). Coping with abortion. *Journal of Human Stress, 10,* 140–145.

Cohen, S., & Wills, T. A. (1985). Stress, social support, and the buffering hypothesis. *Psychological Bulletin, 98,* 310–357.

Cotler, S. B., & Guerra, J. J. (1980). *Assertion training.* Champaign, IL: Research Press.

Doleys, D. M., Meredith, R. L., & Ciminero, A. R. (Eds.). (1982). *Behavioral medicine: Assessment and treatment strategies.* New York: Plenum.

Druss, R. G., & Douglas, C. J. (1988). Adaptive responses to illness and disability: Healthy denial. *General Hospital Psychiatry, 10,* 163–168.

Fernandez, E., & Turk, D. C. (1989). The utility of cognitive coping strategies for altering pain perception: A meta-analysis. *Pain, 38,* 123–135.

Folkman, S., & Lazarus, R. S. (1980). An analysis of coping in a middle-aged community sample. *Journal of Health and Social Behavior, 21,* 219–239.

Haan, N. (1977). *Coping and defending: Processes of self-environment organization.* New York: Academic Press.

Hargie, O. (Ed.). (1986). *A handbook of communication skills.* New York: New York University Press.

Horowitz, M. J. (1979). Psychological response to serious life events. In V. Hamilton & D. M. Warburton (Eds.), *Human stress and cognition: An information processing approach* (pp. 235–263). New York: Wiley.

Janis, I. L. (1983a). The role of social support in adherence to stressful decisions. *American Psychologist, 38,* 143–160.

Janis, I. L. (1983b). Stress inoculation in health care: Theory and research. In D. Meichenbaum & M. E. Jaremko (Eds.), *Stress reduction and prevention* (pp. 67–99). New York: Plenum.

King, A. C., Winett, R. A., & Lovett, S. B. (1986). Enhancing coping behaviors in at-risk populations: The effects of time-management instruction and social support in women from dual-earner families. *Behavior Therapy, 17,* 57–66.

Kirkham, M. A., Schilling, R. F., Norelius, K., & Schinke, S. P. (1986). Developing coping styles and social support networks: An intervention outcome study with mothers of handicapped children. *Child: Care, Health and Development, 12,* 313–323.

Klingman, A. (1985). Mass inoculation in a community: The effect of primary prevention of stress reactions. *American Journal of Community Psychology, 13,* 323–332.

Leavy, R. L. (1983). Social support and psychological disorder: A review. *Journal of Community Psychology, 11,* 3–21.

Mader, T. F., & Mader, D. C. (1990). *Understanding one another: Communicating interpersonally.* Dubuque, IA: William C. Brown.

Marsh, P. (Ed.). (1988). *Eye to eye: How people interact.* Topsfield, MA: Salem House.

Martin, R. A., & Lefcourt, H. M. (1983). Sense of humor as a moderator of the relation between stressors and moods. *Journal of Personality and Social Psychology, 45,* 1313–1324.

Matheny, K. B., Aycock, D. W., Pugh, J. L., Curlette, W. L., & Silva-Cannella, K. A. (1986). Stress coping: A qualitative and quantitative synthesis with implications for treatment. *Counseling Psychologist, 14,* 499–549.

McLaughlin, M., Cormier, L. S., & Cormier, W. H. (1988). Relation between coping strategies and distress, stress, and marital adjustment of multiple-role women. *Journal of Counseling Psychology, 35,* 187–193.

Menaghan, E. G. (1983). Individual coping efforts: Moderators of the relationship between life stress and mental health outcomes. In H. B. Kaplan (Ed.), *Psychosocial stress: Trends in theory and research* (pp. 157–191). New York: Academic Press.

Nack, W. (1986, February 26). This case was one for the books. *Sports Illustrated,* pp. 34–42.

O'Leary, A. (1985). Self-efficacy and health. *Behaviour Research and Therapy, 23,* 437–451.

Richmond, V. P., McCroskey, J. C., & Payne, S. K. (1987). *Nonverbal behavior in interpersonal relations.* Englewood Cliffs, NJ: Prentice-Hall.

Scheier, M., & Carver, C. S. (1987). Dispositional optimism and physical well-being: The influence of generalized outcome expectancies on health. *Journal of Personality, 55,* 169–210.

Schill, T., & O'Laughlin, S. (1984). Humor preference and coping with stress. *Psychological Reports, 55,* 309–310.

Schultz, B. J., & Saklofske, D. H. (1983). Relationship between social support and selected measures of psychological well-being. *Psychological Review, 53,* 847–850.

Shapiro, J. (1983). Family reactions and coping strategies in response to the physically ill or handicapped child: A review. *Social Science and Medicine, 17,* 913–931.

Sorbi, M., & Tellegen, B. (1988). Stress-coping in migraine. *Social Science and Medicine, 26,* 351–358.

Stevens, M. J., & Pfost, K. S. (1984). Stress management interventions. *Journal of College Student Personnel, 25,* 269–270.

Stone, A. A., & Neale, J. M. (1984). New measure of daily coping: Development and preliminary results. *Journal of Personality and Social Psychology, 46,* 892–906.

Suls, J., & Fletcher, B. (1985). The relative efficacy of avoidant and nonavoidant coping strategies: A meta-analysis. *Health Psychology, 4,* 249–288.

Taylor, S. E. (1983). Adjustment to threatening events: A theory of cognitive adaptation. *American Psychologist, 38,* 1161–1173.

Vaillant, G. E. (1977). *Adaptation to life.* Boston: Little, Brown.

Wiedenfeld, S. A., O'Leary, A., Bandura, A., Brown, S., Levine, S., & Raske, K. (1990). Impact of perceived self-efficacy in coping with stressors on components of the immune system. *Journal of Personality and Social Psychology, 59,* 1082–1094.

Witmer, J. M. (1986). Stress coping: Further considerations. *The Counseling Psychologist, 14,* 562–566.

Witmer, J. M., Rich, C., Barcikowski, R. S., & Mague, J. C. (1983). Psychosocial characteristics mediating the stress response: An exploratory study. *The Personnel and Guidance Journal, 62,* 73–77.

Yablin, B. A. (1986). Maximizing the disabled adolescent: Family challenges and coping techniques. *International Journal of Adolescent Medicine and Health, 2,* 223–231.

Zich, J., & Temoshok, L. (1987). Perceptions of social support in men with AIDS and ARC: Relationships with distress and hardiness. *Journal of Applied Social Psychology, 17,* 193–215.

Zuker, E. (1983). *Mastering assertiveness skills: Power and positive influence at work.* New York: American Management Association.

CHAPTER 11

Progressive Muscle Relaxation: Premises and Process

THE REAL TASK IS TO SUCCEED IN SETTING MAN FREE BY MAKING HIM MASTER OF HIMSELF.
ANTOINE DE SAINT-EXUPÉRY

While teaching off-campus courses in stress management and personal health, I have encountered several interesting and unusual cases for which relaxation offered relief. One involved a person I'll call Elaine. She suffered from chostochondritis, or Tietze's syndrome,[1] an affliction that leaves the front walls of the chest inflamed and irritated. The effects of the inflammation can be very powerful and frightening. People afflicted with chostochondritis may think they have a heart problem or a serious stomach disease. Women are more frequently afflicted than men, and the condition may intensify with tension and overwork.

When I first met her, Elaine had been suffering from this condition for nearly a year. During that time, she had obtained medical diagnosis and treatment. X-ray examination of the chest, stress tests, electrocardiograms, and other examinations revealed no physical cause. The attending physician diagnosed the condition as chostochondritis and recommended that Elaine use a heating pad whenever possible and take three aspirins four times daily. After complying with this medical regimen for a time, Elaine reported that "the chest pains continued. It was as if I were having a heart attack many times a day, although I was relieved to know this wasn't my problem."[2] Further tests for stomach and colon disease were also negative, and the doctor prescribed a stronger drug. Unfortunately, nothing seemed to work.

At the beginning of the stress management class, I assigned each student the task of researching a stress situation or personal health problem. Then each student was to design a program to reduce stress or improve health or both. Meanwhile, we began training the relaxation response.

During class discussions, we were able to piece together some vital bits of information about times and places when Elaine's chest pain seemed most likely to strike. She worked as a real estate appraiser and reported that stresses, both mental and physical, occurred frequently. Almost always, the most severe

---

[1]Technically, the term *Tietze's syndrome* designates the condition when local swelling occurs, something that does not occur in chostochondritis.
[2]Personal statement supplied by the student with permission to publish.

inflammation occurred during these periods of severe work stress. Because of this, the condition seemed to occur much more regularly than not. The recognition that stress was somehow related either to the onset or the intensification of the condition suggested that it might respond to a stress management technique such as progressive relaxation.

Therefore, we used a structured approach to introduce relaxation in relation to the condition. First, Elaine practiced relaxation, using techniques described later in this chapter, until she could induce relaxation very rapidly. Simultaneously, she monitored the frequency, intensity, and duration of the attacks. Finally, Elaine was instructed to begin the relaxation response whenever she recognized the presence of stress during the day. Over a five-week period, she reported that the frequency of attacks decreased to near zero. Even when an occasional attack occurred, it was much less intense and was over much quicker than those she had suffered prior to the training. This outcome is nearly as important as the decrease in frequency of attacks. Elaine's case showed how effective the relaxation technique can be. In approximately seven weeks, it had eliminated a painful affliction that had lasted nearly a year.

This chapter will provide an overview of the rationale for and practice of **progressive muscle relaxation (PMR).** Several methods of stress reduction build on this skill, including **cue-controlled relaxation, differential relaxation,** and desensitization.

PROGRESSIVE MUSCLE RELAXATION: THE PROMISE

Few techniques have proven as powerful and generally applicable as the relaxation technique. It has withstood the test of time, as well as stiff competition from the new kid on the block—*biofeedback.* The advantages of relaxation are many. Relaxation can be used in the privacy of one's home or exported to the office. It can enter the boardroom or the courtroom. You can take it on the road during rush-hour traffic or settle jittery nerves at 30,000 feet. Without fanfare and public recognition, it debuted at Wimbledon, restoring smoothness to tense muscles and accuracy to a champion's service.[3] It also got a novice skier down a terrifying ski slope in Utah.

Relaxation procedures can be used to treat migraine (Sorbi, Tellegen, & du Long, 1989), hypertension, insomnia, tension headaches, test anxiety, performance anxiety, flight phobias, and Raynaud's disease (Pinkerton, Hughes, & Wenrich, 1982). Reviews of clinical applications reveal that relaxation is also useful for children suffering from stress-related symptoms (Smith & Womack, 1987). Bruning and Frew (1987) suggest that relaxation is a stress management technique in its own right, with the power to lower arousal indicators of stress. Thomas Burish and his research group used relaxation training to reduce the side effects of chemotherapy in cancer patients (Burish et al., 1988). This is only a partial list of applications.

[3]This procedure, differential and graduated relaxation, will be discussed later in this chapter.

There are numerous relaxation techniques. These include PMR, autogenic training, the relaxation response, Transcendental Meditation, and hypnosis. Autogenic training, described in Chapter 12, came from Johannes Schultz's work during the early 1950s. Autogenics is an imagery-based procedure (Schultz & Luthe, 1959). The relaxation response (not to be confused with PMR) derives from Herbert Benson's (1975) interest in Transcendental Meditation. We will discuss autogenics and the relaxation response in Chapter 13. Hypnosis can be regarded as a relaxation technique only with a very broad definition of relaxation. Still, some clinicians use hypnosis in this way. I note these variations on the relaxation theme to make an important point: *The particular form of relaxation you develop is probably unimportant.* I say "probably" because we cannot state with confidence that all relaxation procedures are equivalent or interchangeable (Smith, 1988). Nonetheless, most research shows that they have similar results in practice. The most important issue is that you develop at least one tension-reduction skill to a level of practical proficiency.

The technique described here, progressive muscle relaxation, has other names, including progressive relaxation and deep muscular relaxation. It has grown steadily in popularity since its founder, Edmund Jacobson, first wrote about it in 1938. Jacobson took great care in developing progressive relaxation. In addition, many clinicians added to and refined the practice while providing a massive body of supporting data. Because of this, it is now possible to provide clear, detailed instructions on how to practice and apply PMR. Learning relaxation, then, does not require one-on-one, high-cost therapy. With careful attention to a few guidelines and some diligent practice, most people can begin to practice PMR in a short time.

It is important to note that relaxation training involves more than just learning how to relax. It includes learning to spot signs of stress in mind and body and to connect these signs to the conditions present in your environment. Ultimately, it also includes learning to apply the skill selectively to a variety of situations and individual muscle groups.

FROM PROMISE TO PREMISE

Relaxation training relies on a simple assumption: You cannot be relaxed and tense simultaneously. In spite of the apparent simplicity of this statement, there is much more to it than that. Tension and relaxation are body states that correspond to two parts of the nervous system, the sympathetic and the parasympathetic. Because we discussed the operation of these two autonomic components in Chapter 5, here we will just review the elements that pertain to the relaxation technique.

Recall that when we are in an aroused state, as when threatened, afraid, angry, or excited, the sympathetic nervous system is in control. This is the *fight-or-flight* system, or the emergency system. Blood rushes from the digestive tract to provide energy to important muscle groups, such as the arms and legs. Heart rate increases, and blood pressure usually rises as well. During aroused states, the body burns energy at a tremendous rate. Breathing rate increases, and sweating may occur. Sympathetic arousal, then, is a tearing-down process.

During sympathetic arousal, *muscle tension increases dramatically.* This tension is not an all-or-nothing affair, though. Depending on the type of stress, only certain muscle groups may tense. Which group tenses usually depends on factors unique to your body and your way of dealing with stress. Some people feel tension in the back, some in the forehead, some in the neck, and so on. Also, muscle tension varies on a continuum from slight to extreme depending on the severity of the stressor.

Conversely, when we are in a quiet, contented mood or asleep, the parasympathetic system is in control. Heart rate slows, blood pressure normally drops, and breathing becomes slow and easy. Blood returns to the center of the body for digestion and energy storage. Muscle tension decreases, and people generally report a feeling of muscular heaviness or relaxation. This is a building-up or restoring process.

Parasympathetic processes are the opposite of sympathetic processes. In technical terms, these two systems are reciprocally inhibitory; that is, they inhibit each other alternately. In less technical terms, when one system is loud, the other system must be quiet. When one is dominant, the other must be subordinate. Both systems cannot be highly active at once. Again, in behavioral terms, you cannot be tense and relaxed simultaneously.

This relationship seems intuitively obvious, even simple. Jacobson recognized this but took it a step further. He claimed that we could directly control the balance in the autonomic nervous system. In making this claim, though, he challenged established scientific theory. The prevailing scientific view held that the autonomic nervous system, which controls nearly all life-support functions, is an *involuntary* system. Scientists assumed it was involuntary because the processes continue whether we are asleep or awake. On the surface, this logic seemed acceptable.

Still, a long history of observations and research began to expose the label's fallacy. One line of evidence came from joint American and Indian research teams who studied the remarkable Yogis. These investigations revealed that Yogis could produce extraordinary changes in body processes. They survived burial for two or three days through heart and respiratory control. They regulated body heat to withstand freezing temperatures with scant clothing. They altered brain waves through self-induced trances. The research team agreed that the Yogis showed clear control capability, even though the mechanisms were not immediately obvious (Anand, Chhina, & Singh, 1961; Bagchi & Wenger, 1959).

The dilemma was clear: What should be done with the theory of the involuntary nervous system? True to the scientific spirit, numerous investigators conducted more controlled studies and confirmed that these responses could be controlled voluntarily (Kamiya, 1969; Miller, 1969). It was Jacobson who put two and two together in the relaxation training program. Very simply stated, *relaxation is a voluntary behavioral method of controlling the alternating relationship between the excited and calm sides of your autonomic nervous system.* You can put the parasympathetic system back in control through practiced relaxation. When the sympathetic system is loud—your stomach is tied in knots, your muscles are tense, or a headache makes your head feel like a drum—you can quiet it down behaviorally.

A COGNITIVE-BEHAVIORAL VIEW OF RELAXATION

Before moving on to relaxation procedures, we must discuss a recent theoretical controversy about what occurs during relaxation. Jonathan Smith (1988) challenged the popular notion that relaxation primarily reduces arousal. Smith believes that this arousal model of relaxation is more incomplete than incorrect. He also questioned the interchangeability assumption proposed by Benson (1975). This is the notion that various relaxation techniques are interchangeable and will lead to identical outcomes. Smith's **cognitive-behavioral theory of relaxation** attempts to round out the incomplete arousal model of relaxation.

Smith proposed that three cognitive processes are involved in relaxation: focusing, passivity, and receptivity. Focusing is the ability to maintain attention to a single stimulus for an extended period. Passivity is the ability to stop customary goal-directed activity or analytic pursuits and become quiescent for a period. Receptivity is the ability to tolerate and be open to uncertain or paradoxical experiences. According to Smith, learning relaxation involves altering cognitive schemata in many ways.

These cognitive schemata include the notion that being a productive, valued member of family and society requires constant activity, wage-earning, and social involvement. Inactivity is nonproductive, if not a sign of laziness. In this view, we exaggerate the value of those behaviors that directly lead to goal attainment. We devalue, if not ignore, indirect behaviors, such as restoring energy and creativity through diversions. As relaxation progresses, convergent cognitive structures emerge that support the value of focusing, passivity, and openness. In addition, divergent cognitive structures that interfere with relaxation slowly dissipate.

Positive relaxation experiences provide support for convergent structures. As practice continues, the ability to control arousal provides more positive feedback. In addition, the person becomes aware of differences between relaxation and tension both sensorily and cognitively. Cognitive structures emerge, allowing one to label and articulate changes that accompany relaxation. Simultaneously, the person abandons irrational or incorrect cognitive structures that interfere with relaxation. The result is a changed set of beliefs about self and the value of activity versus passivity. In Smith's model, arousal is controllable, but it is only one component in a complex process of cognitive change.

Although Smith believes a family resemblance exists between the relaxation techniques, he also thinks the techniques differ greatly in demands on the cognitive system. Progressive muscle relaxation is concrete and undemanding, whereas meditative techniques are more demanding. He suggests that the more demanding techniques are also more threatening and take longer to learn. Still, people who begin with a concrete method probably will progress to more complex cognitive structures. Until recently, though, clinical research showed little concern for theoretical niceties such as those contained in Smith's view.

FROM PREMISE TO PREPARATION

Clinicians believe four conditions are important prerequisites for successful relaxation practice:[4] setting, mood, preparation, and medical precautions.

Setting

Where you practice relaxation can affect success and consistency. First, *select a comfortable room where you can isolate yourself from family or friends for a while.* The room should be properly ventilated in the summer and adequately warm in the winter. Use a comfortable chair that provides support for the entire body. A recliner is ideal, but avoid the fully reclined position; the temptation to sleep may interfere with learning. Some clinicians insist on a hard, straight-backed chair for initial training. The reason is that *you should practice relaxation for the first few weeks with an optimal level of self-awareness and observation.* Extended use of the technique requires that you can recognize the difference between muscle tension and relaxation. That awareness cannot come if you are nearly asleep.

The room in which you practice should be quiet and free from distractions. Disconnect the telephone if possible or ask a family member to answer the phone immediately. Try not to worry about missed phone calls. Recognize that you have a right to privacy and a right to time for yourself. You can choose not to have that privacy invaded.

With family members, it is probably best to appeal to their understanding by explaining what you are doing and why it is important. Enlisting family support can help reduce the likelihood of chance interruptions. This may work well with older children but not as well with younger children. Here, a simple matter of timing may suffice. Try to practice during their naps or after they have gone to bed in the evening.

An important condition for early success is consistency. *Practice relaxation exercises twice daily at roughly the same time each day for the first three to four weeks.* This will increase the likelihood of success and speed development of the skill. Be flexible in applying this rule. Some books recommend even more daily practice, up to four times per day. Experience suggests that such a recommendation is hard to follow because of its sheer impracticality. Further, no evidence suggests that you will progress faster with more sessions.

Finally, *use background music during practice if you wish.* The right type of music can foster a sense of tranquility and aid relaxation. Quiet classical or

---

[4]A detailed set of instructions appears in the Appendix. Other methods for presenting instructions (audiotapes, for example) are also discussed there.

easy-listening music is probably preferable. Clinics often use "nature" music, such as sounds of wind and seashore and calls of whales and porpoises. Whatever you choose, play it at a low volume so you will not be attending to the music more than to the relaxation exercise.

Mood

Approaching daily practice in the right frame of mind is important both to objective success and to the subjective sense of satisfaction. The following are the most important rules for setting the mood.

Cultivate a sense of passive attention Learning relaxation well requires a balance between attention and quiescence. The key to using relaxation anywhere is that you can read muscle tension whether it is loud or soft. Jacobson designed the sequence of instructions to attain this outcome, especially in the early stages of practice. Muscle tension is the body's red-light warning system that indicates when you are under stress. Passive attention is necessary for learning to discern when tension is present. Strained attention relegates everything else to secondary importance and adds more tension to the system. Passive attention can be likened to listening with an inner or third ear; it goes on with no conscious thought.

Do not try to make relaxation happen This is not a task like jogging. You do not have to sweat and strain to master relaxation. It is not a technique to beat into submission. It is, instead, a technique that comes quietly and gently.

Do not hurry Relaxation is not like lunch hour, to be rushed through to get back to more important things. It is more like prayer and meditation. It is like lying on a beach soaking up rays or lounging in a boat listening to the lapping and rocking of gentle waves. At these moments, time is the least important condition of existence. As you become more skilled, you may come to regret that tranquility must be abandoned for the clamor of the real world. Getting through the exercises is not what is important: Experiencing the moment is.

Do not use drugs Although certain drugs may help you relax, drugs will interfere with the primary goal of relaxation training: learning to recognize muscular tension that signals stress. Tranquilizing drugs, for example, depress normal brain function. Thus, it may be more difficult to recognize *real signals* of body tension as opposed to *noise* generated by the drugs. Developing sensitivity to body signals will be harder, not easier. If you are on medication by doctor's order, wait until you are off the medication to begin relaxation.

Train first; apply later A major mistake in developing a technique like relaxation is trying to use it on big jobs right away. Then, when it doesn't work, for whatever reason, one tends to blame the technique and quit. This can lead to frustration and possibly feelings of helplessness and hopelessness. Master the technique and its extensions before moving on.

Do not be afraid of different feelings   The practice of relaxation can produce anxiety and other novel sensations. Among those who learn relaxation, about 40% experience some anxiety. To explain, the experience of very deep relaxation can produce a feeling of loss of control and strong feelings of fear. It appears that the thought of losing control frightens some people. We do not know how to explain *why* they feel this way, only *that* they do. The feeling generally passes quickly as they experience the benefits of relaxation. Relaxation may not be the method of choice when a person has a history of extreme anxiety reactions (Heide & Borkovec, 1983).

Clients also report feeling they will not be able to come back. The sensation of deep relaxation seems like a hypnotic trance with no one around to guide them back. In reality, coming out of relaxation is no more difficult and no more aversive than waking up from a nap. In many ways, the heavy feeling and tranquil state of mind are similar to feelings in a nap state. Although the sensations are different, you may come to welcome and enjoy these sensations before long.

Medical Precautions

Persons with physical conditions such as severe back injuries, recent muscle strains, or broken bones should exercise caution. *Ask your physician if it is safe to engage in an exercise that will place a moderate strain on bones and muscles.* With strains or broken bones, you may have to wait for complete healing before beginning your practice. For severe back injuries, procedures such as autogenics (see Chapter 12) or Benson's relaxation response (see Chapter 13) may be suitable. Benson's technique is meditative, passive, and intuitive and thus eliminates any muscle tension exercise.

Also, persons with a history of heart difficulty should seek advice from their physician before beginning. Problems may occur when there is a history of heart difficulty combined with a current severe cold, especially a cold with chest congestion. Deep-breathing exercises could be painful, leading to anxiety, which in turn could aggravate a heart condition.

RELAXATION: THE PROCESS

Relaxation exercises follow a sequence of alternating tension and relaxation in 16 muscle groups. Table 11-1 shows a typical sequence beginning with the hands and arms. This sequence can be altered to suit personal preference. Some people feel more comfortable working from head to feet, while others may work a reverse sequence from feet to head. There is no evidence that one sequence is better than another. Also, the number of muscle groups may vary depending on grouping. Some clinicians suggest that the tongue and jaw muscles should

TABLE 11-1
Sequence and Timing for Self-Directed Progressive Muscular Relaxation

---

Sequence guide for relaxation practice

---

1. Preferred arm
2. Alternate arm
3. Preferred hand
4. Alternate hand
5. Shoulder muscles
   a. Preferred-hand side
   b. Alternate side
6. Neck muscles
7. Forehead, eyes, scalp
8. Jaws and mouth (tongue, optionally as extra step)
9. Breathing—chest and trunk
10. Stomach
11. Lower back
12. Buttocks
13. Preferred thigh
14. Alternate thigh
15. Preferred foot and calf
16. Alternate foot and calf

Additional reminders:
 2 sessions per day, same time, same place
 3 repetitions for each muscle set
10–15 seconds for tension sets
15–20 seconds for relaxation sets
45–75 minutes for the first few sessions
Sessions will be greatly reduced in length after the first few sessions.

---

be treated as separate groups. Again, there is no evidence that this is crucial to success.

Tension-relaxation cycles should be about 30 seconds each, with slightly more time given to relaxation than to tension. Early sessions may require approximately 45 to 75 minutes to finish. Later, much less time is needed for relaxation. Experienced practitioners can reach complete body relaxation in about 5 to 15 minutes. Reducing time also requires shortcut techniques, described later in this chapter.

As a first step to making relaxation a useful stress management technique, it is important to spend the allotted time studying the difference between tension and relaxation. *These differences in muscle sensations exaggerate the signals that occur during stress.* Studying these contrasts develops sensitivity to signs of tension and adds to the utility of relaxation.

Frequently, people report feeling pressured, but they do not know why they feel that way. They also do not seem to know the source of the pressure.

This may be because they do not hear the warning signals from their body. Even when they do hear, some do not understand the connection to what is going on around them. When you can detect subtle changes in muscular tension, you can also look for the event that triggered it. When the alarm sounds, the natural response should be: Who is present? What is the situation? What is the theme of the conversation? Money? Sex? Control? How am I responding? Defensively, aggressively, angrily? Has this cycle happened before? In this way, the red-light warning system can help us detect the sources of stress.

A TENSION-SCANNING EXERCISE

To aid this learning, carry out a simple exercise for a full week. Make a mental note each day that you have one personal project to do: namely, *tune in* to signs of muscular tension. During this week, observe body tension reactions all day, not just during relaxation. Carry a small notebook or diary with you. Whenever you spot signs of muscular tension, record the time, place, and people involved. If you cannot do so immediately, then record it as quickly as possible without disrupting your normal routine.

The event may be loud and long or quiet and short. It may involve many muscle groups or only an isolated muscle. Yet it will result in noticeable change. Look for signs of tension: neck muscles cramping, shoulder muscles knotting up, lower back muscles tightening, stomach knotting, forehead muscles tensing, jaws clenching, teeth grinding, fists doubling, breathing increasing, and heart pounding. The objective is to learn how to identify tension signals in the real world before you become distressed or physically sick.

MOVING ON:
WHEN CAN I DO SOMETHING WITH IT?

One practical problem is how to know when it is suitable to move on. First, allow at least two weeks for basic practice before proceeding. Second, gauge the depth of relaxation and your satisfaction with it. In clinical research, formal procedures exist to do this, but this is unnecessary in practice. You should experience both deep relaxation and personal pleasure with relaxation before applying the skill. Third, monitor the amount of time it takes to become relaxed. You should become relaxed in less than 30 minutes before trying advanced procedures.

GETTING RELAXED THE FAST WAY

If you had to spend 30 minutes to become relaxed every time and needed a recliner and quietness, you might question how useful the technique could be. As you will see, you can reduce tension quickly and quietly through a combination of techniques that make a total package of relaxation training.

First I will describe a method of relaxing entire groups of muscles together. Then we will discuss a method called *cue-controlled relaxation*. With this method, a single word that you associate with relaxing can be your password to reduced tension. Later, I will describe how to relax one muscle group by itself through the technique of differential and graduated relaxation.

RELAXING A GROUP OF MUSCLES

The 16-step sequence described earlier relaxed each muscle as though it were separate from any other muscle. It is possible, however, to relax groups of muscles together. Typically, we use five stages to reduce the time to relaxation. Two stages reduce the number of muscle groups; three stages reduce the amount of voluntary muscle tension.

From Sixteen to Eight Steps

For the first few days, relax (1) both arms together, (2) both hands together, (3) both shoulders and neck muscles, (4) the forehead with scalp, jaws and mouth together, (5) both chest and stomach muscles, (6) lower back and buttocks together, (7) both thighs, and (8) both calves and feet together. The 16-step procedure is now 8 steps. This phase usually requires about five days. Table 11-2 shows the steps to take.

At first you may encounter difficulty with tension-relaxation contrasts. The arms, hands, and legs are probably the easiest. Continue to study the contrasts in tension and relaxation. Some people have difficulty with the head muscles because several very different muscles are in this group. If you encounter this, continue to relax the muscles in this group as separate muscles. Practice with the other combined muscle groups until you are successful, then return to the head muscles.

Now Softer on the Tension

The next step is to reduce the intensity of tension in the tension-relaxation cycle. Instead of tensing the biceps very tightly, tense them a moderate amount. For all muscle groups, lower the amount of tension without reducing the amount of time in the tension cycle itself. Do not change the relaxation cycle in any way.

To help with this step, imagine muscle tension on a 100-point scale. The high end of the scale corresponds to the highest tension. The low end corresponds to the deepest relaxation. For the first step, imagine what your muscles would feel like at the 75-point mark on the scale and try to tense to about that 75% level. The scale is very subjective and personal, with no absolutes.

This step may seem paradoxical, but we alluded to the rationale earlier. Ultimately, you should be able to sense tension whenever and wherever it occurs.

TABLE 11-2
Guide for Reduction Steps in Relaxation Practice

First reduction set	*Second reduction set*
1. Both arms	1. Both arms and hands
2. Both hands	
3. Shoulder and neck	2. Shoulders, neck, and head
4. All head muscles	
5. Chest and stomach	3. Chest, stomach, lower back, and buttocks
6. Lower back and buttocks	
7. Both thighs	4. Thighs, feet, and calves
8. Both feet and calves	

Additional Reminders:
 2 sessions per day, same time, same place
 3 repetitions for each muscle group
10–15 seconds for tension sets
15–20 seconds for relaxation sets
25–35 minutes for the first few sessions
Sessions will be reduced in length after the first few sessions.
Reduce tension about 25% after you reach the main criterion and before going on to the second set. Reduce tension about 25% more at the end of the second reduction set.
Reduce tension about another 25% and practice to criterion. Go on to cue-controlled relaxation.

To do this, you need to sense subtle tension just as easily as nagging tension. When you can spot the whispers of stress as readily as the screams, you will begin to realize the benefits of relaxation. Reducing tension voluntarily in these exercises will teach you to discriminate degrees of tension.

There is another important reason for reducing tension. The portability of relaxation depends on your ability to become relaxed quickly. When you have finished reducing the muscle groups to four, you should have phased out the intense tightening routine. From that point, you will return to the tension cycles only when you need a booster.

From Eight Muscle Groups to Four

Table 11-2 also shows the second reduction set. The procedure is the same as before. Try to relax all the muscles in a group together. Again, if you have any difficulty with a group of muscles, go back to the previous mastery step for that muscle group. The idea is to be flexible; the rules are not absolute. There is nothing wrong with using nine muscle groups in the first reduction phase or five muscle groups in the second phase. Allow yourself freedom to read your body, and adjust the groupings so they feel right. This phase should take another five to seven days.

Even Softer on the Tension

At the end of the first reduction phase, you reduced voluntary tension to about 75% of maximum. The goal now is to reduce it even further. Try to imagine how your muscles would feel when tensed to about 50% on the scale. For another week, use this 50% standard for the tension phase.

Now Ever So Softly

The last step is to reduce the level of induced muscle tension to about 25% of the original level. Try to imagine the 25% level on the scale, and tense to that level. This may take another three to five days. You should still reach deep relaxation, and you should become relaxed as quickly as before. You may find that you can achieve deep relaxation in 5 to 15 minutes. If so, congratulate yourself and feel well rewarded for your efforts.

To review, progressively reduce the number of steps to reach relaxation by grouping muscles together. Also reduce the amount of voluntary muscle tension as follows.

1. Reduce from 16 muscle sets to 8 muscle groups over five to seven days. When you can relax as quickly and almost as deeply as before, go to step 2.
2. Reduce the amount of artificially induced muscle tension to about 75% of the original level. Practice until you can relax as quickly and deeply as before, then go to step 3.
3. Reduce from 8 muscle groups to 4 muscle groups over five to seven days. Practice until you can relax quickly and deeply, then go to step 4.
4. Reduce the amount of artificially induced muscle tension to about 50% of the original level. Practice until you can relax as quickly and deeply as before, then go to step 5.
5. Reduce the amount of voluntarily induced muscle tension to roughly 25%.

TERRIFYING SLOPES: RELAXATION TO THE RESCUE

Life can have its terrifying moments, even when you are having fun. Such was the case when I combined a business trip with some skiing pleasure on the slopes at Park City, Utah. Although I had been on skis just once before, the morning went wonderfully. After lunch I somehow ended up on a slope that completely disappeared from view. It had beautiful moguls—many, many moguls, tightly packed and small. For me, it was too much too soon. The end was a humbling slide on my posterior, skis in hand, while supportive souls in the lift above found their afternoon lightened by this comic sight. Yet the real terror was still ahead.

A quick search of the trail map revealed a green-marked trail, the beginner's route down the mountain. I settled back, relieved that I would have a pleasant cruise to the bottom where I could count my ego losses, reconstruct my self-image, and prepare for a frontal assault on the mountains another day. At first the trail looked like a gentle, slowly winding descent down the mountain. Of course it wasn't really the easy trail. It was only the easiest from that part of the mountain.

My partner and I skied past a rope tied with red flags and signs warning of danger. Beyond was a sheer, ice-packed slope that looked as though it went straight down. It had just one purpose: to convey any object in a straight line as fast as possible to the bottom. Only later did I learn that it was the downhill race course. For now, that sheer cliff was beyond the rope, and here where I was skiing, that beautiful trail still stretched out gently in front of me. It vanished around a cluster of trees ahead. That could only mean one thing—the *real* trail must continue somewhere beyond and to the side of this ice sled. But, disappearing around the trees wasn't half of it. The trail wound around those trees and disappeared—right onto the top of that downhill course. Now there was no way back, around, or down . . . except!

My terror was complete. I had never seen anything like this. My partner gave a brief reassuring smile and a "See you at the bottom" salute. He pointed his skis down the slope and gracefully rounded a ridge at the bottom before I could even consider what to do. If only I could be off this mountain that fast.

My problem was with my body and my mind. Both had to be calmed before I could get down that hill. My mind was a jumble of thoughts. My body felt like muscular pretzels. Every inch was in knots except my knees, which wouldn't stand still for anything.

I went through two processes to get down that mountain: thought stopping and muscular relaxation. The mental process combined rational problem solving and an emotional control process to drive the frightening, self-defeating thoughts out of my head. The relaxation process was to get my body under control. If you watch professional skiers, you realize how fluid and loose they look. Whether it is Michael Jordan doing a spectacular slam dunk, or Boris Becker making a reflex shot at the net, muscular tension is the athlete's enemy.

Because I had practiced the technique before, it took just a few minutes to achieve relaxation, even on this mountain slope. I concentrated on the major tense spots—my stomach, shoulders, and legs. Finally, I planned a path down the mountain that included several traverses. This helped mentally as well because I recognized that I could control my speed with this technique. I must have spent several minutes transfixed in the middle of that course thinking and relaxing. Then I began the trip down. The first traverse and turn was tense, but I felt the ski edges bite and carve. My confidence went up, and the next turn was crisp and clean. It now seemed more like fun, and before I knew it, there was the bottom of that once terrifying slope. I must have felt some degree of arrogance, then, because I turned and gave a defiant salute to the mountain. I also praised myself for a victory over both the physical elements and the fear that only moments before had been my oppressor.

These are obviously not the conditions in which you should practice relaxation the first time. Once you have developed the skill, though, you may be surprised where you can take relaxation. This incident illustrates the use of two different procedures: cue-controlled relaxation and differential relaxation. In the next few pages, we will examine these techniques to see how they might operate in stress management.

RELAXING WITH A WORD

Most instructions for relaxation suggest that you use a cue word with breathing; for example: "Breathe out, and as you do, say 'Relax.'" This instruction forms the core of cue-controlled relaxation. The secret of the technique is simple: the repeated connection between a cue and a response makes it possible for the cue to produce the response automatically. A familiar example may help to illustrate this point.

When you were born, many cues, such as words, did not have any real power to control or change your behavior in and of themselves. Through a long process of learning, words become connected to important events in such a way that they now alter your behavior as directly as the events themselves did.

"Stop!" and "No!" mean nothing to an infant. Along the way, many connections will be made between such commands and something dangerous the child is doing. When children first touch a hot stove, they encounter a powerful incentive to withdraw the hand—burning pain. Pain usually leads to quick and permanent learning. If the parent is nearby, the child may hear a loud "No, no!" just before touching the stove. If so, a quick yet permanent connection may be built between the command and the dangerous event. Over time, many repeated connections between a cue (such as parents' warning words) and some dangerous event (such as running into a heavily traveled street) will occur. Children's ability to control their behavior will increase as they internalize additional examples of cue-response connections. It may not happen on the very first try, but it will come with time.

You may have seen another step in the development of personal control after an incident of this type. The child approaches the stove again and reaches toward the stove. Then the child stops, looks at the parent, and says "No" aloud. The word is now an internalized controlling cue. The child does not need to be burned or punished repeatedly to avoid hot stoves and onrushing cars.

The process of using a word to control relaxation is much the same. Relaxation is the response we want to control. The cue word is the signal that triggers the response of relaxation. At first, the cue word may have only a general meaning. After you repeatedly link the cue to relaxation, you can use it to induce relaxation directly. Instead of several tension-relaxation cycles, you simply say the word and relax.

What's the Word?

The particular word used is not important, although you should avoid words that occur in routine conversation. Some people use words like *peace, quiet, easy,* or *warm.* Some select a word that is similar to a **mantra,** a sacred, privileged, and secret word. Whatever word you choose, make sure that, when you breathe out, you use that word only.

Beginning Cue-Controlled Relaxation

Learning cue-controlled relaxation is usually easier than the steps you have taken to learn relaxation. There is nothing special to do except practice breathing out and using the chosen cue word. You will find abbreviated instructions in the Appendix.

Repeat the cue-controlled sequence for approximately one week. Start each relaxation period with breathing–cue-word cycles. Complete each period by using the tension-relaxation cycles to achieve relaxation if necessary. When you can reach about 50 to 75% of the relaxation you normally reach with the tension-relaxation method, you can move to the next step. You should not expect to achieve the depth of relaxation that you achieve from tension-relaxation cycles. The uses of cue-controlled relaxation do not demand complete relaxation because complete relaxation would be detrimental to its everyday use.

Using Cue-Controlled Relaxation

In addition to knowing how to produce cue-controlled relaxation, you need to know where and when to use it. Earlier in this chapter, I suggested you keep a diary noting times, places, and people involved when you felt tension. If you did this, you should have some useful information by now to tell you where and when to practice cue-controlled relaxation. First, categorize the diary incidents of stress on two dimensions (home and work or home and school, whichever is appropriate). Then go through the events and evaluate the corresponding levels of tension (high or low). The correct classification of home, school, or work should be automatic. The correct classification for level of tension is entirely a subjective judgment.

To classify tension, start with the event that produced the most intense muscle tension. Then find the event that produced the lowest muscle tension.

Use these extremes to scale and categorize the remaining events. After you do this, you are ready to apply cue-controlled relaxation to a real situation.

Select a situation from the low-tension/home category. It is best to pick one that happens regularly so you can practice more and sooner. The next time the event occurs, prompt yourself to use cue-controlled relaxation. Take a deep breath, hold for a moment, and release it completely while you say to yourself your personal cue word. Nobody needs to know that you are cuing relaxation. In fact, it is probably best to avoid telling other people what you are doing. In the middle of an intense exchange, it might irritate others more than relieve them. You should notice a decrease in the intensity of your arousal. Most people report a *rush* of relaxation and a reduction in anxiety.

The positive effects should be even more pronounced in interpersonal relationships and problem-solving situations. Amid interpersonal conflict and crises, extreme arousal and tension reduce our ability to think clearly and to respond sensitively (Bandura, 1989). Arousal may also interfere with our ability to read verbal and nonverbal nuances in messages from others involved in the conflict. We may become defensive, responding to protect our ego and personal needs instead of listening to the needs revealed by others. Then the outcome is predictable. We miss possible solutions to the problem or overlook important clues to what the other person is really saying. Thus, we may bring tension back into the situation. Decreasing tension by cue-controlled relaxation should help prevent this defensive posturing and garbled communication.

It should now be obvious why complete relaxation is not the goal of cue-controlled relaxation. Complete relaxation would not be constructive in the middle of an interpersonal conflict or a crisis. It helps your spouse or supervisor little for you to say "Excuse me for a few minutes while I relax." During a major exam, you want to control extreme tension, but you still want some arousal. The goal is to bring tension back to an optimal, moderate level. After gaining success with a home stressor, go on to other situations for practice; just make sure they come from the low-tension category.

CUE-CONTROLLED RELAXATION
AT SCHOOL OR WORK

After success at home, go back to the diary and identify stressful situations that occur regularly at school or work. The principle is the same as before: Find a situation that will allow you to practice cue-controlled relaxation with a high degree of frequency, but one that does not have high tension. One such situation for students is the midterm exam.

When you recognize that tension is developing, use cue-controlled relaxation. Go through the same procedure as before: Take a deep breath, hold it momentarily, let the breath go, say your personal cue word to yourself, and relax. If necessary, repeat the cycle.

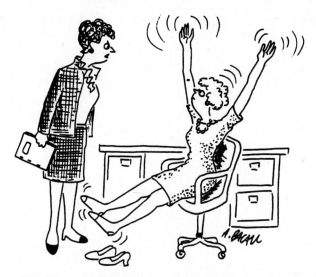

"Would you mind not going through your stress-reduction
exercises while I'm reprimanding you?"

SOURCE: *New Woman,* 1986: Reprinted with permission of A. Bacall.

Make a mental note of the effect. If you succeeded in relaxing, work with this situation until you feel you can control your tension as needed. Then do the same with other events in that category. If you did not feel a sense of moderate relaxation and some relief, reexamine the incident. Perhaps the situation was more stressful than you originally judged. Perhaps this particular episode was more stressful than it usually is. If the former, reassign the situation to the *high-tension* category and pick another event. Return to this one later. If the episode became more stressful than usual, continue with it, especially if you attained at least some degree of relaxation.

After you succeed with both home and school (or work) low-tension stress situations, move on to the high-tension stressors. It may be helpful to reexamine the situations you originally placed in the high-tension categories. First, judge whether you can make finer distinctions among the events. If so, separate the moderate stressors and work with them in the same way as before. Finally, pick a tough stressor from the school or work list. After you succeed with one of your toughest stressors, you should be close to having a useful stress management technique.

A final word of caution is in order. Cue-controlled relaxation is not a panacea. It will not make up for lack of training in areas of technical or professional expertise on the job. It will not solve problems of insensitivity, lack of impulse control, or incompetence in other people. No matter how reasonable, calm, and in control you are, this will not necessarily make other people more reasonable, calm, and in control. However, cue-controlled relaxation may help you assess when circumstances are out of your control. Then, instead of dumping pressure on yourself, you may recognize that long-term and group goals need to be negotiated. Further, you may see when you need to go to someone else for help. It is important to recognize that admitting you need outside help does not mean admitting defeat; it is more properly recognizing the limits of human abilities, an important part of realistic self-appraisal. The popular "Serenity Prayer" expresses the message well: "God grant me the serenity to accept the things I cannot change, the courage to change the things I can and the wisdom to know the difference."

DIFFERENTIAL AND GRADUATED RELAXATION

This section deals with differential and graduated relaxation, a technique that can be used in private or in public to reduce stress-induced tension and physical fatigue. This technique is widely used by professional athletes, such as tennis players, to reduce muscle tension and restore fluidity to serves and volleys. The technique depends on two essential skills: the ability to scan muscles to judge which muscle group is tense, and the ability to relax that muscle group to the level that is desirable and suited for the situation. While this may seem like a tall order, you will see that you have done much of the work already.

Mental Scanning for Tension

Scanning your body for tension should be almost second nature by now. Mental scanning for tension should be like a CB scanner, quietly but automatically scanning body channels until it finds a signal. Reducing tension on a graduated scale should be possible as well because you have practiced reducing tension to 75%, then 50%, and finally 25% of maximum tension.

Relaxing One Muscle Group

An example may help show how differential relaxation can be used. When driving in heavy traffic to meet a deadline, I sometimes find my right shoulder muscle growing very tight. I might just ignore it at first, but I soon realize that tension will make me more tired and may interfere with concentration. It also takes the pleasure out of driving.

In a situation like this, we do not want to reduce general arousal, as should occur with cue-controlled relaxation; we just want to reduce the tension in that one muscle group. Most importantly, we want to control the depth of the relaxation. Too much relaxation while driving could be dangerous. Similarly, when playing tennis or basketball, we want to maintain some muscle tension, but we want fluid tension. This is why the procedure is called *differential and graduated relaxation.*

To develop this skill, look again through your diary and judge whether one muscle group becomes tense more frequently than others. Then practice relaxing that muscle group only. Tense one muscle by itself, then relax. Make sure you are working only on that muscle and do not worry about the rest of your body. When you can achieve deep relaxation, work on graduated levels of relaxation. Try to scale tension relaxation as you did before and reduce tension first to 75%, then to 50%.

It is not necessary to produce deep relaxation with this procedure. Most clinical studies suggest that you will not be able to do that anyway. If you achieve relaxation even in the 50% range, you are probably doing very well. A 50% reduction in muscle tension will usually suffice for practical application of the technique.

Two other techniques can be combined with relaxation for better control. One is to attach a novel cue word to the muscle group. If you are typically only concerned with one muscle group, this can be quite effective; just be sure to select a cue word other than the one you use for general relaxation. Combine deep breathing and the cue word with practiced relaxation of that muscle group. With enough practice, you can reduce tension in one muscle the same way you reduce general tension—with a word. You can regulate the depth of relaxation by repetitions of breathing and cue control.

A second technique is to use visual imagery. Form a mental picture of something unique—for example, see yourself with that shoulder muscle in a whirlpool bath, with warm jets of water pulsing the muscle. See yourself receiving a massage. This is similar to the autogenic procedure, which makes extensive use of visual imagery.

When you tense the muscle during practice, the image should not be present. Just as you relax, call up the image and make it as strong as possible while you continue to relax. Another technique is to prepare slides or cut pictures from a magazine to pin on the wall. Close your eyes during the tension phase. Open your eyes and look at the picture during the relaxation phase. Try to lock the picture in your mind so it can be called up quickly and vividly. If you know you are good at imagery, this technique may be right for you. If you have difficulty forming mental images, it might be better to stick with the cue-word technique.

After some practice at home, the next step is to apply it on the go. Use your diary again. Do you still have events to deal with that are suitable targets? Maybe you play bridge regularly and find your neck muscles tense during keen competition (or because your partner does not always play well). This social situation might be a good candidate for differential relaxation.

Differential relaxation can be used in many situations. As noted earlier, this technique has found widespread acceptance among professional athletes, who need to maintain fluid muscle control even in the midst of intense competition. You can use it while driving, flying, or skydiving. Mountain climbers even use it while climbing. You might find it more useful on the tennis court or in a staff meeting.

To conclude, be sure the relaxation procedure you use is situationally appropriate. You would not want to go into a deep state of relaxation while driving. After a long, pressure-packed day at the office, deep relaxation may be very pleasurable. Differential relaxation may not be desirable in a staff meeting if general anxiety is the problem; cue-controlled relaxation would be better. Intense cramping in the neck during an exam calls for differential relaxation. The next chapter discusses extensions of the imagery technique and how to desensitize specific fears.

KEY TERMS

cognitive-behavioral
   theory of relaxation
cue-controlled
   relaxation

differential (and
   graduated)
   relaxation

mantra
progressive muscle
   relaxation (PMR)

REFERENCES

Anand, B. K., Chhina, G., & Singh, B. (1961). Some aspects of electroencephalographic studies in Yogis. *Electroencephalography and Clinical Neurophysiology, 13,* 452–456.

Bagchi, B. K., & Wenger, M. A. (1957). Electrophysiological correlates of some Yogi exercises. *EEG Clinical Neurophysiology* (Supplement No. 7), 132–149.

Bandura, A. (1989). Human agency in social cognitive theory. *American Psychologist, 44,* 1175–1184.

Benson, H. (1975). *The relaxation response.* New York: Avon Books.

Bruning, N. S., & Frew, D. R. (1987). Effects of exercise, relaxation, and management skills training on physiological stress indicators: A field experiment. *Journal of Applied Psychology, 72,* 515–521.

Burish, T. G., Vasterling, J. J., Carey, M. P., Matt, D. A., & Krozely, M. G. (1988). Posttreatment use of relaxation training by cancer patients. *The Hospice Journal, 4,* 1–8.

Heide, F. J., & Borkovec, T. D. (1983). Relaxation-induced anxiety: Paradoxical anxiety enhancement due to relaxation training. *Journal of Consulting and Clinical Psychology, 51,* 171–182.

Jacobson, E. (1938). *Progressive relaxation* (2nd ed.). Chicago: University of Chicago Press.

Kamiya, J. (1969). Operant control of the EEG alpha rhythm and some of its reported effects on consciousness. In C. T. Tart (Ed.), *Altered states of consciousness* (pp. 519–529). New York: Wiley.

Miller, N. E. (1969). Learning of visceral and glandular responses. *Science, 163,* 434–445.

Pinkerton, S. S., Hughes, H., & Wenrich, W. W. (1982). *Behavioral medicine: Clinical applications.* New York: Wiley.

Schultz, J., & Luthe, W. (1959). *Autogenic training: A psychophysiological approach to psychotherapy.* New York: Grune & Stratton.

Smith, J. C. (1988). Steps toward a cognitive-behavioral model of relaxation. *Biofeedback and Self-Regulation, 13,* 307–329.

Smith, M. S., & Womack, W. M. (1987). Stress management techniques in childhood and adolescence: Relaxation training, meditation, hypnosis, and biofeedback: Appropriate clinical applications. *Clinical Pediatrics, 26,* 581–585.

Sorbi, M., Tellegen, B., & du Long, A. (1989). Long-term effects of training in relaxation and stress-coping in patients with migraine: A 3-year follow-up. *Headache, 29,* 111–121.

CHAPTER 12

Cognitive and Imagery Techniques: Autogenics, Desensitization, and Stress Inoculation

ALL OUR INTERIOR WORLD IS REALITY—AND THAT PERHAPS MORE SO THAN OUR AP-
PARENT WORLD.
MARC CHAGALL

Tom was a 28-year-old who had suffered several years with severe colitis.[1] For nearly seven years, he had gone from doctor to doctor seeking a physical remedy. He had even checked into a prominent Midwestern medical facility for a lengthy series of tests. Still, the answer seemed to elude him, while the abdominal pain and diarrhea frequently disabled him. The first time he called me, it was for help with the colitis. Soon it became obvious that Tom's colitis was just one branch in a maze of symptoms, a complex set of anxieties and fears that prevented him from enjoying life to the fullest.

In addition to colitis, Tom had a phobic fear of meeting customers in the store where he worked. His most debilitating fear, though, was the obsession that he would be stricken by a heart attack while out with friends. This fear stemmed from a previous social engagement when he became highly aroused in the presence of a young woman. Tom found the intensity of the arousal very frightening, but that was not the worst of it. He felt guilty because of his passion and feared the woman would reject him. The result was a terrifying panic attack with hyperventilation, which can feel like a heart attack. Unfortunately, Tom gave the worst possible interpretation to the symptoms—that he had a serious heart problem. From this he reasoned that he could not ask anyone to marry him, and, at 28, became a recluse with little or no social life.

This was not the end of the symptoms, however. Tom could seldom relax and had extreme difficulty sleeping. He also had a pervasive pattern of obsessional thinking that influenced all his actions. While at work, he was obsessed with the thought that he had left the gas range turned on or the windows open at his apartment. He thought the landlord would find out and evict him. At night, Tom worried that he had left a machine on at work that would destroy the store. At times these thoughts overwhelmed him, and he would leave home in the middle of the night and walk nearly one mile to the store to reassure himself that the machine was off.

---

[1]"Tom" is a pseudonym. While Tom was my client, he related numerous specific fears that sometimes incapacitated him. Colitis is also called "irritable bowel syndrome."

Dealing with pervasive anxiety, deep-seated fears, and panic requires more than just relaxation. It requires some way of restructuring irrational thoughts and attitudes that prompt self-defeating, self-restricting behaviors. In this chapter, we will describe **autogenics,** a variation of the relaxation technique. We will also discuss **desensitization,** a technique for dealing with specific fears and obsessional thought patterns. Finally, we will examine the process of **stress inoculation training (SIT),** a technique that prepares a person to deal with stress in advance.

IMAGERY: THE CORE OF RELAXATION

In many clinical studies of relaxation and meditation, investigators have tried to discover what clients are doing internally, what they are thinking or saying to themselves to bring on deep, quieting, satisfying states of relaxation. A common thread that ran through client reports was the clients' use of mental pictures or images. For example, one person might picture a peaceful, sunlit beach and hear the soft lapping of waves and cries of sea gulls. Another might imagine being on a mountain peak looking out over a vast, beautiful, unspoiled wilderness while listening to the wind murmur through the spruce. Still another might imagine the face of a friend or lover.

Eastern meditators use a variety of imagery techniques to gain control over mind and body. During religious ecstasies, they produce a brain wave called **alpha,** a slow (12 to 14 Hz) wave form that occurs between the alert waking state and the first stages of sleep. Joe Kamiya (1969), a pioneer biofeedback researcher, showed that people could learn to control alpha rhythms with **biofeedback.** During his research program, Kamiya noted that many subjects used some form of visualization to keep alpha high. It may have been the images used more than the specific biofeedback procedure that allowed them to control alpha. Runners and other athletes also report that visualization helps in training and competition.

AUTOGENICS: IMAGERY-BASED RELAXATION

Autogenic therapy (*autogenic* means self-produced) is a relaxation technique that emphasizes imagery and self-suggestion. Autogenics is the relaxation method of choice in Europe, where the German psychiatrist Johannes Schultz introduced it in 1932. According to Schultz and his protege, Wolfgang Luthe (1959), autogenics is a means of maintaining the internal psychophysiological balance of the body. Schultz and Luthe also maintain that autogenics allows a person to plumb the depths of the unconscious. Its major appeal, though, is that autogenics is a simple procedure for beginners wanting to learn a basic tension-reducing method. Still, it is complex enough to permit more adept users to use the esoteric facets that presumably tap the recesses of the psyche. A cautionary note is important here: Advanced autogenics usually requires professional guidance to use it safely and effectively!

The training procedure for autogenics bears some resemblance to procedures for deep muscular relaxation, but some differences exist both in practice and in application. Relaxation training is a very active muscle exercise procedure that teaches the person to recognize differences between tension and relief. In autogenics, the goal is to develop an association between a verbal (thought) cue and the desired body state of calm; there are no active physical exercises as such. Thus, while autogenics focuses on body posture, imagery, and self-instructions, the body remains passive.

Preparing for Autogenic Training

Just as one takes certain steps to prepare for relaxation, Schultz and Luthe recommended several conditions for successful autogenic training:

1. A high degree of motivation and willingness to follow the instructions exactly.
2. An adequate degree of self-direction and self-control.
3. Use and maintenance of correct body posture.
4. Reduction of external stimuli and mental focusing on internal physical and mental states.
5. Use of monotonous, repetitive input to the various senses.
6. Concentration on somatic processes to produce an inward-focused consciousness as opposed to an outward-focused consciousness.

If the person meets these six conditions, he or she will soon attain a feeling of passivity, an almost vegetative state of mental activity that melts into altered consciousness.

The last two conditions are really outcomes of autogenic training, not steps in preparation. They are signs of success when the person adheres to the instructions.

7. The emergence of an overpowering, reflexive psychic reorganization.
8. The occurrence of disassociative and autonomous mental processes, leading to an alteration of ego functioning and dissolution of ego boundaries (Pelletier, 1977).

A pupil of autogenic training must be prepared to accept the altered state of awareness, look for it, and perhaps even long for it. Otherwise, its appearance may be regarded as something to be feared and rejected instead of welcomed. This could interfere with continued progress in autogenic training, if it does not result in the pupil's discarding the technique altogether.

Luthe (1969) discusses a type of reflex motor tremor that occurs during early training called the **autogenic discharge.** Crying spells may also occur during training. These are a type of emotional catharsis for pent-up mental tension. The resemblance of the reflex motor tremor to relaxation—the strange sensations that some people report—is apparent.

Maintaining passive concentration during the exercises is important to continued progress in training. Therefore, when these foreign sensations occur, do not try to fight them. Just let them pass as part of the process, as signs of progress, not failure.

The preparation rules discussed for relaxation also pertain here. That is, choose a time and place for comfort and isolation. Reduce external distractions by removing the phone or having calls intercepted. Remove tight-fitting clothes or jewelry, and prepare your mood for passive attention to the exercises.

Autogenic Body Postures

In relaxation training, the recommendation was to use a recliner in a partial reclining position. In autogenics, a person may use one of three body positions, none of which matches the prescribed relaxation posture. These three are (1) lying down, (2) seated with back support, and (3) seated without back support.

In the first position, you lie on your back on the floor with pillows or blankets to cushion the head and knees. If you use a pillow under your head, you should not throw your head forward onto your chest. A shallow pillow will cushion without misaligning your head and body. Arms should be at your side, with hands near your thighs and palms turned up. Your legs may be slightly apart, with toes pointed away from the body. Avoid using a bed so you do not fall asleep during training.

The second position requires a chair with a high, straight back. A chair with arms is fine, but not necessary. Position yourself back in the chair so both your back and your head are supported. Keep your head aligned straight over your neck and back; avoid letting it fall to either side, because correct alignment with the body axis is important to success. Arms can be supported either on the arms of the chair or in your lap if you do not use an armchair.

The third position uses a stool or low-backed chair. With either type of seat, sit forward on the stool or chair. Support your arms on your thighs, your hands dangling loosely over your knees. Your head may come forward over your chest but should not touch the chest. Keep your feet about shoulder-width apart and just slightly forward of the knees.

The image of the doll suggested by Schultz and Luthe may help you visualize this position. Imagine you are a big rag doll puppet with a string attached to the top of your head. The string pulls you upright in the chair. Because you are a rag doll, you will be completely limp, legs and arms dangling with no tension. Then, imagine that the string breaks. What would happen to the doll? The head, neck, and shoulders would collapse forward. This is the posture you want. Take care that your head and chest do not roll so far forward that you restrict breathing.

In the seated positions, you will not attain the degree of muscular relaxation that occurs while reclining because the muscles must continue to support the body. Still, you can obtain adequate relaxation if you concentrate on proper body position. If you sense that you are tensing to support yourself in a seated posture, check to be sure that your alignment is correct. Whichever position you choose, stick with that position in the early stages of training until you see the results. The only exception to this is that some exercises specify a particular position. Later, you can switch from one position to another.

Learning autogenics is broken down into two phases; phase 1 has six elementary exercises, and phase 2 has six advanced exercises. Specifically, the basic exercises emphasize body sensations to establish balance and rhythm in the autonomic system. In the second phase, imagery exercises emphasize mental capacity to form, hold, and manipulate mental images of external objects. Do not rush through the exercises, and do not move to the second set until you have reached the criterion described at the end of instructions for the first set.

The Six Primary Exercises of Autogenics

Autogenic training begins with six staged exercises that concentrate attention on different parts of the body or on different sensations. Here are the basic exercises and instructions that support the practice of autogenic relaxation.

Stage 1: Arm and leg heaviness Concentrate first on the arm that is your active arm. (If right-handed, start with the right arm; if left-handed, start with the left arm.) Repeat silently to yourself as you concentrate on the arm:

"My right (left) arm is heavy."

Do this about three to six times in a 30- to 60-second period. Close your eyes if you wish. When finished, shake yourself out of any lethargy and open your eyes. In autogenic terms, this is *cancellation*. Then switch to the other arm. Repeat the instruction, using the rule of three to six repetitions in each 30- to 60-second interval. Then repeat the process for each leg using the instruction:

"My right (left) leg is heavy."

Finally, do the limbs together using the sequence indicated in these instructions:

"Both my arms are heavy."
"Both my legs are heavy."
"My arms and legs are heavy."

Remember to use *cancellation* after each sequence before moving to the next stage.

Stage 2: Arm and leg warmth In the second stage of the exercise, concentrate on the sensation of warmth. It is not uncommon for people to experience feelings of warmth during the previous heaviness exercises. Now, the specific focus is on warmth, which feels like a spreading sensation of warmth throughout the body. Repeat the general procedure used in Stage 1, but with the instructions modified to suit the desired outcome as follows:

"My right (left) arm is warm."
"My right (left) leg is warm."
"Both my arms are warm."
"Both my legs are warm."
"My arms and legs are warm."

If it helps, use a mental image such as the warm sun on a beach, or imagine soaking in a hot bath.

With each exercise, be patient until you experience the comfortable, pleasant sensations of warmth and heaviness. You may need anywhere from four to eight weeks to learn to produce warmth in the limbs (Pelletier, 1977). It may be several months before you can produce the entire range of experiences with ease and speed.

The speed with which you develop the skill depends on how consistently you practice. In autogenic training, regular practice is one to six sessions *per day*, with each session lasting from 10 to 45 minutes. Expect early sessions to take 40 to 45 minutes. The norm is two to three daily sessions, but you may use more if you have time. Still, you will make rapid progress by practicing twice daily. Later, you may experience the full benefits in as few as 10 to 15 minutes.

Stage 3: Heaviness and warmth in the heart   In the third stage, extend the heaviness and warmth exercises to heart processes. The instruction is:

"My heartbeat is regular and calm."

Do this for 2 to 3 minutes, repeating the instruction at regular intervals. You may want to hold your hand over your heart so you can feel changes occurring. Also, for this exercise, you may use the reclining position. Remember, always use cancellation between each instruction and stage.

Stage 4: Paced respiration   After focusing on heaviness and warmth in the heart region, the exercises concentrate on measured or paced respiration. Paced breathing can have a very calming effect on the mind. With intense attention, it takes on a rhythmic, trancelike quality. Many groups have used breathing as a means to enhance muscular relaxation and mental tranquility. You can alternate between the two self-instructions listed here:

"It breathes me."
"My breathing is calm and relaxed."

Repeat these instructions four to five times in about a 90- to 150-second period. Mental visualization of an image may also help. For example, you might visualize waves rolling in on the beach and pace your breathing to each wave that breaks.

With this exercise, you may notice significant gains in anywhere from one to five weeks.

Stage 5: Abdominal (solar plexus) warmth   In the fifth exercise, you try to induce warmth in the abdominal region. The focus of attention is the solar plexus, the upper abdomen just above the stomach but below the heart. The instruction used for the heart can be used with only minor modification:

"My solar plexus is warm."

It is important to note that you are not trying to warm the surface of the skin. The intent is to produce warmth deep inside the upper abdominal cavity. Warming the solar plexus has a soothing effect on the activity of the central nervous system. It will also enhance muscular relaxation, and it may cause drowsiness. These effects may be related to parasympathetic nervous system activity. For example, imagining warmth in the abdomen may induce increased blood flow to the center of the body and reduce muscle tension. Thus, the verbal cues of autogenics may behaviorally switch the autonomic system from sympathetic arousal to parasympathetic calmness.

Stage 6: A cool forehead   The last basic exercise is to practice cooling the forehead. The instruction is:

"My forehead is cool."

The other exercises have focused on warmth or heaviness, but this one tries to induce a feeling of coolness on the forehead. This exercise may require the prone posture. If you work at this exercise too quickly, you might experience light dizziness or even fainting. Start slowly, then, with no more than two to three repetitions over about 20 to 30 seconds. Later, you can build up to four or five repetitions lasting 2 to 4 minutes.

Sometime during the first year, most people reach a point where they can complete all six exercises in less than 5 minutes. As noted earlier, you should not expect this to occur in less than about two months. Some exercises may not feel right until much later, while others, such as breathing, may feel right much sooner. When you reach this point of proficiency, though, you should stay in the state of autogenic meditation for 30 minutes to an hour.

Beginning Autogenic Visualization

Although basic exercises use very little imagery, visualization is an integral part of advanced autogenics. According to Schultz and Luthe, the purpose of visualization exercises is to capture and hold images long enough to assess their effects on consciousness. Some clinicians feel the assistance of an autogenic therapist is necessary at the beginning of this sequence. Therefore, the following discussion will be descriptive only. It is not intended as a guide to the practice of advanced autogenics.

Looking at your forehead   The first exercise rolls the eyeballs upward as though looking at the back of the forehead. Many meditators use this eye position. It usually increases brain alpha and enhances a trancelike state.

Immersing the mind in color   In the second exercise, the pupil picks a favorite color and tries to "see" that color. Imagine a room without form or dimension. Then imagine that room bathed in a favorite color. The color fills the entire visual field and saturates the mind. If pupils master this exercise, they are ready for more complex images.

Autogenic therapists suggest that different colors have different effects. For example, purples, reds, yellows, and oranges may induce warmth. Blue and green, on the other hand, more frequently induce coolness. Still, the colors most likely to induce a mood may depend on personal factors.

From this point on, the pupil can begin to visualize more complex shapes and colors. For example, pupils might visualize bright white clouds against a blue sky. Then they could visualize moving clouds. Next comes simple geometric forms such as squares, triangles, and circles. After this, pupils can try many different manipulations. They can fill the forms with color and change them. They can zoom in so the forms fill the entire mental frame, then draw back to view them from a distance. The intent is to become familiar with the ability of the mind to manipulate images of form and color.

Focusing on objects   In this exercise, the autogenic student chooses an object to visualize against a dark void. They might pick a vase, the mandala,[2] the Oriental symbol of unity, Greek theater masks, or silhouettes. The choice of object is personal but should be kept simple. This stage of training can take much more time than previous stages.

Transforming abstractions   This exercise concentrates on some abstract idea, such as truth, love, justice, or freedom. The intent is to obtain a mental image of an idea and transform it into a concrete symbol. You may hear a word, such as love, and see a symbol that represents unity better than any dictionary could. This is the meaning of transforming abstractions. This stage takes about two to six weeks.

Transcending feelings   Previous exercises involved some form of visual or auditory imagery. This exercise requires the pupil to concentrate on a feeling, an arousing emotion, just as though something external started it. Imagery still plays a role, but imagery is only a tool in this exercise. It is the feeling that

[2]The mandala, or circle, is a universal religious symbol.

is important. Seeing oneself on top of a mountain peak overlooking a vast wilderness may be associated with joy, contentment, or ecstasy. Vivid erotic fantasies may occur as though one is a part of the scene.

The intent of this exercise is to explore the role that personal involvement plays in emotionally loaded transactions. It provides practice in detecting switches from reality to fantasy. If successful, we could begin to plumb psychic depths and gain insight into conflicts and tensions that we create. Then we should be able to manage stressful events more effectively. Finally, we should be able to maintain better physiological balance conducive to good health.

Visualizing others   In the last stage of imagery practice, the task is to visualize other people. At first, pupils should focus on innocuous people at some personal distance. Then they may visualize more important people, such as peers, colleagues, and family members. With progress, these significant others include parties to previous conflicts. As pupils visualize these troubled transactions, they should work to achieve a vivid image of the person and the setting. The intent is to revive the former emotions. This training provides valuable insights into feelings toward others. It may also help change one's attitudes toward others and thus, one's perceptions of them.

In sum, autogenic exercises intend to provide a means of self-regulation and self-study. Through the power of imagery, a person can attain a balance between the arousing influence of the sympathetic and the calming effect of the parasympathetic. One line of speculation suggests that this is because the right side of the brain, which controls the autonomic nervous system, is also the creative, holistic, imagery-processing side of the brain. Thus, we may have a way to tell the autonomic system how fast we want the body to run. The exercises may also provide a way to bring intense feelings closer to the surface so we can neutralize, if not eliminate, the seeds of conflict that keep the body aroused.

Autogenics for Coping and Wellness

A word of caution is needed before we discuss autogenic successes and failures. A recurrent script in clinical practice reads something like this. A new therapeutic technique seems to bring hope for helping people resolve personal dilemmas. A rush of research on physical and mental ailments takes place, and we hear glowing reports of great success. Soon someone "markets" the technique with great fanfare, and people jump on the bandwagon. After more careful and dispassionate observation, others find the practice is far less of a panacea than formerly claimed, but it has a special clinical niche that it fills with some success. Unfortunately, great expectations followed by a negative press and eroding confidence can destroy the credibility of the practice even for that special niche.

At first, numerous studies showed that autogenic practice can have a positive effect on health problems. Luthe (1969) provided an example in the treatment outcomes for 78 patients. These patients received eight weekly sessions of group training. The clients presented several complaints, including anxiety, phobic, and hysterical disorders. Of the 78 patients, 10 (12%) showed very good improvement, and 20 (26%) showed little or no change. The remaining 48 clients showed good improvement. Luthe and Blumberger (1977) summarize many successful applications of autogenic therapy.

In reviewing research on autogenics, we may be astonished by the success it has enjoyed over the years. Yet, we may be disconcerted by the elixirlike quality of the claims for autogenics. Investigators claim success for autogenics in rehabilitation of neurologically impaired patients or in curing cancer (Simonton & Simonton, 1975). They suggest that autogenics is a viable treatment for epilepsy or alcoholism, for reducing smoking, for curing sexual dysfunction, and for tension headaches (Anderson, Lawrence, & Olson, 1981) or hypertension (Charlesworth & Nathan, 1982). Foerster (1984) reported success with a group of leukemia patients restrained in a germfree environment. In contrast to the claims of cure contained in the Simonton and Simonton study, Foerster wanted to help patients accept their treatment and adjust to the restraint with the least distress possible.

Charlesworth, Murphy, and Beutler (1981) also used autogenic training to help nursing students manage anxiety associated with their medical training, including reducing test anxiety. They reported modest success in achieving these goals. Their treatment was a multimodal package combining autogenics with several other components (such as relaxation, imagery, and desensitization). In this context, it is impossible to separate the contributions of the different components.

Clinicians now are more skeptical of the exuberant claims for autogenics. Still, this should not lead to its casual dismissal because despite its failures with certain disorders, autogenics still may have a niche to fill as a valuable coping technique.

MANAGING SPECIFIC FEARS

While relaxation and autogenics can be used for many stress and health problems, another group of stress problems requires different approaches. This is especially true for extreme anxiety and specific fears, as illustrated with Tom's situation. For these people, it is more than just being anxious or fearful. It is knowing that anxiety and fear always exist that keeps them captive in a world with invisible bars. It is knowing that no matter how silly or irrational their thoughts may be, they cannot be driven from consciousness. It is wrestling with the mental distress, behavioral restrictions, and social confinement that fear brings.

Fear of any kind produces behavioral changes, physical reactions, and thought processes. Behavior motivated by fear is usually some type of escape or avoidance behavior seeking to get away from the feared object or event. Physical reactions range from cold sweat and light-headedness to chest pains, nausea, and fainting. Thought processes include recurring images of a feared scene, feelings of unworthiness and being out of control, and fear of going crazy.

There are different types of fears. First, *simple fear* is alarm or fright at some real or imaginary danger. The most severe fear is a **phobia,** the irrational but persistent fear of some specific object or situation. **Anxiety** is the feeling of impending doom without knowing when, where, and how the doom will occur. When it is severe, anxiety can render a person incapable of speech, movement, or coherent thought (Scrignar, 1983). **Panic attacks** are the most severe anxiety reactions. During a panic attack, the person experiences a sudden onset of terror or apprehension of doom (American Psychiatric Association, 1987). In addition, physical changes occur, including sweating, faintness or dizziness, shaking, nausea, rapid pulse, shallow breathing, and hyperventilation.

The most common phobia is **agoraphobia.** The word is from the Greek, *agora,* for marketplace. It is fear of the marketplace, of open, public places. Agoraphobia often makes an individual housebound. **Social phobias** involve an irrational fear of situations that expose the person to public observation and possible embarrassment. A very common social phobia is fear of speaking or performing in public. Another common social phobia afflicts men who are afraid to use public urinals. Simple phobias include fear of animals, such as dogs or snakes; fear of closed spaces, such as elevators and tunnels; and fear of heights, such as tall buildings and flying. As Scrignar (1983) pointed out, simple fears are not really simple. They can interfere with travel, personal relationships, vocations, and even recreation.

Anxiety seems to be the core of obsessive-compulsive disorders. An obsessive-compulsive disorder has two components. First, recurrent and persistent thought patterns (obsessions) emerge that cannot be voluntarily stopped. Second, repetitive behavior patterns (compulsions) seem to occur almost automatically.

Tom's obsessive thought was that he had not shut off the gas stove. Several times he walked to work only to have fear compel him to walk home, check the stove, and return to work late. His solution was simple, if ineffective: get up an hour earlier to check the stove more often—sometimes 15 to 20 checks—and still get to work on time.

MANAGING SPECIFIC FEARS WITH DESENSITIZATION

In recent years, desensitization has proven very effective in dealing with recurrent fears. One clinical group even automated it to improve efficiency in treatment delivery (Thomas, Rapp, & Gentles, 1979). Joseph Wolpe (1958), a South African psychiatrist, developed the procedure in the 1950s. Wolpe worked for several years with phobic and obsessive-compulsive clients using traditional psychoanalytic therapy. He became concerned about his low rate of success in curing his patients. Other clinicians noted their own lack of success as well.

After reading a wide range of experimental literature, Wolpe became convinced that phobic and obsessive-compulsive disorders could be treated using recently developed behavioral theories. The behavioral model argues that phobic and compulsive disorders are learned disorders that can be unlearned. Wolpe (1958) detailed the desensitization procedure in his now classic book, *Psychotherapy by Reciprocal Inhibition.* Reciprocal inhibition means that the two branches of the autonomic nervous system stop each other in turn. When the sympathetic system is aroused, the parasympathetic is quiet, and vice versa.

Wolpe accepted the idea that relaxation is a behavioral switch that turns off sympathetic arousal, but he went far beyond this. He reasoned that the power of an event to incite fear can be controlled by manipulating the intensity of the feared event. This, he proposed, can be done through mental imagery. If the person relaxes while imagining the feared object, the object will become associated with relaxation instead of fear. Gradually, more intense images of the feared object could be presented until the person can stay relaxed while imagining the most feared object. The term *desensitization,* then, means removal of the sensitizing power of a feared object. In this way, we can countercondition or unlearn fear.

THE THREE KEYS TO DESENSITIZATION

Desensitization requires three elements: training in deep muscular relaxation, construction of a hierarchy of feared objects or events, and the person imagining the feared objects while in a state of relaxation. In the previous chapter, we discussed the rationale and procedure of relaxation training. The next few pages will explain the remaining two keys to the method.

Constructing a Ladder of Fear

The second step in desensitization is to build a stimulus hierarchy. Think of this as a ladder of feared objects. The low rungs hold less feared objects, and the highest rungs hold the most feared objects. The rationale for building this hierarchy can be explained as follows.

Fear of objects can be controlled by maintaining physical distance. If you are afraid of heights, the solution is to stay off tall buildings. If you are afraid of snakes, you stay away from areas that have snakes. You restrict the amount of time spent in elevators if you are afraid of closed in spaces.

Psychologically, fear decreases as objects or events become less and less similar to the original. For example, assume someone is deathly afraid of rats or mice. The person might maintain physical distance from rodents by having frequent visits from the local exterminator. The person could also stay away from pet shops or laboratories, where rats and mice might be on display. Now assume that this person goes to a theater to see a movie. Much to the viewer's dismay, the action takes the characters into a dark basement where rats run across their feet. A movie with rats may be too realistic and result in tension. Now suppose

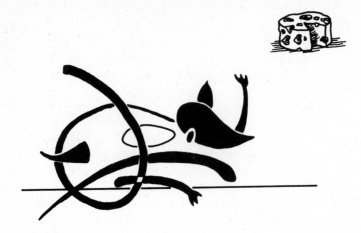

FIGURE 12-1
An abstract representation of a rat
SOURCE: Brooks/Cole.

I showed this person an abstract representation of a rat (Figure 12-1). In all likelihood, the person would experience very little anxiety because the artwork is so different from the real thing.

In more formal terms, this is the principle of **stimulus generalization.** Simply put, stimulus generalization occurs when someone responds in the same way to similar objects. The more similar the objects, the more likely the same response will occur. Rats, mice, and possibly gerbils could all produce the same fear response. Rabbits and guinea pigs probably would not because of major differences in appearance and meaning. The abstract rat would be even more unlike the real thing than a rabbit or a guinea pig.

Thus, the likelihood that similar objects will produce a response is not all or nothing. It is a generalization gradient that describes objects in terms of degree of similarity. Figure 12-2 shows one fear gradient of generalization. Objects at one end of the scale, rats and mice, are very similar. At the other extreme are less similar objects. The vertical scale shows the probability of a fear response. As objects become less and less like rats and mice, the fear response is less and less likely to occur.

Building a ladder of fear, a stimulus hierarchy in technical terms, is building a generalization gradient. We place objects on all rungs of the ladder in order of increasing fear, with the real thing at the top of the ladder. Figure 12-3 shows examples of fear ladders for flying and for public speaking. By starting at the lowest level, you can control fear and keep it at a distance psychologically, so that calm prevails instead of tension.

Generally, we cannot use the real objects or events; that is where visualization comes in. As we well know, the mind can replay images of feared objects. These images are the mental videotapes of anticipated encounters. They contain threat and arouse fear as though the object is there. As noted earlier in this book, research shows that the brain does not distinguish between a real and

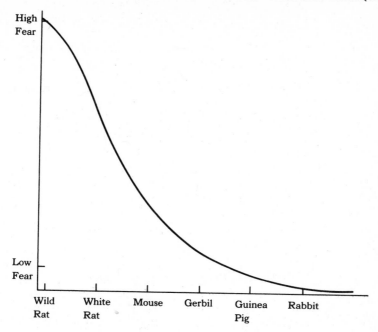

FIGURE 12-2
A stimulus generalization gradient for the feared stimulus of rats

an imagined event (John, 1967). This is why the process of imagining a feared event can produce the positive effects observed in this procedure. Desensitization uses a controlled, voluntary replay of images to maintain psychological distance from the object and thus keep fear at manageable levels.

When we imagine the object on the lowest rung of the fear ladder while staying relaxed, stimulus generalization also works in our favor. The association between calmness and the first object spreads to the second rung on the ladder. Then the second object arouses less fear than it did before, even though we have not yet paired it with relaxation. As we climb the ladder, we can handle more feared items because we have already desensitized them somewhat by the spread of relaxation from lower rungs. Finally, we can handle the most feared event. At this point, we have desensitized the object, and fear should no longer occur when the object is present.

Here are some rules of thumb for building a hierarchy or fear ladder. First, keep the length of the ladder at about 15 rungs. You could brainstorm until you have about 20 to 25 items at first. This is important because you may have to drop some items later. Second, place the most feared object or event at the top of the ladder. Third, try to think of an object far enough from the top so that it will produce very little tension. Put this event on the bottom rung of the fear ladder. It is important, though, that the object has some similarity to the high-fear object. You cannot just select any object to fill this bottom rung. Finally, select objects to fill the middle rungs.

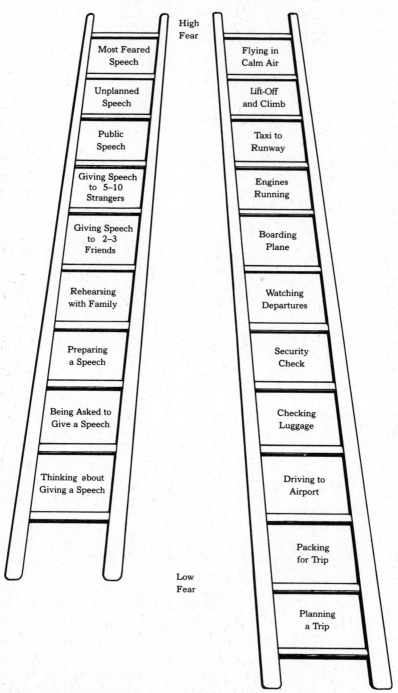

FIGURE 12-3
Fear ladders for the common fears of flying and public speaking

After you finish the fear ladder, go through the objects—from bottom to top—as you have placed them on the ladder. Try to visualize each object or event as vividly as possible. Note the amount of tension you feel, and decide whether you placed all the items in the right order. If you find a pair in which the lower object produces more tension than the next higher one, reverse the order or think about using a new object to fill that rung.

If you want to be really precise, assign the lowest rung on the ladder a scale value of 1 and the top rung a value of 100. Then assign values to the other objects to reflect the relative increase in fear you feel when going from low to high. Clinicians call this the **subjective unit of distress (SUD).** For example, the distance from the first object to the second may deserve a scale value of 5 units because it requires only a small jump in fear. The next object might deserve a scale value of 15 because moving up requires a larger jump in tension. You can play with these values until you have rated all the rungs on the scale, but each rung should be spaced about the same distance apart on the fear scale.

Some pairs of items may be too close to each other on this scale. If so, go back to the pool of objects you chose at the beginning. The objective is to have about 15 items, with equal distances between each object in terms of the amount of fear produced. Just as climbing a ladder should require the same amount of effort to move equal distances from rung to rung, subjective distress should change the same amount as you move up the fear ladder.

You might express fear of dogs on a continuum from seeing a dog at a distance to petting a dog. Fear of leaving home might be expressed in blocks or miles and in the number of family members present versus being alone. Claustrophobia can be scaled in terms of the size of the room and the amount of time spent in the room. You might scale fear of flying in terms of making flight arrangements, going to the airport, watching planes take off, boarding a plane but not flying, taxiing to the runway but not taking off, and taking off in a plane. These are examples of common fear ladders.

Before you take the third and final step, a few comments are necessary on how to present the items to yourself. As noted before, you do not typically work with real objects. There are methods that do this, and even Wolpe's technique can be modified to do this. When we conduct desensitization with the real object, it is called **contact desensitization** or **in vivo desensitization.** The latter means desensitization performed in the natural environment.

The two methods commonly used to present the fear stimuli are emotive imagery and pictorial representation. Which is better for you probably depends most on how visual or how concrete you are. If you have good powers of visual imagery, you should start with emotive imagery. If you need more concrete stimuli and do not consider yourself a good visualizer, the pictorial method may be best.[3] Either way, the method should not change the outcome.

Emotive imagery   The technique of **emotive imagery** is the old stand-by for desensitization. Imagine a feared scene from the ladder as though you

---

[3]You can also use autogenic exercises to increase your ability to visualize.

are drawing a mental picture of it or playing a mental videotape. Make a conscious effort to picture the scene as vividly as possible, as though you were viewing a movie on the screen of your mind. The scene usually has emotion associated with it, but be passive in this regard. In other words, you should not try to force a feeling into the scene, nor should you try to block feelings that well up.

In the clinical setting, it is the clinician's job to prompt images with verbal phrases that help make the mental image more vivid. This luxury is not available in your home. Some people find that a verbal cue for each rung of the ladder written on a sheet of paper is all that is necessary. Others record prompts on a tape recorder to have an electronic stand-in for the clinician. Whatever the method, know what objects or scenes you want to use before you begin relaxation. It is easy to do this because you need to visualize no more than three to four objects from the fear ladder in any given session.

Pictorial representation   The method of **pictorial representation** uses drawings, pictures, or slides to present feared scenes. It is possible to mix drawings and pictures. Drawings make it easy to obtain some remote symbols of feared objects. Some years ago, a student of mine was distraught about a rodent phobia she had had since she was about 6 years old. With my direction, she carried out a self-conducted desensitization program beginning with only line drawings and pictures. For the lower rungs of the fear ladder, she used line drawings like the abstract rat in Figure 12-1 and cartoons of rats and mice. Blurred and dark pictures of rats were just below the middle of the ladder. She placed more vivid color pictures just above the middle. Pictures of people holding rats were near the top. Scenes of this nature can be presented by either slides, drawings, or photos, although I do not recommend mixing slides with drawings or photos. It is best to keep the presentation method and medium as uniform as possible.

Pairing Relaxation and Fear

At this point you are ready to take the third, final step—to practice relaxation while imagining the objects on the fear ladder. To proceed, first prepare your quiet retreat as though you were going to engage in a regular relaxation session, but omit background music for desensitization sessions. Then choose the three or four images you will use for the session. Next, induce a deep level of relaxation and maintain it for a short time.

When you feel comfortably relaxed, stir yourself enough to imagine the first item on the fear ladder. Concentrate on the image so it becomes as vivid as possible. While you try passively to remain relaxed, scan your body to spot any rise of tension. Hold the image for approximately 1 minute. After this time, if you feel no disturbance in relaxation, stop the image and continue to relax for a few seconds. Repeat the imagery of the first rung one or two more times, then go on to the second rung of the fear ladder. Repeat the process through the set of objects selected for the session.

Should you experience disruption in relaxation at any time while imagining an object, *stop the imagery immediately!* Reinstate deep relaxation and enjoy it for about 1 to 2 minutes. Next, go down the ladder one rung to the previous object. Imagine the scene again while relaxing. If you have already progressed to about the third or fourth image, stop on that positive note and wait another day to resume. If the disruption occurs early in the session, you may try the image again or return to an image from the previous day's session that you successfully imagined. Sometimes you have to back down the ladder two steps, but usually you can manage setbacks by going back just one step.

Do not worry about these slight regressions, they are typical of the process. They only suggest that you moved up the ladder too quickly or that you tried to take a bigger emotive step than you thought. After two or three tries, if you cannot get past this event, you may need to insert one or two more rungs from your first pool of items.

In each session, you should work with no more than three or four scenes and present each image two to three times. Typically, it takes about three weeks to desensitize all the objects on the hierarchy. This depends, though, on the nature and intensity of the fear. Some hierarchies might be completed in as little as one week, whereas others might take six weeks or more.

When you have finished the procedure, test yourself in the real world. It is advisable, though, to *proceed slowly.* To the extent possible, try lower items of the hierarchy in the real world first. After testing yourself at this level, test yourself with more items from the upper range before trying the item highest on the ladder. This is equivalent to in vivo desensitization. Although this may be necessary with severe phobias, desensitization through emotive imagery is typically enough to eliminate fear of the real event.

COGNITIVE RESTRUCTURING

Cognitive restructuring is most closely associated with the work of Albert Ellis (1962). Ellis assumed that irrational, self-defeating thoughts and beliefs, combined with catastrophizing behavior, lead to increased personal distress. To eliminate this distress, Ellis believed that the cognitive system must be restructured with positive, self-supporting, and reasonable patterns of thinking. Decker, Williams, and Hall (1982) compared cognitive restructuring to a no-treatment control group after a 12-week training program. They showed that the treatment effectively reduced stress and irrational beliefs. Unfortunately, their study used intact groups instead of random assignment. Also, a no-treatment control does not eliminate the explanation of suggestion and expectation. That is, because subjects expected to receive a treatment that had potential for success, this expectation could account for the improvement. One way to offset this problem would be to use an attention-placebo control group.

Heimberg (1989) reviewed several methods, including cognitive restructuring, used to remove social phobias. Most studies showed substantial improvement after treatment. However, the designs used were rarely strong enough to

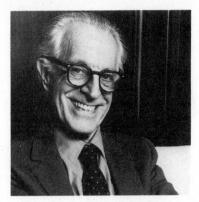

Albert Ellis developed rational-emotive therapy, which has been applied to cognitive coping skills.
SOURCE: Courtesy of Albert Ellis.

conclude that cognitive restructuring produced the change. The outcomes might also be explained by reduced fear of self-evaluation, lowered self-awareness (or manageable self-consciousness), and habituation of somatic arousal. These outcomes also result from desensitization and relaxation components, which are often unsystematically mingled with cognitive restructuring.

One major component of cognitive restructuring is self-talk or **self-statement modification (SSM).** Self-statement modification assumes that anxious people carry on private monologues that include "I can't" or "I'm bad" statements. David Dush and his associates conducted a meta-analysis of 69 studies that focused on self-statement modification as the primary method of treatment (Dush, Hirt, & Schroeder, 1983). Most of the studies reviewed dealt with test anxiety, speech anxiety, and unassertiveness.

The analysis suggested that SSM produces substantial gains compared to no-treatment controls, but only modest gains compared to placebo controls. When clients received personal treatment, the gains were almost double that achieved when clients were treated in groups. The authors noted another interesting outcome. Gains were extremely large in all studies conducted by Meichenbaum compared with studies by other investigators using Meichenbaum's variation of SSM. This may reflect expertise, investment, or interest. The authors also noted that the effects of SSM have declined over the years, which may add strength to the interest explanation for differences in treatment outcomes.

Another result confirms earlier clinical analyses: Self-referred clients showed much larger gains than volunteers or referred clients. This finding, that personal motivation is important to success in therapy, is an extremely robust finding, having been replicated over many years and many studies. It was also found that short-term interventions proved effective, casting doubt on the cost-effectiveness of long-term treatments. Desensitization was effective, but not as effective as SSM. Finally, relaxation training did not prove successful compared with SSM for this group of problems.

STRESS INOCULATION: PREPARING FOR STRESS

When confronted with diseases of epidemic proportions, medicine developed inoculation procedures. Doctors injected vaccines into the body in controlled amounts. The body, through the autoimmune system, reacted to the presence of the germ cells by developing antigens to fight the disease. In other words, the body acquired immunity to the disease so that any future exposure would not be as likely to make the person sick.

Stress inoculation, the brainchild of Donald Meichenbaum (1977), adopts the same notion, but the "germ" is psychosocial stress and the vaccine is exposure to low doses of stress in controlled conditions.[4] Meichenbaum believed that if people receive low doses of psychosocial threat combined with skills to deal with that threat, they develop resistance to the effects of stress. Later, when exposed to stress, they seem to have an immunity, and psychosocial stress does not seem to disturb them.

There are now many success stories in preventing stress among adult patients facing surgery or childbirth or preparing for painful medical tests. People with phobias, test anxiety, social shyness, speech anxiety, depression, anger, and chronic pain also respond positively to stress inoculation training (Janis, 1982). It appears to help those who are in conflict after making difficult career decisions and those who have decided to file for divorce. Further, it may be helpful in dealing with problems of recidivism in dieting and nutrition, smoking, and alcohol consumption (Janis, 1982).

Stress inoculation training (SIT) involves three distinct phases:[5] education, rehearsal of coping skills, and graded exposure to stressors combined with practice of coping skills (Meichenbaum, 1977). The goal of the educational phase is to provide understanding of the nature of the stress response and normal stress reactions. This information must be specific to the major current or anticipated stressor.

For example, people facing surgery or the death of a loved one can obtain information on what to expect. They can prepare for the emotional and physical reactions that are likely to occur. Surgical patients seem to endure better any disruptive emotional and physical effects, whether anticipated or real, when they have such information (Janis, 1982). With reassurances provided in SIT, they can shed feelings of self-efficacy. Because of this, stress inoculation may change the extent to which a person feels in control of a threatening situation.

In the second phase, SIT teaches specific techniques to deal with particular situations. The techniques may include, among others, relaxation, cognitive rehearsal, thought stopping, and self-instructions. Georgiana Tryon (1979)

---

[4]Seymour Epstein was among the first to emphasize self-pacing and exposure to small doses of threat. He helped develop coping skills in men who routinely engaged in dangerous activities such as parachuting and combat flying.

[5]West, Horan, and Games (1984) point out that the terminology of stress inoculation has changed even in Meichenbaum's work. The tems *coping skills* and *exposure* are used in reference to the second and third stages. More recently, the tems *conceptualization, skill acquisition,* and *application* have been used for the three stages.

reviewed thought-stopping research covering a wide range of designs. Much of the research occurred in clinical settings with less than adequate controls and small samples or samples of size one. The target of the treatment usually was obsessive thoughts. While the technique has shown some success, it remains unproven that thought stopping is the most effective means to deal with intrusive thoughts.

Meichenbaum listed a variety of self-instructions that can be used in various situations. For example, in preparing for some type of provocation, a person might mentally rehearse these statements:

"This is going to upset me, but I know how to deal with it."
"Try not to take this too seriously."

When the situation is a confrontation, an appropriate self-instruction might be:

"If I get mad, I'll just be banging my head against the wall. So I might as well just relax" (Meichenbaum, 1977).

Cognitive rehearsals effectively change perceptions and attitudes that initiate and perpetuate stress interpretations.

The third phase involves applying the new coping skills to a graded series of imaginary and real stress situations. For example, assume a manager has had difficulty providing candid periodic evaluations of employees. The manager might prepare for an upcoming meeting by imagining an evaluation session in process. Aspects of the situation that produce fear might be desensitized, and tense interactions might be met with cue-controlled relaxation. The manager might mentally rehearse self-instructions for interactions that often undermine the integrity of the process. In this way, when the real sessions take place, the manager is more likely to conduct them in a calm, professional fashion.

Does Stress Inoculation Work?

Novaco, Don Meichenbaum's associate, provided some of the best examples of stress inoculation. Novaco (1977) suggested that we fan the flames of anger with self-statements made in tense situations. For example, police dealing with rioters or involved in crowd control are under immense pressure. Anger may kindle very quickly. One impulsive move prompted by frustration can lead to counter-attack and disastrous consequences. The riots during the 1968 Democratic Convention in Chicago amply illustrate this point.

In Novaco's educational scheme, he conceptualized anger in terms of a sequence of events that involve cognitive appraisal and physical arousal. When physical arousal occurs, the brain probably will interpret the arousal as due to real danger or threat. When this happens, one tends to label the opponent in a negative, perhaps even demeaning, way. Then the antagonists may play out anger-attack scripts in the mind. This drives the physical system to even higher levels of arousal. The higher the arousal, the more likely that some word or action will trigger the anger-attack schema.

In the second phase, Novaco taught relaxation training and self-instructional rehearsal. The person learns how to self-prompt with statements about the sequence of events that will occur. He or she also learns thought-stopping statements to interrupt the labeling process and the arousal spiral. Finally, in the third phase, the person imagines various anger-arousing situations. Then, he or she cognitively rehearses coping with such provocations through relaxation, deep breathing, and self-statements (Meichenbaum, 1977).

Much of the information provided earlier in this book is equivalent to the first inoculation phase. Its primary purpose was to inform you of the internal processes and situations that lead to stress interpretations and reactions. Information on methods makes up the second part of this book. This is the foundation of coping skills necessary to manage stress. The third phase, graded exposure, is something you must do yourself.

How Does Stress Inoculation Work?

Researchers are still evaluating SIT. One research group compared SIT to a standard psychotherapy procedure combined with medical interventions (Foley et al., 1987). The group's clients, 40 multiple sclerosis patients, received a five-week training program. The SIT group showed significantly lower depression, state anxiety, and subjective stress. Members of the SIT group also improved their problem-focused coping efforts. They maintained the first three improvements at 6 months, but their problem-focused coping had declined. The psychotherapy group did not show any change on these measures.

It is possible that type of training may interact with client characteristics. This principle is well understood in college life, where the method of delivering instruction may interact with characteristics of the student. One theory of anxiety suggested that people experience anxiety differently. That is, some people may experience anxiety largely as cognitive distress, whereas others may experience anxiety primarily as somatic disturbance and arousal (Heimberg, 1989). If so, cognitive interventions may be better for those who experience anxiety primarily in the cognitive mode. Relaxation or arousal-reducing therapies may be better for those who experience anxiety in the somatic modality.

This notion received some support from the work of Elizabeth Altmaier and her colleagues (Altmaier, Ross, Leary, & Thornbrough, 1982). They assigned subjects to either a cognitive restructuring treatment, a coping relaxation treatment, a typical stress inoculation program, or a no-treatment control. They also assessed differences in cognitive-somatic anxiety, but they assigned subjects to treatments without regard to type of anxiety. Their results partially confirmed the hypothesis. Cognitive anxiety subjects responded favorably to stress inoculation and cognitive restructuring, whereas relaxation was least effective for them. Somatic anxiety subjects, though, responded about equally well to all treatments.

Much of the early research treated SIT in total and took reported successes at face value. A research team led by Daniel West carried out a detailed analysis on the components of stress inoculation training (West, Horan, & Games, 1984).

They reasoned that because SIT is a complex program combining multiple treatments, any single treatment or combination of treatments could account for positive outcomes. West's team randomly assigned 60 acute care nurses to five groups, one of which was a control group. They designed the four experimental groups to isolate the relative contribution of the different SIT components. One group received education only. The second group received education plus coping skills training. The third group received education plus exposure, and the fourth group received the customary three-step procedure. The dependent variables included state-trait anxiety, assertiveness, job tension, burnout, life satisfaction, and blood pressure measures.

The results of this study were very instructive. First, compared to the control group, all the treatment groups improved on the dependent measures. Second, *the component most consistently associated with positive outcomes was the coping skills training step.* Coping skills subjects improved significantly compared with subjects who received no coping skills training. Further, all dependent measures improved in coping skills groups. Yet, when coping skills were excluded, only two measures changed. These changes were still visible at follow-up. For subjects not receiving coping skills training, however, the improvements obtained on only two measures had disappeared at follow-up. The authors concluded that coping skills training is the major active ingredient of stress inoculation training.

SUMMARY

In this chapter, we discussed four techniques that use imagery and cognitive representations of stress situations. Autogenics, a variation of deep muscular relaxation, is relatively passive and incorporates explicit imagery exercises. Developing imagery skills helps in applying autogenics to anxiety and stress problems. Further, autogenics can enhance the practice of other stress management skills, such as desensitization and stress inoculation, that also include significant imagery components.

Desensitization may be used to treat anxiety, fear, and panic disturbances. It can be tailored to individual situations and fears. Desensitization can be carried out in the privacy of one's home and requires no equipment other than the capacity to use mental visualization. It is a natural extension of relaxation training for dealing with specific fears.

Self-statement modification is a cognitive restructuring procedure. It tries to replace negative, self-defeating internal talk with positive, self-enhancing talk.

Stress inoculation is the preventive, immunizing branch of stress management. It teaches people, first, how to anticipate stress transactions, then, how to defuse the potential for stress by rehearsing statements and behaviors that can be carried out in real-world situations. By building up doses of mentally rehearsed stress conditions, the individual can deal more effectively with a variety of stressful situations.

KEY TERMS

agoraphobia

alpha

anxiety

autogenic discharge

autogenics

autogenic therapy

biofeedback

cognitive restructuring

contact desensitization

desensitization

emotive imagery

in vivo desensitization

panic attacks

phobia

pictorial
  representation

self-statement
  modification (SSM)

social phobias

stimulus generalization

stress inoculation
  training (SIT)

subjective unit of
  distress (SUD)

REFERENCES

Altmaier, E. M., Ross, S. L., Leary, M. R., & Thornbrough, M. (1982). Matching stress inoculation's treatment components to clients' anxiety mode. *Journal of Counseling Psychology, 29,* 331–334.

American Psychiatric Association. (1987). *Diagnostic and statistical manual of mental disorders* (3rd ed., rev.). Washington, DC.: Author.

Anderson, N. B., Lawrence, P. S., & Olson, T. W. (1981). Within-subject analysis of autogenic training and cognitive coping training in the treatment of tension headache pain. *Journal of Behavior Therapy and Experimental Psychiatry, 12,* 219–223.

Charlesworth, E. A., Murphy, S., & Beutler, L. E. (1981). Stress management skill for nursing students. *Journal of Clinical Psychology, 37,* 284–290.

Charlesworth, E. A., & Nathan, R. G. (1982). *Stress management: A comprehensive guide to wellness.* Houston, TX: Biobehavioral Press.

Decker, T. W., Williams, J. M., & Hall, D. (1982). Preventive training in management of stress for reduction of physiological symptoms through increased cognitive and behavioral controls. *Psychological Reports, 50,* 1327–1334.

Dush, D. M., Hirt, M. L., & Schroeder, H. (1983). Self-statement modification with adults: A meta-analysis. *Psychological Bulletin, 94,* 408–422.

Ellis, A. (1962). *Reason and emotion in psychotherapy.* New York: Stuart.

Foerster, K. (1984). Supportive psychotherapy combined with autogenous training in acute leukemic patients under isolation therapy. *Psychotherapy and Psychosomatics, 41,* 100–105.

Foley, F. W., Bedell, J. R., LaRocca, N. G., Scheinberg, L. C., & Reznikoff, M. (1987). Efficacy of stress-inoculation training in coping with multiple sclerosis. *Journal of Consulting and Clinical Psychology, 55,* 919–922.

Heimberg, R. G. (1989). Cognitive and behavioral treatments for social phobia: A critical analysis. *Clinical Psychology Review, 9,* 107–128.

Janis, I. L. (1982). *Stress, attitudes, and decisions.* New York: Praeger.

John, E. R. (1967). *Mechanisms of memory.* New York: Academic Press.

Kamiya, J. (1969). Operant control of the EEG alpha rhythm and some of its reported effects on consciousness. In C. T. Tart (Ed.), *Altered states of consciousness* (pp. 519–529). Garden City, NY: Anchor Books.

Luthe, W. (1969). *Autogenic therapy.* New York: Grune & Stratton.

Luthe, W., & Blumberger, S. R. (1977). Autogenic therapy. In E. D. Wittkower & H. Warnes (Eds.), *Psychosomatic medicine: Its clinical applications* (pp. 146–165). New York: Harper & Row.

Meichenbaum, D. (1977). *Cognitive-behavior modification: An integrative approach.* New York: Plenum.

Novaco, R. W. (1977). A stress inoculation approach to anger management in the training of law enforcement officers. *American Journal of Community Psychology, 5,* 327–346.

Pelletier, K. R. (1977). *Mind as healer, mind as slayer: A holistic approach to preventing stress disorders.* New York: Dell.

Schultz, J., & Luthe, W. (1959). *Autogenic training: A psychophysiological approach to psychotherapy.* New York: Grune & Stratton.

Scrignar, C. B. (1983). *Stress strategies: The treatment of the anxiety disorders.* New York: Karger.

Simonton, O. C., & Simonton, S. (1975). Belief systems and management of the emotional aspects of malignancy. *Journal of Transpersonal Psychology, 7,* 29–47.

Thomas, M. R., Rapp, M. S., & Gentles, W. M. (1979). An inexpensive automated desensitization procedure for clinical application. *Journal of Behavior Therapy and Experimental Psychiatry, 10,* 317–321.

Tryon, G. S. (1979). A review and critique of thought stopping research. *Journal of Behavior Therapy and Experimental Psychiatry, 10,* 189–192.

West, D. J., Horan, J. J., & Games, P. A. (1984). Component analysis of occupational stress inoculation applied to registered nurses in an acute care hospital setting. *Journal of Counseling Psychology, 31,* 209–218.

Wolpe, J. (1958). *Psychotherapy by reciprocal inhibition.* Stanford, CA: Stanford University Press.

CHAPTER 13

The Concentration Techniques: Meditation and Biofeedback

ONE NIGHT . . . BEING KEPT AWAKE BY PAIN, I AVAILED MYSELF OF THE STOICAL MEANS OF CONCENTRATION UPON SOME DIFFERENT OBJECT OF THOUGHT . . . IN THIS WAY I FOUND IT POSSIBLE TO DIVERT MY ATTENTION, SO THAT PAIN WAS SOON DULLED . . .
IMMANUEL KANT

The systematic approaches to relaxing and treating anxiety, described earlier in this book, are mostly products of modern technological culture. They mesh well with the Western penchant for scientific study and treatment of mental and physical health problems. Still, a long tradition of altering and controlling internal body states reaches back to the dawn of recorded history. The most prominent of these, the Yogi tradition of deep **meditation,** has its roots in ancient Hindu society. We cannot discuss at length the sequence of events that led from the Western "discovery" of Eastern yoga to practical coping methods. But even the most cursory historical sleuthing reveals a fascinating story with intriguing vignettes and startling insights.

THE MYSTERIOUS GOD-MEN OF INDIA

From the time the British landed in India to current times, reports filtered out of India about Yogis who could control their bodies to a degree never before believed attainable. For nearly half a century, Western scientists observed these mysterious "god-men" of India (Brent, 1972). What they explored and observed with scientific methods led to changes in our notions of how the mind and body interact.

For example, there were sensational reports of gurus who could reduce heart rate to the point of total cessation. In a type of suspended animation, they could be buried alive for days (Hoenig, 1968). The mystery of how they could control heart function is now partially solved, but having explained it does not detract from the sheer wonder that they could do it at all (Anand, Chhina, & Singh, 1961). Other reports told of Yogis who could control blood flow to their bodies so they could withstand severe temperatures.

What is the secret behind these Yogi practices? And what can we learn, if anything, that is useful for modern living? To answer the first question, we must look at Yogi meditative practice. In the process, we will study **Transcendental Meditation (TM),** a meditative procedure widely recognized in Western cultures. In addition, I will describe Herbert **Benson's** (1975) **secular meditation.**

To answer the second question, we must look at how the West has placed meditation under the scientific microscope. One outcome of this laboratory close-up is **biofeedback,** once touted as a high-tech alternative to years of religious discipline. In the last section of this chapter, we will discuss the more common biofeedback procedures. Finally, we will consider empirical evidence on the merits of biofeedback and how it may complement the other coping techniques described.

THE HIGHROAD OF MEDITATION

In ancient Hindu society, meditation was the highroad to spiritual enlightenment. Religious literature shows that meditation often occupied a position on a par with sacrifice and prayer. It was a means to an end, a concentrative method for withdrawing from the world of illusion, escaping the cycle of rebirths, and obtaining union with the oversoul.

The Yoga System of Meditation

One prominent system that featured various meditative practices was Yoga, which literally means "union." The first systematic record of the Yoga way of life is the *Yoga-Sutras,* a manual written by Patanjali about 200 B.C.[1] The *Yoga-Sutras* reveal a moral philosophy with strict ethical and moral codes of conduct. It prescribes an ascetic lifestyle and teaches a set of rigorous physical and mental exercises.

The practice of Yoga is an eightfold pathway beginning with ethical teachings to (1) restrain antisocial and selfish behavior and (2) ensure positive conduct.[2] Then the student of Yoga learns (3) postures, (4) control of breathing, and (5) withdrawal of the senses.[3] The physical path of postures and strenuous exercises has become associated with Hatha Yoga. Breathing exercises consist of learning how to inhale, hold the breath, and exhale with control (Behanan, 1964). Through these exercises, a person can gain control of the body and then also control the mind. Still, control of the mind is the province of (6) meditation, (7) contemplation, and (8) isolation.[4] The intent of Yoga in this life is to recondition the mind to release creative energy and free the person from chains of unconscious impulses and bondage to the senses.

---

[1]A controversy exists among scholars of the East as to the exact time frame of Patanjali's life and the date of the *Yoga-Sutras.* The dates range from the third century B.C. to the fourth century A.D. This date comes from the thoughtful analysis of Dasgupta in *A History of Indian Philosophy.*
[2]The negative ethical code was *yamas* and the positive ethical code was *niyamas.* These were the first two steps in Yogi practice.
[3]The postures are *asanas,* breathing rituals are *pranayamas,* and withdrawal is *pratyahara.*
[4]Meditation is *dharana,* and contemplation is *dhyana.* Isolation is the final release, called *samadhi.*

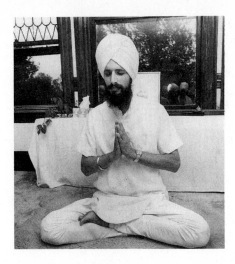

Yoga meditation usually involves sitting in the lotus position and focusing concentration on a sacred word or some object to bring the mind under control.
SOURCE: Jerry Berndt/Stock, Boston.

Science Tunes In to Meditation

While philosophers wrote about the Yoga system for years, the Western scientific community discounted, if not ignored, most of the claims for altering heart rate, changing body temperature, fire walking, needle penetration without bleeding, and altering consciousness. Scientific interest dawned in the 1950s, when investigative teams set out to verify the claims. Before this, however, a French cardiologist, Thérèse Brosse, traveled to India in 1935, anticipating later efforts to understand Yoga methods. Brosse carried a portable electrocardiograph to measure Yogis as they tried to control their heart activity. One of the published EKG records showed heart potentials approaching zero. Her work gave credibility to the scientific study of Yoga practice and had a major impact on the next team that made a similar trip, over 20 years later.

The team of Wenger and Bagchi (1961) traveled in India for five months in early 1957. The purpose of their trip was to test "various claims of voluntary control of autonomic functions and [record] physiological changes during Yogic meditation" (p. 312). In observations of 45 Yogis, they observed temperature control, voluntary regurgitation, heart control, increased systolic blood pressure, and lower skin resistance. They concluded that the Yogis were controlling heart processes through muscular control and breathing but not through any direct control. Later studies of a Yogi at the Menninger Clinic in Topeka, Kansas, supported this conclusion (Green, Green, & Walters, 1972).

Wenger and Bagchi also attempted to measure arousal in the sympathetic nervous system in beginning and advanced students of Yoga. The Yoga school claimed for centuries that the practice of meditation benefits both the mental and physical life of the practitioner. If this claim is true, Wenger and Bagchi reasoned, there ought to be some correlate in lowered activity of the sympathetic system. Wenger and Bagchi compared the physiological recordings of the Yoga group to an American control group. The results were somewhat surprising. On 7 of the 11 measures, the Yoga group showed *higher* sympathetic activity during yoga meditation than the American control group. If meditation was aiding in coping with stress, it was not apparent in these observations. Still, Wenger and Bagchi recognized the limitations of their method and urged others to carry on research to understand the changes associated with meditation.

Western society has been most fascinated with **alpha,** a brain wave consistently produced by Yogis during periods of meditation. Zen monks practice a form of meditation derived from the Indian Buddhist tradition. They also show increased alpha during meditation (Kasamatsu & Hirai, 1963). More will be said about the alpha rhythm later in this chapter.

TRANSCENDENTAL MEDITATION: A WESTERN MANTRA YOGA?

During the 1960s, political, social, and religious activism were at a fever pitch. It was the decade of Students for a Democratic Society (SDS), hippies, communes, resistance to the war effort in Vietnam, and Transcendental Meditation (TM). TM is an adaptation of Mantra Yoga tailored to Western sensibilities. The Maharishi Mahesh Yogi, TM's founder, cut out nonessential elements of traditional Yoga practices. He also stripped TM of theological significance so it could be marketed as a secular practice. He and his organization took steps to ensure that no one connected TM with hypnosis, autosuggestion, or any of the then-popular encounter groups.[5] At one time, TM may have had between 500,000 and 1 million followers, and they had a university with its own curriculum.

The practice of TM is remarkably simple, although the formal initiation ceremonies make it seem mysterious and complex. The normal format of instruction includes three sessions. After an opening information session, students attend a more detailed instructional session at which a commitment to practice TM occurs. The final session is an initiation ceremony where the guide aids students in choosing their **mantra,** a secret word that should not be divulged to anyone else. From this point on, the person practices TM alone.

The guidelines for practicing TM are sparse. A person practices about 20 to 30 minutes per day twice a day. The preferred time for practice is just before breakfast and just before the evening meal. During meditation, the person takes a seated position on a bed or on a floor cushion. TM prefers the lotus position, the posture of "physical centeredness." Research shows that this position is the most relaxed of any seated position (Shapiro & Zifferblatt, 1976). Practice usually

---

[5]A TM instructor once gave a presentation over three sessions to introduce and initiate a group of people into TM. I attended the meetings to observe and plan research involving TM. The statements on the origins of TM represent the position of TM as presented in these meetings.

occurs in a setting free of distractions. During meditation, the person typically closes his or her eyes and repeats the mantra continuously. The purpose of this mental focusing is to prevent thoughts of object attachment or concern with mundane matters. Thus, the use of the mantra is similar to the practice of visual focusing used in other circles. Zen monks concentrate on a **koan,** an unsolvable riddle, to help focus the mind but also to drive the mind beyond itself (Kapleau, 1966).

TM Under the Microscope

Shortly after TM appeared in America, the team of Robert Wallace and Herbert Benson (1972) put TM under the scientific microscope. They used instruments that permitted continuous recording of blood pressure, heart rate, temperature, skin resistance, and EEG. They also measured oxygen consumption and carbon dioxide elimination. Another measure, blood-lactate, was of special interest because of its presumed connection to anxiety.

Wallace and Benson observed 36 subjects whose experience in the practice of TM ranged from one month to 9 years. After a brief period to adapt to the laboratory situation, each person provided data over three 20- to 30-minute periods before, during, and after meditation. The results showed reduced oxygen use, a marked decrease in blood-lactate, increased skin resistance, and intensification of the alpha wave. These results closely paralleled those obtained in the earlier field studies of Yoga and Zen monks.

Based on their observations, Wallace and Benson suggested that TM is a fourth state of consciousness, which they called a "wakeful, hypometabolic" state. It is different from any of the three primary states of consciousness— waking, sleeping, or dreaming—although it shares some similarities with each. Wallace and Benson called it "hypometabolic" because energy expenditure goes down. Because several physiological indicators related to stress and anxiety decreased during meditation, Wallace and Benson argued that TM could be used to ensure better mental and physical health. Dillbeck and Orme-Johnson (1987) conducted a meta-analysis of 31 studies that used TM. They also found consistent evidence for lowered somatic arousal combined with increased alertness as compared with eyes-closed resting.

Numerous reports during the 1970s extolled TM's virtues. It was the mental super cure for drug dependency and smoking. It could increase IQ, control depression, reduce anxiety (including death anxiety), aid self-actualization, and manage job stress (Boerstler, 1986; Delmonte, 1984; Dillbeck, Aron, & Dillbeck, 1979). Vietnam veterans could manage posttraumatic stress syndrome using meditation (Brooks & Scarano, 1985). Another study, using a variant called *mindfulness meditation,* showed success in self-regulation of pain (Kabat-Zinn, Lipworth, & Burney, 1985). A best-selling book praised TM and suggested that a fulfilled society would result if everyone practiced TM (Bloomfield, Cain, Jaffe, & Kory, 1975).

Subsequent research led to skepticism about the claims for TM, including the notion that meditation produces a unique state of consciousness. One study showed that meditators spend significant time in sleep stages and in alpha, which do not necessarily qualify as unique states of consciousness (Pagano, Rose, Stivers, & Warrenburg, 1976). Another study failed to find any reduction in physiological indicators of anxiety during a stress test (Lintel, 1980). Holmes and colleagues found that meditators had lower somatic arousal, but they also showed that TM did not reduce arousal more than simply resting (Holmes, Solomon, Cappo, & Greenberg, 1983).

Puente and Beiman (1980) tested TM head to head against self-relaxation, PMR combined with cognitive coping skills, and a waiting-list control. TM clients had higher cardiovascular stress responses following treatment than before and their cardiovascular stress responses were worse than the waiting-list group. Both relaxation groups showed significant decreases in their cardiovascular stress responses (Puente & Beiman, 1980). Thus, if TM has any positive effects, they apparently cannot be attributed to a unique ingredient. TM's benefits are more likely the result of a nonspecific component similar to that found in other relaxation procedures.

Many TM studies suffered from methodological flaws, which only added to the skepticism. They often lacked control groups or failed to control for expectation effects by using an untreated control but not a placebo control. Finally, the studies frequently mixed meditation with other forms of relaxation training, which makes it difficult to assess the contributions of TM itself.

Still, some people point to the fact that TM is easy to learn and practice. Further, the results may be as good as from any general relaxation procedure (Throll, 1982). Therefore, there is no good reason not to use it. As with other methods, however, TM is not a panacea: It cannot be all things to all people for all situations. In addition, TM does not have the clinical track record of PMR, especially when PMR is combined with cue-controlled, differential relaxation and desensitization.

THE RELAXATION RESPONSE: SECULAR MEDITATION

After studying TM for some time, Herbert Benson became convinced that the active agent in TM is general relaxation. From this, he reasoned that we do not need either the physical exercises of PMR or the initiation rites of TM to relax. Benson (1975) then developed the secular meditation procedure described in *The Relaxation Response.*

In brief, Benson (1975) felt that four basic ingredients are necessary to cultivate the relaxation response. In his view, these elements contain no cultural, religious, or philosophical prejudices, thus the name *secular meditation.* The four elements are as follows:

1. a quiet environment
2. an object on which to focus mentally

3. a passive attitude
4. a comfortable position (pp. 78, 79)

A quick inspection shows secular meditation's similarities to both progressive muscle relaxation and autogenics. A quiet setting is vital for any of the relaxation-concentration exercises described earlier. A comfortable position is also important, although the actual position probably is not important. In PMR, it was a semireclined seated position. In autogenics, it could be any one of three positions. Benson recommends a sitting position, but other positions may be used, including the lotus position. However, any position that is conducive to sleep should be avoided.

In TM, mental focusing results from silently repeating the mantra, the sacred word. Many other methods also result in focused attention. Autogenics used color and form. In PMR, it was alternating states of tension and relaxation. Symbols, such as the mandala, may be especially good choices for mental focusing. The Eastern symbol of unity might serve just as well. Another ancient practice is to focus on the navel, the forehead, or the inside of the eyelids. Arthur Deikman (1969) used a blue vase in his work. You can choose nearly any word, sound, symbol, or object and obtain the same relaxing result. Benson recommended a rhythmic breathing cadence with the word "one" repeated each time you breathe out.

Benson also recommended use of a thought-stopping technique to control intrusive thoughts during early practice sessions. For a short time, repeat the word *no* each time the intrusive thought occurs. This should enable you to eliminate unwanted thoughts easily and return to focused concentration. If the cue word is strong, you could eliminate the intrusive thought with breathing cycles: each time you breathe out, repeat the cue word.

All relaxation procedures emphasize a passive attitude. In fact, attitude seems to be the most important thing in producing alpha during meditation (Shapiro & Zifferblatt, 1976). Attempts to make relaxation happen will only destroy the effort. Simply allow it to happen. Even if you do not attain deep relaxation at first, do not struggle to do so. Continue in quiet contemplation until the end the session. Deeper states of relaxation will come eventually.

Benson's secular method may produce the same positive benefits that occur with PMR, autogenics, and TM. Benson (1975) says that the relaxation response "can act as a built-in method of counteracting the stresses of everyday living which bring forth the fight-or-flight response" (p. 111).

Although clinical research has not tested secular meditation as extensively as PMR, it may be possible to extend the procedure somewhat. For example, Benson's procedure recommended using a cue word in connection with breathing. This was the backbone of cue-controlled relaxation, the ability to relax anywhere. Intuitively, secular meditation could follow the same procedure and thus cover the same range of stressful situations. Still, we must emphasize that we do not know precisely the effective ingredient of cue-controlled or differential relaxation. Further, little research exists to suggest whether secular meditation can be used effectively in this way. Thus, the generality of secular meditation is mostly a matter of guesswork, and any extensions must be attempted on a strictly experimental basis.

BIOFEEDBACK: ELECTRONIC EUPHORIA OR PRACTICAL TOOL?

Even as field and laboratory investigations exposed meditation to critical analysis, other researchers were looking at new ways of producing altered states of consciousness. There seemed to be two different lines of reasoning that supported this effort. One view was largely rooted in theory building. It assumed that science ought to do its best to explore and explain the conditions that lead to physiological and brain-wave changes in meditation. A second practical, if not mystical, view suggested that there ought to be some way to produce the changes more directly without going through 20 years of asceticism. Yet it was not clear how this could be done. Then several investigators thought they had found the answer in biofeedback. Through 1985, over 2400 journal articles and 100 books provided the best laboratory and clinical evidence available (Hatch & Riley, 1986).

Putting Information Back into the System

Biofeedback has historical roots in *cybernetics,* or communication and control science. The mathematician Norbert Weiner (1954) defined *feedback* as regulating a system by putting back into the system information about its past performance. Biofeedback uses a special type of information—information about the performance of the biological system. Whenever we obtain information about how our body is working by making internal signals externally visible, we are using biofeedback. George Fuller (1977) defined biofeedback in a more formal sense as "the use of instrumentation to mirror psychophysiological processes of which the individual is not normally aware and which may be brought under voluntary control" (p. 3).

An Overview of Biofeedback Procedures

In practice, biofeedback has very few components. First, we must decide on the physiological system to be changed. Then we must identify a body signal produced by that system. Finally, we must use a detection device that can read, amplify, and display the body signal. (See Figure 13-1). We may adjust the output of the detection display from time to time so we force larger and larger changes in the body response. When the learner reaches the desired state (for example, reliable production of alpha or elimination of headaches), we typically fade out the feedback system. Then we try to transfer control of the body response to cognitive or behavioral cues or both.

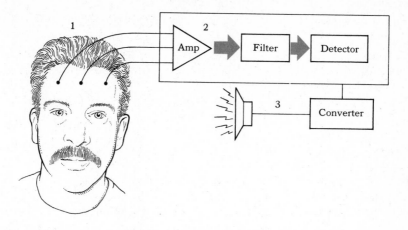

FIGURE 13-1

A biofeedback system usually includes (1) a sensing device that reads body signals, such as electrodes; (2) a filter/amplifier system to select the right signals and convert the body signal into an electrical signal; and (3) a display device to make the signal visible to the person.

Body signals can be displayed with lights or meters, with sounds or strip charts. Any method is acceptable as long as it tells a person when the desired internal state is present. Some clinicians devised novel displays of body messages. In one case, a model train provided feedback. The train ran when alpha was present and stopped when alpha disappeared. Another team, working with children who were polio victims, used muscle signals to light up a clown's face (Stern & Ray, 1977). No matter how we choose to display body signals, the purpose is the same: to enable the person to connect the internal change to a behavior, a thought, or an image. By engaging in the same activity later, it may be possible to reproduce the internal state voluntarily.

LISTENING TO YOUR BODY

There are now numerous biofeedback techniques that make many internal responses visible. The procedures most often used are electromyography **(EMG)**, electroencephalography **(EEG)**, skin **temperature,** galvanic skin response **(GSR), blood pressure,** and heart rate **(cardiovascular)** feedback.

Listening to Muscle Tension

As muscles contract, they give off an electrical signal that can be detected through small electrodes. Electromyographic feedback amplifies this signal and provides information on the amount of muscle tension. Visual feedback is most often a dial somewhat like an ammeter that shows when a battery is charging (high tension) or discharging (low tension). We typically provide auditory feedback in one of two ways. In the first method, a single tone goes on when muscle tension is too high and off when muscle tension drops to an acceptable level. In the second method, a tone is on when muscle tension exceeds a certain level and increases in loudness as muscle tension increases. As muscle tension drops, so does the loudness of the tone, until it turns off when muscle tension is under the desired level again. This method is very effective when used to aid relaxation training.

Electrode placement depends on the physiological response to be changed. (See Figure 13-2.) If the intent is to aid general relaxation, either the trapezius muscles of the shoulder or the forearm site is appropriate. If the intent is to reduce tension headaches, then clinicians prefer the frontalis muscle location on the forehead. EMG biofeedback has proven very useful in the treatment of **tension headaches** and neuromuscular rehabilitation of stroke victims. It may be useful in the treatment of lower back pain, but the efficacy of biofeedback for chronic low back pain is still in doubt (Nouwen & Bush, 1984).

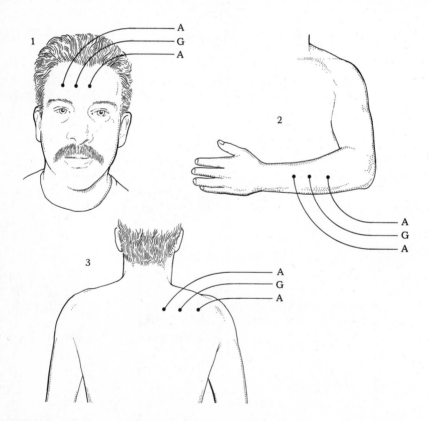

FIGURE 13-2
Location of measuring electrodes for EMG biofeedback in muscle tension at (1) the frontalis muscle, (2) forearm, and (3) the trapezius. The labels on the electrodes indicate the active (A) and ground (G) electrodes.

EEG Feedback: The Alpha Wave Revisited

The brain emits tiny electrical discharges just as muscles do. In 1928, Hans Berger showed that these minute currents could be amplified and displayed in graphic form on a machine that he invented, the electroencephalograph (EEG). The process is still somewhat troublesome, however, because of the care that must be taken to get accurate recordings.

In most clinical settings, EEG recordings come from electrodes placed on the surface of the skull. This means that the electrodes pick up the combined activity of thousands, if not millions, of cells located just below the electrode. Uniquely different brain waves—alpha, beta, theta, and delta—reflect different states of consciousness. Alpha reflects a relaxed, meditative state; beta is present during alert waking stages. Theta reflects states such as daydreaming or a hypnogogic state, and delta waves reflect deep sleep.

Sensing devices can be "tuned" to see a certain brain wave. Assume, for example, that clinicians want to feed back information on the alpha wave. They set the detection device so it filters out any brain wave below 8 Hz and above 12 Hz. When the filter detects a brain wave within this window, that brain wave can be amplified and used to turn on a tone or a light. For EEG feedback, an auditory signal is most frequently used.

EEG recording is difficult to carry out at home. Care must be taken in placement of electrodes, and they must be coated with a special electrolytic gel to get good readings. Although new techniques now make the process easier and more reliable in the clinic, these techniques are not likely to filter down to the home market for some time.

Most importantly, EEG biofeedback has few clinical uses. It may be useful in the treatment of insomnia and epilepsy. Some studies showed improvements in concentration, attention, and shifting awareness. Yet the potential for self-management seems even more limited than for clinical applications. Even the hoped-for electronic euphoria, equivalent to the Eastern mystical trance, did not appear.

Temperature Biofeedback: Keeping Cool

The body regulates temperature by changing the amount of blood in the extremities of the body. Surface blood vessels expand or contract in response to environmental conditions and internal demands. When the vessels relax, they permit more blood to flow, thus raising body temperature. When the vessels contract, they restrict the volume of blood, thus lowering body temperature.

The Yogis of India apparently had very fine control of blood flow. In one report, a Yogi could raise the temperature of the right earlobe by several degrees and simultaneously drop the temperature of the left earlobe by an equal amount. Clinical applications usually target finger temperature. This method may be used to treat **migraine headaches** and a rare disorder called **Raynaud's disease** (Blanchard & Haynes, 1975; Rose & Carlson, 1987). Further, it may be useful to treat irritable bowel syndrome, a disorder associated with distress (Blanchard, Schwarz, & Radnitz, 1987).

In temperature biofeedback, the detection device is a small electrode, called a thermistor, that measures finger termperature. Feedback may be visual or auditory or a combination of the two. Multicolor displays that change to yellow and red as the temperature goes up are very effective. Care must be taken to move the electrodes from finger to finger and from hand to hand as learning takes place. This is to ensure that the person learns a global response that warms the whole hand. Huge temperature changes may be possible in a single finger. But unless the person can warm the entire hand, the change will not be enough to alter the main symptom that needs to be controlled, such as migraine.

Visual imagery, such as that used in autogenics, aids in the process of changing skin temperature. The Menninger Clinic reported using autogenics in combination with biofeedback. They suggested that the cognitive aspects of autogenics can be guided by biofeedback while biofeedback aids in producing the desired physical change more rapidly (Green et al., 1973).

The Telltale Skin

When a person has an emotional reaction, a subtle but telltale change occurs in the skin. The skin's resistance goes down so that it conducts an electric current more readily. This is the principle behind the lie detector test. The galvanic skin response (GSR) may measure several different underlying processes; it may be related to increased moisture, sympathetic activity, or other processes.

Few biofeedback procedures depend on the GSR. Clinicians typically use it to help people who are insensitive to internal changes. Finally, it may be helpful for sorting items in a desensitization hierarchy.

Changing Cardiovascular Activity

Obtaining a reliable measure of cardiovascular activity is in some ways even more difficult than obtaining reliable brain-wave measures. People have learned how to control blood pressure and heart rate. Unfortunately, the gains are often statistically significant but clinically meaningless. These methods seemed at first to have great utility for people with hypertension, cardiac arrhythmias, and other heart problems, but the instrumentation was complicated and expensive. Also, most gains obtained with biofeedback, such as reduction in blood pressure, could be obtained through relaxation or EMG biofeedback or both (Lustman & Sowa, 1983). It seems, then, that a practical, useful cardiovascular biofeedback system is still years away; and even should it become available, it might not produce clinically meaningful changes.

BUT IS IT GOOD FOR ANYTHING?

Among the many questions raised about the promise of biofeedback, three are crucial. The first is whether people can learn to alter specific internal functions with biofeedback. The answer is an unqualified yes. The second question is whether biofeedback is useful for treating a variety of stress and health problems. The best answer is a qualified maybe. The third question is whether biofeedback's success comes from unique properties not present in other procedures. The answer is, mostly, no. The more scientists examined biofeedback, the more it appeared to share common elements with relaxation and cognitive restructuring procedures. The following is a brief summary of biofeedback's major successes and failures.

Biofeedback for High Blood Pressure

At first there was great hope for biofeedback as a treatment method for high blood pressure. Typically, subjects can reduce both systolic and diastolic blood pressure to a degree that is not due to chance factors. Still, the results are often not clinically meaningful because the amount of change is so small and/or the training does not have a long-term effect. Where large changes do occur, it is usually because blood pressure was extremely high at the outset. In addition, the new blood pressure levels generally are still above safe levels.

Biofeedback may help subjects reduce blood pressure more than relaxation does, but both procedures lead to lower levels (Engel, Glasgow, & Gaarder, 1983). One study showed that biofeedback and relaxation are equally effective and that both maintain lowered blood pressure up to a year after treatment (Walsh, Dale, & Anderson, 1977). Blanchard's research group conducted studies of hypertensive patients on medications (Blanchard et al., 1989; Blanchard et al., 1986). The group obtained a highly significant result showing that thermal biofeedback was successful in 65% of the cases, compared with 35% of those on relaxation training. Interestingly, their thermal biofeedback training combined autogenic phrases for warming hands. Still, professionals disagree on the issues of permanence and superiority.

Excedrin Headache #27 or EMG Headache #1?

The use of biofeedback for treating headaches has been very popular. Most frequently, the targets are either tension headaches or migraine headaches. Tension headaches may occur because of prolonged muscle contractions that result from some type of stress. Migraine headaches are most often attributed to vasoconstriction (Cohen et al., 1983). Typically, clinicians used EMG biofeedback for tension headaches and skin temperature biofeedback for migraine headaches (Budzynski, Stoyva, & Adler, 1970). One extensive study compared relaxation and biofeedback in treatment of three headache groups—migraine, tension, and a third group whose members suffered both migraine and tension headaches at different times. Relaxation alone led to significant improvement in all three groups, but biofeedback led to significant additional gains. In the tension-headache group, 73% improved greatly, and 52% in the migraine group improved greatly (Blanchard et al., 1982). Further studies by Blanchard's group showed that successful treatment with long-term maintenance can be attained with very little contact (Blanchard et al., 1988).

Recent evidence reviewed by Stanley Chapman (1986) called into question the prevailing notion that migraine calls for thermal biofeedback and tension headache calls for EMG biofeedback. He noted that migraine patients improve as much with EMG biofeedback as they do with thermal biofeedback. Also, the bulk of evidence does not support the contention that biofeedback is superior to relaxation in the treatment of headaches. Most negative outcomes occurred in studies with better controls, clearer diagnostic criteria, and longer adaptation periods and baselines. Finally, Chapman suggested that investigators provide little evidence that their subjects have really learned biofeedback when they maintain that biofeedback has been the effective agent.

In spite of the successes, there is still reason to doubt that biofeedback is necessary. For example, a study by Theodor Knapp (1982) showed that both biofeedback and cognitive coping skills can reduce frequency, duration, and intensity of migraines. In addition, the patients reduced medications after either treatment. The Colorado group headed by Thomas Budzynski concluded one report by noting that "EMG training [for tension headaches] alone is not effective in all cases" (Budzynski, Stoyva, Adler, & Mullaney, 1973). Robert Stern and William Ray (1977) suggested that the real benefit of biofeedback in the treatment of tension headaches may be that it teaches people to recognize signs of tension in body muscles so that they can begin relaxing immediately. Thus, biofeedback is probably not essential for control of headaches, but it may be an important element in education. Silver and Blanchard summed up the situation even more bluntly: In clinical tests comparing biofeedback to other procedures, there is no consistent advantage for any treatment (Silver & Blanchard, 1978).

A Cure for Cold Hands and Feet?

Raynaud's disease involves greatly restricted peripheral blood volume that causes the person to feel uncomfortably, if not painfully, cold. Usually this coldness occurs in the hands or feet or both, although the face and tongue also may feel cold at times. Both cold outside temperatures and emotional stress can trigger attacks (Pinkerton, Hughes, & Wenrich, 1982). As the attack progresses, the affected area may change color from whitish to cyanotic blue to bright red.

Clinicians often use temperature biofeedback to treat Raynaud's syndrome. One research group compared finger temperature biofeedback with frontalis EMG biofeedback or autogenic training (Freedman, Ianni, & Wenig, 1983). The patients treated with finger temperature biofeedback showed a significant reduction (92.5%) in symptoms compared to the other two groups (32.6% and 17%, respectively). This difference was still significant one year later at follow-up. Rose and Carlson (1987) discovered one promising treatment strategy, biofeedback with a cold stress condition, developed by Freedman's group. On the negative side, David Holmes (1981) conducted a thorough review of the literature on biofeedback, including the treatment of Raynaud's disease. He concluded that scientific support for the effectiveness of biofeedback in the treatment of Raynaud's disease, migraine, or hypertension is inconsistent.

There are many other uses for biofeedback to treat other ailments and medical conditions, but reviewing all these uses is beyond the scope of this book. Stern and Ray's (1977) book, *Biofeedback: Potential and Limits,* is an easy-to-read yet comprehensive review of biofeedback research.

BIOFEEDBACK: THE FINAL SCORE

In spite of the attention and great expectations, biofeedback has not lived up to its promise as a treatment technique or as a coping procedure. Independent reviews of biofeedback have provided comparable sobering conclusions. Turk's research group concluded that biofeedback has no demonstrated superiority over procedures such as relaxing or cognitive coping skills training. In addition, these procedures can be carried out with much less cost and effort than biofeedback (Turk, Meichenbaum, & Berman, 1979). Turk's group also noted that many biofeedback clients use cognitive controls and instructional sets to obtain successful outcomes.

Carol Schneider (1987) tried to provide evidence for the cost-effectiveness of biofeedback. Unfortunately, her review clouded issues by using relaxation training as the primary intervention, assisted by biofeedback as a learning strategy. The review also mixed studies that have clear cognitive stress management components; this makes it difficult to evaluate the contribution of each discrete treatment component. Cost-benefits assessment in this quagmire cannot be applied meaningfully to a single component.

Thomas Burish (1981) looked at EMG biofeedback specifically for stress-related disorders. He concluded that biofeedback has not proven effective in reducing either internal or behavioral reactions to stress. As he stated:

> It may be naive to think not only that a biofeedback procedure aimed at changing the EMG level of a specific muscle group will produce a general (i.e., multisystem) relaxation effect, but also that any type of relaxation strategy will *by itself* produce and maintain a permanent change in stress-related symptoms if the nature and intensity of the stressor is not modified. (p. 418)

Lawrence Simkins (1982) asked the rhetorical question "Is biofeedback clinically valid or oversold?" He pointed out that many studies have internal flaws that fail to eliminate alternate explanations, especially the placebo effect. In addition, many studies use small samples and lack adequate controls. Simkins concluded that we probably expect too much from biofeedback. Effective stress management and personal health maintenance must incorporate cognitive, attitudinal, and lifestyle changes as well.

It is important to note that biofeedback can play an important part in teaching people how to read the signals of their body, including signals of tension. On this issue, no disagreement exists. When used as an educational and counseling ally, biofeedback can be very helpful (Schneider, 1987; Winfield, 1983). There is also no dispute that biofeedback *can* produce some positive outcomes. The point is that *it is not absolutely necessary to use biofeedback to produce these positive results.* If we could shift focus from biofeedback as a primary treatment or coping strategy and focus instead on the information gained from biofeedback that can be used in other ways, then this procedure should find an honored and rightful place with the other techniques described here.

SHOULD I TRY BIOFEEDBACK?

Whether you should try biofeedback depends on several factors such as (1) the intended use; (2) the nature and severity of the symptom to be treated; (3) prior treatment history, if any; and (4) the demonstrated usefulness for treating the target symptom. There are various uses for biofeedback. You can obtain more objective ratings of anxiety to help build a fear ladder for desensitization. You can improve your ability to tune in to body signals. You should be cautious, though, if you intend to use biofeedback to alter a symptom that has medical implications. The more serious the symptom, the more cautious you should be. Also, if you have never received treatment for the symptom, you should have a medical examination first.

Any use of biofeedback should first seek evidence that biofeedback is successful for the target symptom. In the absence of this evidence, biofeedback should not be used. If you do decide to use biofeedback, set realistic goals. Do not expect to make global changes in health problems. Also, do not expect biofeedback to cure everything. As suggested before, typically you need to combine biofeedback with lifestyle change and cognitive coping strategies to obtain satisfactory long-term results.

SUMMARY

This chapter reviewed the status of some popular methods for coping with stress and improving health. This included Yoga meditation, the Western version of Mantra Yoga called Transcendental Meditation, and Herbert Benson's variation of TM, called secular meditation. We discussed the claims for meditation in historical and scientific perspective. Meditation may produce certain desirable altered mental and physical states. Still, these changes are not unique to the practice of meditation. Other procedures, such as deep muscle relaxation and autogenics, can produce the same positive results. In addition, extensive supporting research and tested applications do not exist regarding meditation. Thus, it seems more limited in comparison to previously mentioned procedures. Because Benson's secular meditation is easy to learn, we discussed guidelines to begin practicing.

We also reviewed the high-tech solution, biofeedback. The most common types of biofeedback include EMG, EEG, GSR, temperature, and forms of cardiovascular feedback. The stress symptoms most frequently treated with biofeedback include migraine and tension headaches, hypertension, and chronic pain. While biofeedback may yield positive results, most practitioners are no longer as enthusiastic about biofeedback as they once were. Several factors have contributed to this change: biofeedback does not always result in clinically meaningful change; the results do not always last; cheaper and easier techniques are as successful; and other techniques often must be added to obtain satisfactory results. Still, biofeedback may be valuable for education and symptomatic relief if the person takes certain precautions.

KEY TERMS

alpha
Benson's secular
  meditation
biofeedback
blood pressure
  biofeedback
cardiovascular
  biofeedback

EEG biofeedback
EMG biofeedback
GSR biofeedback
koan
mantra
meditation
migraine head-
  aches

Raynaud's disease
tension headaches
temperature
  biofeedback
Transcendental Medita-
  tion (TM)

REFERENCES

Anand, B. K., Chhina, G. S., & Singh, B. (1961). Studies on Shri Ramananda Yogi during his stay in an air-tight box. *Indian Journal of Medical Research, 49,* 82–89.

Behanan, K. T. (1964). *Yoga: A scientific evaluation.* New York: Dover.

Benson, H. (1975). *The relaxation response.* New York: Morrow.

Blanchard, E. B., Andrasik, F., Neff, D. F., Arena, J. G., Ahles, T. A., & Jurish, S. E., et al. (1982). Biofeedback and relaxation training with three kinds of headache: Treatment effects and their prediction. *Journal of Consulting and Clinical Psychology, 50,* 562–575.

Blanchard, E. B., Appelbaum, K. A., Guarnieri, P., Neff, D. F., Andrasik, F., Jaccard, J., & Barron, K. D. (1988). Two studies of the long-term follow-up of minimal therapist contact treatments of vascular and tension headache. *Journal of Consulting and Clinical Psychology, 56,* 427–432.

Blanchard, E. B., & Haynes, M. R. (1975). Biofeedback treatment of a case of Raynaud's disease. *Journal of Behavior Therapy and Experimental Psychiatry, 6,* 230–234.

Blanchard, E. B., McCoy, G. C., Berger, M., Musso, A., Pallmeyer, T. P., Gerardi, R., et al. (1989). A controlled comparison of thermal biofeedback and relaxation training in the treatment of essential hypertension: IV. Prediction of short-term clinical outcome. *Behavior Therapy, 20,* 405–415.

Blanchard, E. B., McCoy, G. C., Musso, A., Gerardi, M. A., Pallmeyer, T. P., Gerardi, R. J., et al. (1986). A controlled comparison of thermal biofeedback and relaxation training in the treatment of essential hypertension: I. Short-term and long-term outcome. *Behavior Therapy, 17,* 563–579.

Blanchard, E. B., Schwarz, S. P., & Radnitz, C. R. (1987). Psychological assessment and treatment of irritable bowel syndrome. *Behavior Modification, 11,* 348–372.

Bloomfield, H. H., Cain, M. P., Jaffe, D. T., & Kory, R. B. (1975). *TM: Discovering inner energy and overcoming stress.* New York: Dell.

Boerstler, R. W. (1986). Meditation and the dying process. *Journal of Humanistic Psychology, 26,* 104–124.

Brent, P. L. (1972). *The god-men of India.* London: Allen Lane.

Brooks, J. S., & Scarano, T. (1985). Transcendental meditation in the treatment of post-Vietnam adjustment. *Journal of Consulting and Development, 64,* 212–215.

Budzynski, T., Stoyva, J., & Adler, C. (1970). Feedback-induced muscle relaxation: Application to tension headache. *Journal of Behavior Therapy and Experimental Psychiatry, 1,* 205–211.

Budzynski, T. H., Stoyva, J. M., Adler, C. S., & Mullaney, D. J. (1973). EMG biofeedback and tension headache: A controlled outcome study. *Psychosomatic Medicine, 35,* 484–496.

Burish, T. G. (1981). EMG biofeedback in the treatment of stress-related disorders. In C. K. Prokop & L. A. Bradley (Eds.), *Medical psychology: Contributions to behavioral medicine* (pp. 395–421). New York: Academic Press.

Chapman, S. L. (1986). A review and clinical perspective on the use of EMG and thermal biofeedback for chronic headaches. *Pain, 27,* 1–43.

Cohen, R. A., Williamson, D. A., Monguillot, J. E., Hutchinson, P. C., Gottlieb, J., & Waters, W. F. (1983). Psychophysiological response patterns in vascular and muscle-contraction headaches. *Journal of Behavioral Medicine, 6,* 93–107.

Deikman, A. (1969). Experimental meditation. In C. Tart (Ed.), *Altered states of consciousness* (pp. 203–223). New York: Wiley.

Delmonte, M. M. (1984). Meditation practice as related to occupational stress, health and productivity. *Perceptual and Motor Skills, 59,* 581–582.

Dillbeck, M. C., Aron, A. P., & Dillbeck, S. L. (1979, November). The Transcendental Meditation program as an educational technology: Research and applications. *Educational Technology, 19,* 7–13.

Dillbeck, M. C., & Orme-Johnson, D. W. (1987). Physiological differences between transcendental meditation and rest. *American Psychologist, 42,* 879–880.

Engel, B. T., Glasgow, M. S., & Gaarder, K. R. (1983). Behavioral treatment of high blood pressure: III. Follow-up results and treatment recommendations. *Psychosomatic Medicine, 45,* 23–29.

Freedman, R. R., Ianni, P., & Wenig, P. (1983). Behavioral treatment of Raynaud's disease. *Journal of Consulting and Clinical Psychology, 51,* 539–549.

Fuller, G. D. (1977). *Biofeedback: Methods and procedures in clinical practice.* San Francisco: Biofeedback Press.

Green, E. E., Green, A. M., Walter, E. D., Sargent, J. D., & Meyer, R. G. (1973). *Autogenic feedback training.* Topeka, KS: The Menninger Foundation.

Green, E. E., Green, A. M., & Walters, D. (1972). Biofeedback for mind-body self-regulation: Healing and creativity. *Fields Within Fields . . . Within Fields, 5,* 131–144.

Hatch, J. P., & Riley, P. (1986). Growth and development of biofeedback: A bibliographic analysis. *Biofeedback and Self-Regulation, 10,* 289–299.

Hoenig, J. (1968). Medical research on Yoga. *Confinia Psychiatrica, 11,* 69–89.

Holmes, D. S. (1981). The use of biofeedback for treating patients with migraine headaches, Raynaud's disease, and hypertension: A critical evaluation. In C. K. Prokop & L. A. Bradley (Eds.), *Medical psychology: Contributions to behavioral medicine* (pp. 423–437). New York: Academic Press.

Holmes, D. S., Solomon, S., Cappo, B. M., & Greenberg, J. L. (1983). Effects of transcendental meditation versus resting on physiological and subjective arousal. *Journal of Personality and Social Psychology, 44,* 1245–1252.

Kabat-Zinn, J., Lipworth, L., & Burney, R. (1985). The clinical use of mindfulness meditation for the self-regulation of chronic pain. *Journal of Behavioral Medicine, 8,* 163–190.

Kapleau, P. (Ed.). (1966). *The three pillars of Zen.* New York: Harper & Row.

Kasamatsu, A., & Hirai, T. (1963). Science of zazen. *Psychologia, 6,* 86–91.

Knapp, T. W. (1982). Treating migraine by training in temporal artery vasoconstriction and/or cognitive behavioral coping: A one-year follow-up. *Journal of Psychosomatic Research, 26,* 551–557.

Lintel, A. G. (1980). Physiological anxiety responses in transcendental meditators and nonmeditators. *Perceptual and Motor Skills, 50,* 295–300.

Lustman, P. J., & Sowa, C. J. (1983). Comparative efficacy of biofeedback and stress inoculation for stress reduction. *Journal of Clinical Psychology, 39,* 191–197.

Nouwen, A., & Bush, C. (1984). The relationship between paraspinal EMG and chronic low back pain. *Pain, 20,* 109–123.

Pagano, R. R., Rose, R. M., Stivers, R. M., & Warrenburg, S. (1976). Sleep during transcendental meditation. *Science, 191,* 308–309.

Pinkerton, S. S., Hughes, H., & Wenrich, W. W. (1982). *Behavioral medicine: Clinical applications.* New York: Wiley.

Puente, A. E., & Beiman, I. (1980). The effects of behavior therapy, self-relaxation, and transcendental meditation on cardiovascular stress response. *Journal of Clinical Psychology, 36,* 291–295.

Rose, G. D., & Carlson, J. G. (1987). The behavioral treatment of Raynaud's disease: A review. *Biofeedback and Self-regulation, 12,* 257–272.

Schneider, C. J. (1987). Cost effectiveness of biofeedback and behavioral medicine treatments: A review of the literature. *Biofeedback and Self-Regulation, 12,* 71–92.

Shapiro, D. H., & Zifferblatt, S. M. (1976). Zen meditation and behavioral self-control: Similarities, differences, and clinical applications. *American Psychologist, 31,* 519–532.

Silver, B. V., & Blanchard, E. B. (1978). Biofeedback and relaxation training in the treatment of psychophysiological disorders: Or are the machines really necessary? *Journal of Behavioral Medicine, 2,* 217–239.

Simkins, L. (1982). Biofeedback: Clinically valid or oversold? *Psychological Record, 32,* 3–17.

Stern, R. M., & Ray, W. J. (1977). *Biofeedback: Potential and limits.* Lincoln: University of Nebraska Press.

Throll, D. A. (1982). Transcendental meditation and progressive relaxation: Their physiological effects. *Journal of Clinical Psychology, 38,* 522–530.

Turk, D. C., Meichenbaum, D. H., & Berman, W. H. (1979). Application of biofeedback for the regulation of pain: A critical review. *Psychological Bulletin, 86,* 1322–1338.

Wallace, R. K., & Benson, H. (1972). The physiology of meditation. *Scientific American, 226,* 84–90.

Walsh, P., Dale, A., & Anderson, D. E. (1977). Comparison of biofeedback, pulse wave velocity and progressive relaxation in essential hypertensives. *Perceptual and Motor Skills, 44,* 839–843.

Weiner, N. (1954). *The human use of human beings: Cybernetics and society.* Garden City, NY: Doubleday/Anchor.

Wenger, M. A., & Bagchi, B. K. (1961). Studies of autonomic function in practitioners of Yoga in India. *Behavioral Science, 6,* 312–323.

Winfield, I. (1983). Counselling with biofeedback: A review. *British Journal of Guidance and Counselling, 11,* 46–51.

PART FIVE

TIME MANAGEMENT, NUTRITION, AND EXERCISE

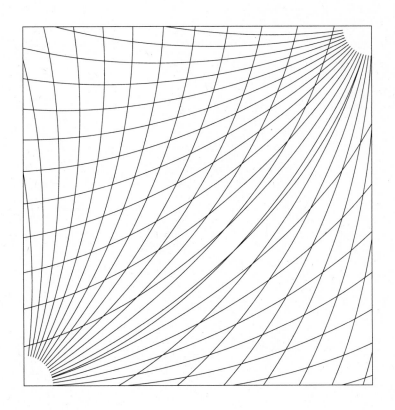

CHAPTER 14

Managing Time-Related Stress

FINDING BETTER WAYS OF DOING WHAT YOU'RE DOING ISN'T WORTHWHILE WHEN
WHAT YOU'RE DOING ISN'T WORTH DOING ANYWAY.
PHILIP MARVIN

Remember those childhood days when time passed without a care? Remember how all those childhood activities, playing house or going fishing, were seldom calculated in terms of time? True, our parents were constantly reminding us of time: "Be home for supper." "Be in by 10:00." "You have to have your homework done by 6:00 or you can't watch TV." No matter. When we were engrossed in pursuits of the imagination, time did not seem to matter.

If anything, time hung heavy. School days could wear on and on. Waiting to become an adult seemed like a trip down the long road of eternity itself. And being an adult meant being on your own and being able do with your time what you wanted.

How times change! Now, time passes too quickly. Now, there is never enough time. If only we could have a 36-hour day! But time is a fixed commodity. Therefore, it is not how much time we have but how we use it that makes the difference. And, perhaps most crucial, it is not so much the absolute standard of time that pushes us, but how we think about time that pressures us.

WHY STUDY TIME MANAGEMENT?

According to Jack Ferner (1980), **time management** is "efficient use of our resources, including time, in such a way that we are effective in achieving important personal goals" (p. 12). Some people have already acquired good time management skills, but others need to spend time developing skills. Several studies have shown that brief courses or workshops in time management can have a positive effect on use of time for teachers (Hall & Hursch, 1982; Woolfolk & Woolfolk, 1986), school principals (Maher, 1986), or hospital managers (Hanel, Martin, & Koop, 1982).

Time management can also produce positive outcomes for students in an academic setting, reducing the likelihood of dropout and raising grade point average by small amounts (Bost, 1984). One study used a critical-incident technique to study this issue. Students ranked setting goals as the second most

355

important factor related to success in college. Time management was ranked the fourth most important factor. Conversely, the students ranked failure to engage in good time management as the second most important factor in academic failure (Schmelzer, Schmelzer, Figler, & Brozo, 1987). What was the most important? It should be no surprise: failure to study.

There are several reasons why time management is also central to the problem of stress and health. First, using some rather simple time management techniques can improve personal productivity. The net effect is to provide more discretionary time for social pursuits, exercise, recreation, and hobbies. Lack of time for personal pursuits tends to be one of the most frequently cited stressors. Providing time for self and family usually has the desirable effect of reducing levels of subjective stress. Barkas (cited in Langfelder, 1987) goes so far as to say that the most important objective of time management is to create more leisure time.

Second, it has become almost a truism that modern society is time driven, if not time obsessed. The Type A behavior pattern is presumably the epitome, the extreme expression of that all-consuming sense of time urgency. Society's preoccupation with time may also be a sign of much that is wrong with the way value is calculated. All too often, value is calculated in terms of money, power, and position, all of which generally require high productivity to attain. And being productive usually means working hard and working long hours. The study of time management may help us rethink some of our attitudes toward time and reduce the sense of time urgency.

But time management should never become a goal in itself. Time management is a tool to be used for a short while to reset priorities and recast inefficient work habits. When the job is done, it should be put on the back shelf until needed again. Time management should never become a chore that must be done every day. Rather, it should help you use time more efficiently. But time management should never manage you. If it does, throw it out!

In the same vein, a number of time management books seem, if anything, to reinforce the Type A pattern. The bottom line is productivity, and the score is measured in dollars. The ethic is more work in less time, ever onward and upward to that next promotion. If there is any concern with those basic human values of caring and sharing, it is not evident. We each need to take time to express all facets of our personality and to appreciate the creative and artistic expressions of others. If time management does not free us for these pursuits, it is a misplaced effort.

TIME IS IN THE EYE OF THE BEHOLDER

Attitudes toward time have changed greatly over the years. They also vary among different cultures and among people in the same society. How we think about time is a critical determinant of whether or not time is viewed as pressure. The following paragraphs describe some of the most common attitudes toward time.

Social-Cultural Context of Time

Even a casual inspection of history suggests that ancient cultures show an almost timeless quality. It is not that they were "nontimed" but that precise timekeeping was not central to their existence. Presumably all this changed with the appearance of clocks in medieval Europe. From that point on, keeping track of time seemed an important pursuit in its own right. If anything, the Industrial Revolution added to this concern because precise timekeeping was viewed as crucial to meeting urgent survival needs.

Another legacy began with Sir Isaac Newton, who viewed each time interval as unique but equal. This view presumably encourages continuous but short-range activity and may obscure long-range goals and futuristic planning. It also seems to foster guilt when nothing that passes as valued activity is observed during an interval.

The importance of time in modern society is further emphasized in research on people who have a high need for achievement. Such people feel annoyed when their watches stop running. For them, a watch is not a luxury but a necessity that keeps them functioning properly. They often feel anxious when they are not certain about the time and wonder how people can get along without watches (Webber, 1972). Boston, the number-one American city in pace, has a phone number to obtain the exact time of day: dial N-E-R-V-O-U-S (Levine, 1989).

Metaphors and Myths of Time

In contemporary society, a number of verbal statements, such as "Time is money," seem to capture the essence of our attitudes toward time. Metaphors for time, or maybe myths, they reflect the implicit, often untested values that focus efforts and guide behavior.

Edwin Bliss (1976) told a wonderful anecdote of a first-grader who observed his father bringing home a briefcase full of work every night. Puzzled over this continuing state of affairs, the little boy asked his mother why it had to be that way. The mother gave a very adult response: "Daddy has so much to do he can't finish at the office and has to work nights." The child's response was simple and uncluttered with the value-laden adult explanation: "Well, then, why don't they just put him in a slower group?" (p. 10).

The behavior of the parents reflects their untested assumptions: Daddy's behavior is normal and necessary; the solution to work problems is to work longer and harder. The following attitudes toward time seem most prominently taught or espoused in modern society:

1. Time is money.
2. Time is a resource.
3. An idle mind is the devil's playground.
4. Wasting time is sinful.
5. I have all the time in the world.

The first statement may be one of the most used, if abused, business clichés. The second may come closest to representing a valid argument for wise use of time. The third and fourth have their roots in the Industrial Revolution as much as in theology. All four are intended to increase personal commitment to use time wisely. The last one is an attitude that works in the opposite direction. Each is in some sense a mental trap, a mindset or perceptual bias that needs to be examined.

Time is money   The central value expressed in this metaphor is obvious, yet is too widely and readily accepted as a creed to live by. Problems arise when the same value interferes with home and social life. Calculating time at home, time with your spouse, with your children, for yourself, for exercise, cannot be calculated in terms of money. If the family is not on an equal footing with work, something is wrong. Counselors have found families torn apart by pressures from an absentee wage-earner who thought that providing material comforts was all-important. In the midst of counseling, revelations made by a neglected spouse and lonely children suggest that they would have gladly done with much less in order to have more time together.

Even in business, time is paramount only in certain occupations. Speculative professions (such as stocks and commodities brokerage or land development) tend to set time on a pedestal. Fortunes may turn on a matter of the minutes or seconds it takes to make a decision to buy, sell, or contract. For many businesses, however, creativity and quality are as important as speed. If time is money, it is so only in a limited arena or to those who prize money above all else.

Time is a resource   The notion that time is a resource is somewhat reminiscent of a statement Will Rogers made about land: "Buy it. It is one thing they're not making any more." Unlike land, we cannot buy, sell, or save time. But like land, time cannot be manufactured. We each come into the world with exactly the same amount of time: 24 hours per day, 8736 hours per year. But if time is conceived as a resource, the proper way to get the most out of it is through wise management. The applicable cliché here is "Work smart, not hard."

Idle minds   The assumption behind this metaphor is that a mind not filled with purposeful thought (directed to engaging in productive activity, deriving income, or serving some pressing social need) must certainly be filled with ideas of a baser variety. Concentration on work and service has come to be synonymous with the active mind. But some of the most creative and brilliant insights have occurred during idle moments, flights of fancy, daydreaming, or dreaming itself. In addition, it now appears that some mental idling serves a useful purpose by providing an outlet for pent-up emotions.

Wasting time is sinful   The hidden trap in this metaphor is the term *wasting*. But what is wasteful? It may well be that you could buy a good rocking chair or cradle for a reasonable price, much less than it would cost you for the lumber and time to build one yourself. But the time spent building one may prove valuable to you in many intangible ways. Taking your mind off job pressures, changing gears mentally, and taking time for yourself all may result from engaging in this type of activity. If the activity is spent with family, teaching a daughter or son some useful skill or hobby, the expenditure of time cannot and should not be calculated in terms of money. If you find yourself saying "I am wasting time," ask yourself this question: "Based on what value?"

All the time in the world   For the most part, this is an illusion of youth. Youth is often filled with perceptions of invulnerability and agelessness. Such perceptions frequently lead to procrastination, which eats up valuable time and results in aimless action. While time obsessions should be avoided, little that is worthwhile in life can be accomplished if time is ignored or treated as though it counts for nothing. The goal of effective time management is to find the harmony or balance in use of time that serves productive, wage-earning needs but still meets personal needs of caring, sharing, and growing.

SEVEN DEADLY SINS OF TIME MISMANAGEMENT

Before discussing how to manage time, it may prove useful to consider how time is mismanaged. Indeed, any time management program should start with a personal inventory of how time is being used. Through this means, you gain a sense of what needs to be changed and what should stay the same. More details on how to do this will be given later in this chapter. For now, consider the following sins of time mismanagement, the acts of omission and commission that drain this resource. The most common are confusion, indecision, diffusion, procrastination, avoidance, interruptions, and perfectionism.

Confusion: Where Am I Going?

When someone complains they are wasting too much time but are not sure where their time is actually going, you can be fairly sure they do not know where *they* are going. Partin (1983) likens this to the airline pilot who radios in that they are "making good time, but [they're] lost" (p. 280). Lewis Carroll's *Alice's Adventures in Wonderland* (1865/1966) contains an interaction between Alice and the Cheshire Cat that aptly captures this time management problem. Alice has come to a fork in the road and is confused about what to do. Spying the Cheshire Cat in the tree, she asks:

> "Would you tell me, please, which way I ought to go from here?"
> "That depends a good deal on where you want to get to," said the Cat.
> "I don't much care where—," said Alice.
> "Then it doesn't matter which way you go," said the Cat. (p. 89)

As one time management specialist points out, time management does not make a lot of sense unless you know where you want to go (Rutherford, 1978). Failing to plot a course for the next few months and years may be the single biggest error in time management.

Indecision: What Should I Do?

The second major error in time management is indecision, or failing to make a decision that needs to be made. It is similar to the approach taken by the ostrich, ignoring whatever does not seem pleasant. It has been noted that there is no such thing as indecision; there is only the decision not to decide. In any case, indecision is the hidden foe of effective time management.

Indecision means that we often end up handling tasks several times instead of once. It also tends to increase our confusion and tension. Further, the higher the position of leadership and management we hold, the more indecision compounds confusion and tension in those around us. Rather than being restricted to the realm of personal outcomes, then, the effects of indecision add to "team" inefficiency as well.

Indecision increases confusion and tension because the decision is easily put off but not so easily put away. It is still there, waiting to be made, playing on the backroads of the mind even while other tasks are pressing. Indecision robs us of the freedom to focus, to relax, to create. Also, the inability to make decisions may be behind other problems in time management such as procrastination, creating and allowing interruptions, and avoidance of duties.

Indecision may stem from many psychological factors. Stress may intrude from some other area of life and erode decision-making capabilities. Or, indecision may be due to lack of interest in the task, a failure of motivation. Indecision may result from a deep-seated fear of making the wrong decision. Finally, it may result from lacking the information necessary to make a good decision; in this case, however, indecision may be acceptable and wise.

Diffusion: Mental and Physical Overload

Diffusion is the attempt to do far more than is necessary, perhaps even more than is possible. It is having too many irons in the fire. Mental diffusion produces ineffective problem solving, lack of concentration, and poor motivation for even the simplest tasks. Trying to keep up with all one's duties then takes its toll on the body in physical fatigue. This tends to further strain the mental system.

Diffusion results from not knowing the limits of your own capabilities. It also results from not knowing when and how to say no to requests from your friends and colleagues. In some cases, the two may be related. That is, the inability to say no may be due to not knowing your own limits.

Charles Kozoll (1982) described the **battered mind syndrome,** widely reported among teachers and administrators, which is quite typical of the effects of diffusion. The major characteristics of the syndrome include (1) many thoughts at once, (2) pervasive worry about what remains to be done, and (3) loss of focus on what can and should be done as pressures continue to mount. In addition, (4) the battered educator seems to operate on the assumption that interruptions will occur often; therefore, involvement in immediate tasks is very shallow (Kozoll, 1982).

Procrastination: That Will Keep for Another Day

Procrastination is the thief of time, the cardinal sin of time mismanagement. Procrastination has been defined as putting off until tomorrow what you should do today. Merrill and Donna Douglass (1980) have identified three types of procrastination: putting off unpleasant things, putting off things that are difficult, and putting off things that involve tough decisions.

Robert Rutherford (1978) discusses two excuses that seem to keep a person from going to work: "I wish" and "I just can't get started" (p. 28). The "I wish" excuse usually entails wishing not to have to do the work or wishing for some type of miracle to do the job. In essence, it removes the responsibility of making something happen. The second wish is a type of self-fulfilling prophecy. It turns self-deceit into reality, which in the end is a self-defeat.

Laura Solomon and Esther Rothblum (1984) were concerned about the observed relationship between procrastination and poor college performance. The results of their study suggested that procrastination is more than just weak study habits and poor time management. One significant component that appeared in a large group of students was task aversiveness. In another, smaller group of students, the factors contributing to procrastination included such cognitive and affective components as irrational ideas, low self-esteem, depression, anxiety, fear of failure, and lack of assertion. Solomon and Rothblum suggested that this group of students would probably need to consider more than just time management in order to get past the procrastination problem.

Eliminating habitual procrastination requires some remedial action. For a while you should note which tasks you keep putting off. Then look for a common pattern in these tasks. Jim Davidson (1978) suggested that you try to find out why you do not like the job. Then, if possible, you could delegate the job to someone else. Otherwise, you might break the job down into smaller units or change the job in some way so it is easier to finish.

One simple rule is to do the things you do not like first. With unpleasant tasks out of the way, you should feel freer to concentrate on the jobs you like. Otherwise, the set-aside job hangs over your head, distracting you and reducing your effectiveness for the job you like. Some people find it helpful to make a contract with themselves. They may reward themselves for finishing less desirable tasks by taking a short extra break or by buying some clothing or a record from money set aside for this purpose.

Avoidance: Escape to Fantasyland

People find many ways of avoiding work. They stretch coffee breaks. They wander the hallways looking for someone to talk to, presumably on business. They read books or sections of the newspaper they really do not need to read. They dwell on trivial aspects of organizing their work. The person who is constantly cleaning the desk or files may really be engaging in escape behavior. Another common escape is daydreaming. Managers sometimes do work they could, and probably should, delegate to someone else while they attend to more important developmental matters. People write and rewrite letters or memos in the name of perfection. In fact, they are probably avoiding some other task they do not want to do. If you catch yourself frequently saying that you are a perfectionist, consider if you are also avoiding by overdoing.

Interruptions: Getting Started Is the Hard Part

One of the most frustrating time-killers is the unscheduled interruption. People who work in walk-in businesses are victims of constant interruptions. But many other offices and businesses have their share of interruptions as well. Phone calls, the boss dropping in for a chat, colleagues stopping by to say hello, and emergencies all represent disruptions to the normal flow of work. Students living in a dormitory face similar problems in trying to manage studies.

According to one study, the average manager is interrupted an average of once every 8 minutes (Davidson, 1978). Another writer even suggested that if the manager is not interrupted at least once every half hour, the manager will arrange for an interruption. This points to the fact that interruptions are not completely uncontrollable. A number of the interruptions that occur could be prevented by decisive action on our own part. As will become evident later, even uncontrolled interruptions can be reduced and made predictable.

Interruptions are perhaps most damaging in complex projects, where larger blocks of time are important to the flow of thought, or in the development of some sequential idea. Computer programming and creative writing are two examples of such projects. Such jobs involve a warm-up period for establishing a rhythm. Frequent interruptions require additional time to reorient and warm up again.

If anything is unscheduled, it is the emergency. While some organizations are structured to respond to emergencies, most are not. A survey of managers showed that fully 12% of their workday was devoted to emergencies. Only 44% of the workday was devoted to planned activities! Another 14% was devoted to customer-initiated activities (Marvin, 1980). The remainder of the manager's day was divided between routine activities and government requirements.

Charles Hummel (cited in Posner, 1982) said that a tension exists between the urgent and the important. Important tasks virtually never have to be done right away, today, or even this week. On the other hand, urgent tasks and crises require instant action. The problem is that the crisis diverts attention from what is important. It takes time away from planned activities and thus disrupts the schedule. But the crisis also becomes an excuse. Work, important work, is not done. It's all right, though, because there was an emergency!

Perfectionism: I Was Raised a Perfectionist

You have probably heard it many times: "I'm a perfectionist." LeBoeuf (1979) points out that a perfect golf score is 18, whereas an excellent golf score is 72. No one seriously expects to attain such perfection in golf, but people will set equally unrealistic standards for other aspects of their life. **Perfectionism** may have a place in life, but perfectionism for the sake of perfection is about as useful as rewaxing the whole car because you missed a tiny spot the first time. This type of perfectionism is really little more than compulsive overdoing.

The problem is to draw the line between the necessary and the excessive, between quality that will return dividends and meticulousness that will never be noticed and will not bring any gain. It is the law of diminished returns: Up to a point, the extra effort will be worthwhile. After that point, no amount of extra effort will produce any gain.

GETTING READY FOR TIME MANAGEMENT

It is one thing to identify time traps. It is another thing to weed them out of one's personal and professional habits. Many people talk about time management, but few are prepared to perform the primary task of identifying how real time is spent. If you feel you are already managing your time effectively, there may be little point in doing a time study. On the other hand, if you feel that some improvement is in order, be prepared to make a commitment for a short time at least. As noted earlier, though, do not think of time management as a lifelong task.

To begin a time management program, you must know what needs to be changed. You can find this out through a time inventory, in which you take stock of how and where you spend your time. This may be done through many formal means. If you wish, you can purchase books solely devoted to time management, with tailored worksheets to help you study your use of time. But in actuality, you can carry out a time study with a few pennies' worth of paper, a pencil, and a few days of attention.

TIME STUDY:
FINDING YOUR TIME MANAGEMENT WEAKNESSES

We quite often think of time as a constant. In purely objective terms, this may be more or less true, but in terms of the subjective perception of time, it is rarely ever true. We tend to misjudge time substantially depending on what we are doing. We elongate tedious or boring periods and foreshorten periods filled with excitement (McConalogue, 1984). As a result, we can be very far off the mark if we depend on our subjective sense of time to tell us how much time we are spending on different activities.

If you find yourself at the end of the day wondering where the time went, you may benefit from a time study. A time study seeks answers to three basic questions: What do you do? When do you do it? How much time does it take?

A simple way to obtain this information is to keep a daily log in which time periods are listed down the left side of the page and days across the top. Use periods as short as 15 minutes or as long as one hour, depending on the type of work you are doing. A 30-minute period will probably work for most purposes.

If you are concerned about time spent at work, chart only the primary working days. If you are concerned about both personal and professional time, use the entire week. Divide each day into two columns, one for the type of activity, the other for the people present. Jot down a short reminder of the activity you carried out during each period and note the people present. If the activity continues for more than one period, you may either fill successive periods with dittos or leave them blank until the activity changes.

After you have collected at least one week's information, begin searching for patterns. First, set out all nonjob blocks of time, including commuting to and from the job. Then identify discretionary time—that is, time under your own control. Finally, label all the nondiscretionary time—time determined by supervisors or requirements of the job or related to family function.

Peter Drucker (1967), one of the pioneers of time management, believed that managers have only about 25% controllable time, whereas the remaining 75% of their time is uncontrollable. After you have set aside the nondiscretionary time, look at the discretionary time to see where improvements or wastes are occurring. But do not label time as nondiscretionary just to be rid of the responsibility of managing it more effectively.

If you see blocks of discretionary time being broken up by interruptions, identify the people (yourself included) or events responsible for those interruptions. You may see a simple plan of action to correct the situation. If you find that a great deal of time is spent in nonproductive commuting, you may be able to transform it into productive time.

POSITIVE TIME MANAGEMENT

Previously, the most common errors of time management were identified. This section and the following section provide some positive steps to eliminate the errors.

Priorities: The Solution to Confusion

"You have to have your priorities straight!" This saying is overworked but nonetheless true. The best solution for confusion is to set goals and reevaluate those goals periodically. There are a few basic guidelines for setting goals. First, establish clear, achievable goals. Second, assign a priority to each goal. Third, identify small tasks, related to your goals, which can be carried out in short work periods. Fourth, set target dates for completion of the smaller tasks. Finally, reevaluate your goals periodically. Even if you have a personal five-year plan, you may need to reevaluate it each year.

Goals should be clear and achievable. While dreams may be the stuff of progress, unrealistic dreams generally produce only disillusionment and lowered resolve. Set your goals for three distinct time frames: long-term, medium-range, and short-term. Long-term goals should answer the basic question: "Where do I want to be in five years and what do I have to do to get there?" Medium-range goals should address the issue of "Where do I want to be next year at this same time?" If you are under 25, you may want to use shorter periods, say three years for long-term goals and six months for short-term goals.

Regardless of your age, you usually have to break short-term goals down into more tangible tasks. First, for each week you should set attainable, concrete objectives that provide for some progress toward the major goal. Second, you should make a daily "to do" list to organize both personal and professional time. These lists do not have to be written formally, but many of the most efficient corporate executives report doing so. They write their "to do" list before leaving the office, later in the evening before retiring, or in the first few minutes after reaching the office. Alan Lakein (1974), author of one of the best-selling time management books, suggested that the major difference between people at the top and people trying to make the top is that the ones at the top know how to use "to do" lists and make one every day.

The Pareto Principle

The **Pareto principle** is named after an Italian economist and sociologist, Vilfredo Pareto, who lived during the late 19th and early 20th centuries. His notion can be summarized in the phrase *the vital few and the trivial many*. In general, the idea is that 20% of your goals contain 80% of the value. The remaining 80% of your goals account for only 20% of the value. To manage time effectively, invest time in proportion to value—in other words, in the few goals with much meaning. Problems appear when the trivial consumes a disproportionate amount of your time.

The way to solve this problem is to list what you want to accomplish in long-term, intermediate, and short-term periods. Then arrange the list from most important to least important. Next, distribute the bulk of your time among the few items at the top of your list. Thus, if your list for the next few months contains ten items, invest the most time in the first two or three and give less attention to the remainder. If the job permits, you may even leave some of the less important items undone.

Peter Drucker said that "Doing the right thing seems to be more important than doing things right" (cited in Bliss, 1976, p. 21). You can be very efficient in what you are doing, but if you are doing the wrong thing, it is still a waste of time. You need to work toward goals that are meaningful. The best way to know which goals are meaningful is to list them, then sort them on the basis of what is important to you—your priorities.

Goals set at one time do not stay valid for all time. Reevaluation is essential to avoid working toward the wrong things. The story of Buzz Aldrin illustrates this point clearly. Aldrin, one of the first astronauts to set foot on the moon, suffered a nervous breakdown shortly after his return to earth. He wrote an autobiographical account of his experiences and revealed what had happened. In essence, he forgot there was life beyond the moon! He had focused his attention so exclusively on going to the moon that he forgot to think about what he would do afterward. Many executives are like this, as Merrill and Donna Douglass (1980) have pointed out. The executive devotes a lifetime to the company, collects some memento of the effort, and retires. "Within 18 months, they are dead. Why? Studies strongly suggest that these executives have much in common with Buzz Aldrin: They have no further goals to live for once they reach the end of their careers" (p. 79).

Pruning and Weeding

The solution to diffusion is to prune out the unnecessary and weed out the unattainable. This may require you to focus on what specific tasks are necessary to reach the goal you have set. For example, many people engage in an incessant round of reading and filing memos, then go through a panic of file cleaning when things pile up. Why file the memo in the first place? When you receive memos announcing meetings or agendas, pitch them right after the meeting. Keeping copies of all correspondence is also a waste of time, especially if the letter was only to seek information.

Most importantly, learn to say no to requests for involvement in other activities. As pleasant as it might be to be all things to all people, it is better to be the best for yourself and your family even if it means being best in a more limited arena of activity. Too much emphasis is placed on being a superperson. In general, trying to live up to such a fiction will probably only drain energy and lead to distractions that interfere with reaching the really important goals.

If you find you are having difficulty saying no, examine the reasons. Is it fear of being left out or fear that you will be less liked? If so, put these hidden assumptions to a test. Recall the times you did say no and examine the outcomes. You will probably find that the results are not as disastrous as you imagined. Is the failure to say no due to lack of assertiveness: you want to say no but cannot? Consider taking an assertion training class or reading a book on assertion.

Getting Started: Breaking the Procrastination Habit

One of the most common causes of procrastination is that the procrastinator views the job as so big and the available time as so small that the job cannot be finished. So why start? The solution is to break the task down into smaller parts. Writing a paper or business report, for example, can be broken into several parts, including background work, reading, organizing, drafting, and rewriting. Even the background work can be broken down into smaller components. A 15-minute period here and there can be used to check facts, figures, and resources. Once the procrastinator views the job this way, he or she will see many more periods of time as useful, and getting started becomes easier.

Structure your work situation to provide cues that help get you started rather than add to inertia and lethargy. Your office should be an office, not a lounge or recreation room. Work cues should facilitate attention without strain while minimizing distractions. It may be nice to have a cozy office, but too many nonwork cues, such as popular magazines and pictures of the family vacation, will only sidetrack you. These cues become conversation pieces when other people come in, extending the interruption even longer. They cry out for attention at the most inopportune times, especially when a hard job is next on your list.

Finally, do not mix functions in your work area. If you must read to fall asleep, do so only in bed, never in your study chair. If you find yourself getting sleepy every time you try to read, you probably have your cues mixed. Your mind is telling you that reading is a signal for going to sleep, when you actually need to be alert. The general idea is to strengthen the cues most conducive to efficient work habits.

Concentrating: Zeroing In on Essentials

Getting started is only one part of the battle in effective time management. Two other issues must also be confronted. One is concentrating on the job long enough to complete some whole unit or stage of the task. The other is sticking with the task until it is done.

The ideas discussed earlier (controlling the cues in your work area and reducing distractions) will help you with concentration as much as with getting started. In addition, you may need to examine two other elements. First, people sometimes have difficulty working at any task for longer than a few minutes. If this is a recurrent problem, use a clock and a self-contract to keep yourself at the task for a set period. Start with a short period of time that is close to what you normally work. Then make a contract with yourself such as "I'm going to work straight through for the next 20 minutes before taking a break." Gradually increase the amount of time by adding 1 or 2 minutes each day. When you are able to concentrate on a task for at least an hour, consider yourself over the hump.

Second, some people try to work too long at a single task. The problem of short-term concentration is that it does not provide for continuity and rhythm, especially in complex tasks. The problem with long-term concentration is that it tends to produce fatigue, lower motivation, and reduced mental efficiency. The way to deal with this is to distribute work sessions and alternate tasks. For example, you can reward yourself with a short break, say 10 minutes, for every hour you work. During this time, you might do some more menial work, return phone calls, or close your eyes and enjoy music on the radio. You might also switch tasks. The new content can help keep motivation and interest at a higher level over longer periods.

A major problem in the normal work environment, as discussed earlier, is dealing with unscheduled interruptions. There are several ways of managing these so that your blocks of time are not broken up. One simple technique is to make an appointment with yourself. If you can block out time on the calendar for your clients, you can also block it out for yourself. If you have an open-door policy, stop this practice and put visits to your office on a more formal appointment basis, or restrict the amount of time the open-door policy is in effect. Then shut the door and focus. Be gentle but firm if people violate the Do Not Disturb sign. Also, do not feel guilty! You have a right to some privacy to complete your work, and you can exercise a measure of control in that regard. If all else fails, consider using a second office either at work or at home.

Dealing with the chronic drop-in can be a problem, but there are some effective solutions. According to Rutherford (1978), every time you respond to drop-ins with idle, pleasant chatter, you sign an implicit or silent contract that encourages them to do it again. In effect, you give them a license to interrupt anytime they want. You can prevent this by advising the interrupter that you are in the middle of a project that needs to be completed and asking them to return later. You can also suggest that you talk at the next scheduled break, or ask if the interruption relates to business and suggest that another time would be more convenient for you. If the behavior persists, you can ignore the person until he or she gets the hint. Or you might tell the person bluntly that the behavior is disruptive and that you do not appreciate unscheduled visits.

Dealing with phone interruptions may be somewhat easier than dealing with face-to-face confrontation. Ask your caller how much time the call will require and either call back or set a time limit. Use a receptionist to screen calls if possible. Perhaps the most effective technique is to simply *batch* calls, both incoming and outgoing. Designate certain times that you will allow a phone call to go straight through and other times when phone calls are to be met with a "not available" response. Then set aside some time, perhaps one of your rest breaks, when you return calls and make some of your own calls you need to make.

Batching can also be used to handle your mail. Set aside one time interval when you open mail and provide responses where needed.

Staying with It: Marking Time and Progress

Perhaps the most effective way to keep yourself at a task is to provide some tangible reward or marker for completion of small steps. You can do this by using a checklist of the total project with each step listed separately. You can then check off each step as it is finished. A daily "to do" list is valuable for just this reason. A project calendar can also provide valuable feedback.

HINTS FOR EFFECTIVE TIME MANAGEMENT

Many suggestions for better use of time do not conveniently fit in any of the preceding categories. The next few pages present a potpourri of ideas, culled from different sources, that may prove helpful for one time management problem or another.

Using Transition or Commuting Time

In the United States, the average time people spend commuting from home to job is approximately 45 minutes per day. In larger metropolitan areas, this increases to approximately 75 minutes per day (Bliss, 1976). Added up over the period of a working year or even a working month, this amounts to a sizable block of nonproductive time. If it is possible to treat the trip as downtime (part of the relaxation you need to recover from the press of job duties), and if you are not falling behind at work, then you may not even need to change your commuting time. On the other hand, if you are finding it difficult to stay on top of your duties, then these moments might provide you with just enough time to take the pressure off at the office and at home. Some activities you can carry out include learning new skills from tapes, dictating notes or ideas on both in-process and new projects, and thinking through time schedules for new projects.

Learning to Delegate

Delegating specific tasks to others can free a lot of time for a manager. If you find it difficult to delegate, consider whether some personal fear prevents you from delegating. Are you afraid you will lose your position? Are you afraid your peers will find out that there is not that much to your job after all? If you are able to pinpoint specific fears, then examine the logic of those fears. Get a friend to help if necesary. If the problem is your lack of trust in your subordinates, examine the basis of that mistrust.

On the positive side, consider the fact that delegating places you in the position of a teacher. You are developing skills and talent in others who might be able to carry on the work of the organization in the future. Your legacy, then, is not just your work but a pool of talent that helps the entire company.

Internal Prime Time

Recall the concept of diurnal cycles and circadian rhythms. We each function on a slightly different internal clock that makes us more efficient at certain times. Know your prime time, when you work the best, and try to structure work so you do the most demanding work in synchrony with your prime time.

Also, study your sleep habits. Many people sleep more than they need to. The norm is eight hours per night, but this may vary from six to nine hours. Evidence exists that sleep over nine to ten hours can have three bad results: it may lower your overall metabolic rate, leading to increased difficulty in maintaining a desirable weight; muscle tone may drop, leading to increased effort in carrying out normal tasks and reducing the ease with which you can exercise; and performance of the mental system may decrease due to lethargy.

If you observe that you are sleeping more than ten hours (the exception being when you are ill), a simple experiment will tell you whether you are sleeping more than necessary. Get up a half hour earlier for a few mornings. If you find you are no more tired at the end of the day and do not feel the need to go to bed any earlier, you can probably get by without the half hour of sleep. You can repeat this process until you reach a point where you sleep enough but do not waste time sleeping. Even if you cut down, you should realize that you will not be cutting down on deep sleep, when the really important biological repair work is done. You will actually be reducing the amount of light sleep that occurs in the morning just before you are ready to wake up. On the other hand, if you are already sleeping less than six to seven hours, you probably should not cut any further. Very few people can get by on less sleep without doing their bodies harm.

Reading for Professional Development

In many technical and professional fields, it is necessary to stick to a routine reading program in order to keep up with important developments. If you tried to read everything, you would be overwhelmed. But even trying to read the bare minimum is a struggle much of the time.

One problem is the habit of reading word for word. On the average, a person will complete college reading at about 350 words per minute. However, repeated reading of very technical information leads to the habit of slower reading, a habit that then is carried over to reading a newspaper or novel. Recent surveys have shown that managers have a constant reading speed of about 250 words per minute, which does not change from one type of material to another (Heyel, 1979). At this rate, it takes anywhere from one to three minutes for each page of text. Even a 20-page article can consume an hour or more, far too much time to be able to keep up. But you do not have to read word for word to get what you need. This will be explained in a moment.

Speed-reading courses claim to be able to increase reading speed to thousands of words per minute. But be assured that what is going on is not word-for-word reading! The visual system is physiologically incapable of processing information at that speed. These exaggerated claims have been shown to be based on a skimming procedure or on some systematic reading procedure (such as reading only the first and last sentence in each paragraph). The most often cited target for speed reading is 600 to 1000 words per minute. Even at this rate, you would still not be able to keep up.

There are ways to whittle the task down to manageable size. First, be selective of what you read. If you have summary or review journals, you may be able to keep up on the high spots of your profession. From the summaries, identify articles or books that contain the detailed information most critical to maintaining and developing your skills.

Then, learn to read with an eye for the forest and not the trees. Develop the ability to scan material and pick out the basic details from an article without having to read the entire article. Most of the time, compulsive, word-for-word reading is based on the fear that something important will be missed. Also, some concepts from memory research can work in your favor.

In general, much of the information you read is lost in the first 24 hours after reading. Only high spots, or story lines, are retained. So why not read that way from the start? Also, if you are reading word for word, you are overriding one of the great powers of the mind—its ability to fill in gaps. You do not need to read all the prepositions, for example, because the mind will just assume that they are there. The message will come through even if you have not read all of the words.

Another way of reducing reading time is to look for organizing themes in the author's style. Some authors provide the main idea at the beginning of a paragraph, elaborate in the middle, and summarize or provide transition at the end. Therefore, you can often obtain the most important information by reading just the first and last sentences of each paragraph. If material is highlighted in the middle, scan it on the way. Also, note other highlights, such as lists of essential points and markers such as *first, second, third,* and *finally.*

Once Should Always Be Enough

Never handle paper more than once. How many times has a letter or memo crossed your desk and you felt you did not have time to deal with it then? Each time you pick up the letter you follow the same sequence: Read it, think about it, decide what to do, decide not to do anything, wait until later, and repeat the sequence. Each time, you add delays and excess mental baggage. If you do this even twice for each piece of correspondence, you can add as much as 25% to your workload. The work you could accomplish in eight hours will take you ten hours or more. If you are taking work home, look at this aspect of your work behavior and consider whether change is needed.

Downtime and Idling

If you are too busy for relaxation, socializing, and exercising, you are just too busy. Downtime is important as a change of both physical and mental pacing. It refreshes the body and revives the spirit. Too often, though, downtime is considered nonproductive, a waste of time. But the usual effect of downtime is that you are able to go back to work after idling and accomplish more in less time.

Edwin Bliss (1976) suggested that being in good physical condition increases the percentage of prime-time working hours.

On the other hand, continuing to work under pressure usually has a snowball effect. Job performance gradually goes down, though often so insidiously that the real reason is overlooked. The conclusion erroneously drawn is that more work and harder work is what is needed, and the snowball grows even bigger.

The idea is to attain a balance between the necessity of work and the value of idling. If you spend 18 hours in front of the tube for sports or soaps, you might be overdoing on the idling end. But allow yourself a minimum of 3 to 4 hours at least two to three times a week when you can shut everything out of your mind and let your mind rest. It may not be the most productive time of your life, but it can still contribute greatly to your overall satisfaction with life and work.

SUMMARY

We identified seven major time traps: confusion, indecision, diffusion, procrastination, avoidance, interruptions, and perfectionism. Confusion stems from lack of a clear vision of where to go. Indecision is the inability to act decisively when required. Diffusion means expending energy on so many activities that all efforts are less focused and efficient than they could otherwise be. Procrastination is unnecessary delay in finishing a task. Avoidance involves using a number of escape behaviors to avoid dealing with unpleasant duties. Interruptions result from unscheduled drop-ins, mismanaged phone calls, and self-initiated stops and starts that detract from continuity on the job. Perfectionism is compulsive overdoing beyond the point of value.

The major means of dealing with these errors in time management are setting goals and priorities within goals. Using cue control for the work environment to increase concentration and reduce interruptions was also discussed. Batching and handling several routine chores at one time is a way of minimizing interruptions. Downtime is important to maintaining mental and physical energy.

KEY TERMS

battered mind syndrome	Pareto principle	time management (defined)
internal prime time	perfectionism	
	procrastination	

REFERENCES

Bliss, E. C. (1976). *Getting things done: The ABC's of time management*. New York: Scribner's.

Bost, J. M. (1984). Retaining students on academic probation: Effects of time management peer counseling on students' grades. *Journal of Learning Skills, 3*, 38–43.

Carroll, L. (1966). *Alice's adventures in wonderland*. New York: Macmillan. (Original work published 1865)

Davidson, J. (1978). *Effective time management*. New York: Human Sciences Press.

Douglass, M. R., & Douglass, D. N. (1980). *Manage your time, manage your work, manage yourself*. New York: AMACOM.

Drucker, P. F. (1967). *The effective executive*. New York: Harper & Row.

Ferner, J. D. (1980). *Successful time management*. New York: Wiley.

Hall, B. L., & Hursch, D. E. (1982). An evaluation of the effects of a time management training program on work efficiency. *Journal of Organizational Behavior Management, 3*, 73–96.

Hanel, F., Martin, G., & Koop, S. (1982). Field testing of a self-instructional time management manual with managerial staff in an institutional setting. *Journal of Organizational Behavior Management, 4*, 81–96.

Heyel, C. (1979). *Getting results with time management* (2nd ed.). New York: American Management Association.

Kozoll, C. E. (1982). *Time management for educators*. Bloomington, IN: Phi Delta Kappa Educational Foundation.

Lakein, A. (1974). *How to get control of your time and your life*. New York: New American Library/Signet.

Langfelder, J. R. (1987). Leisure wellness and time management: Is there a connection? *College Student Journal, 21*, 180–183.

LeBoeuf, M. (1979). *Working smart*. New York: McGraw-Hill.

Levine, R. (1989, October). The pace of life. *Psychology Today*, pp. 42–46.

Maher, C. A. (1986). Improving the instructional supervisory behavior of public school principals by means of time management: Experimental evaluation and social validation. *Professional School Psychology, 1*, 177–191.

Marvin, P. (1980). *Executive time management: An AMA survey report*. New York: AMACOM.

McConalogue, T. (1984). Developing the skill of time management. *Leadership and Organization Development Journal, 5*, 25–27.

Partin, R. L. (1983). Time management for school counselors. *The School Counselor, 30*, 280–284.

Posner, M. J. (1982). *Executive Essentials*. New York: Avon Books.

Rutherford, R. D. (1978). *Administrative time power: Meeting the time challenge of the busy secretary/staff assistant/manager team*. Austin, TX: Learning Concepts.

Schmelzer, R. V., Schmelzer, C. D., Figler, R. A., & Brozo, W. G. (1987). Using the critical incident technique to determine reasons for success and failure of university students. *Journal of College Student Personnel, 28*, 261–266.

Solomon, L. J., & Rothblum, E. D. (1984). Academic procrastination: Frequency and cognitive-behavioral correlates. *Journal of Counseling Psychology, 31*, 504–510.

Webber, R. A. (1972). *Time and management*. New York: Van Nostrand Reinhold.

Woolfolk, A. E., & Woolfolk, R. L. (1986). Time management: An experimental investigation. *Journal of School Psychology, 24*, 267–275.

CHAPTER 15

Behavioral Health Strategies:
Nutrition and Exercise

RUNNING HAS GIVEN ME A GLIMPSE OF THE GREATEST FREEDOM THAT A MAN CAN EVER
KNOW, BECAUSE IT RESULTS IN THE SIMULTANEOUS LIBERATION OF BOTH BODY AND
MIND.
ROGER BANNISTER

On the surface, nutrition and exercise may seem unrelated to stress. But a positive personal health program is as much a part of stress management as relaxation training, autogenics, anxiety management, or cognitive restructuring.

Good health increases resistance to stress by improving a person's capacity for responding to demand. This is true whether the demands are challenging and exciting or threatening and anxiety provoking. Conversely, poor health places a load on the psychophysiological system, thus increasing vulnerability to stress. Beyond this, nutrition can alter mood and neural sensitivity, which in turn can change our reactions to stressors (Spring, Lieberman, Swope, & Garfield, 1986). Further, exercise may function to reduce stress (Crews & Landers, 1987) and as an antidepressant (Dubbert & Wilson, 1984). Often it provides a natural high (Clingman & Hilliard, 1987), and it may be a buffer against illness (Kobasa, Maddi, & Puccetti, 1982).

UNHEALTHY BEHAVIOR

Many statistics support the contention that Americans engage in a wide range of unhealthy behaviors, including smoking, overeating, improper diet, lack of exercise, and excessive use of drugs. For example, recent figures show that each year Americans take nearly 5 billion doses of tranquilizers to calm down. They take another 5 billion doses of barbiturates to unwind and sleep, and another 3 billion doses of amphetamines to perk up (Posner, 1982).

Although nearly 30 million Americans quit smoking in the decade between 1965 and 1975, largely through their own efforts (Schachter, 1982), approximately 35% of adults still smoke. One figure that causes increasing concern is the large increase in teenage girls and working women who now smoke. This increase more than offsets the numbers of those quitting. In addition, smokers are less likely to begin exercise programs and more likely to quit exercise programs than are nonsmokers (Martin & Dubbert, 1982).

374

We consume an excess of fats and do not take in enough carbohydrates. This factor contributes to increased frequency of obesity and coronary disease. Of the ten leading causes of death, diet is a contributing factor in five, including heart disease, cancers, strokes, diabetes, and atherosclerosis[1] (National Center for Health Statistics, 1988). In addition, we spend about $3 billion each year on overfortified packaged nutrients that may have adverse side effects (Gershoff, 1990).

Recent estimates suggest that nearly 34 million Americans, approximately one fourth of the population, are overweight (McGinnis & Nestle, 1989). Although a Gallup poll in 1984 showed that approximately 59% of the adult population engaged in daily exercise, over twice the number in 1961 (Gallup, 1984), the remaining 41% are probably active only at levels too low in intensity and frequency to provide for cardiovascular fitness (Herbert & Teague, 1989). Approximately 50% of those who begin an exercise program drop out in less than a year (Kendzierski & Lamastro, 1988). Among those who engage in physical exercise, many have an "Olympic" syndrome, going into exercise programs too fast and too hard and pushing themselves to limits far beyond what is necessary for good health.

The purpose of this chapter, then, is to provide basic principles to establish and maintain a good personal health program. There are many ways to construct such a program, but here we will focus on nutrition and exercise. Later in this chapter, we will discuss cognitive-behavioral self-control techniques, which can be used to change a variety of unhealthy behaviors.

EFFECTS OF STRESS ON METABOLISM AND DIET

Because stress has a general arousing effect on a person, stress has the potential to change both energy expenditure and energy intake. First, stress increases the rate of metabolism, the rate at which the body changes food supplies into energy. This leads to increased levels of sugar, free fatty acids, and lactic acid in the blood. Stress also has indirect effects on metabolism due to the influence of the pituitary. These include changes in water balance, suppression of the immune system, and increased carbohydrate and protein metabolism. The net effect of stress is that the body uses energy at a faster rate.

The pattern of eating also may change. Whether a person will be affected and how significantly his or her behavior will change depends on a variety of factors such as learning, emotionality, and personality. Some learn that food is a means of escape when one is sad or depressed, whereas others learn that food is less desirable under these same conditions. The former may not only eat more, but may eat more frequently while under pressure. The latter may want to eat only subsistence meals or not want to eat at all. Externally controlled people are likely to respond by eating more; internally controlled people are less likely to do so.

---

[1]Of the remaining five, excessive alcohol consumption contributes to three—unintentional injuries (auto accidents, for example), suicide, and chronic liver disease.

When the typical stress response includes eating more and eating more frequently, the person will find weight control very difficult. The person may even reach weights that qualify as obesity. When the pattern is to eat less, especially to such extremes as going without food for days, the body may be depleted of energy reserves at an even faster rate. Any dramatic change in eating patterns should be a warning to look for stressful events at work, at school, or in the family.

EFFECTS OF DIET ON STRESS

Arousal can change metabolism and eating behavior, but dietary habits can also change sensitivity to stressors. In this sense, eating right is just as important as managing stress because vulnerability to stress increases with poor diet. There are two ways in which this happens.

First, excess amounts of sugars deplete vitamins and minerals. This can have negative side effects because vitamins and minerals are essential to keep body systems, especially the nervous system, working properly. Depletion of certain B vitamins (thiamine, niacin, and B12, for example) increases nervous system reactivity, irritability, and nervousness. In other words, you increase vulnerability to stressful events by taking in too many sweets.

Second, numerous foods commonly taken in large amounts have the potential to increase stress sensitivity. For example, coffee, cola, chocolate, and other products containing caffeine are frequently abused. Heller (1987) estimated that almost 200 over-the-counter drugs contain caffeine. "Cold-caffeine" colas are on their way to replacing coffee as the "wakeup drink," and one soft drink manufacturer has developed a higher-caffeine version for morning use.

One cup of drip-brewed coffee contains approximately 100 to 150 mg of caffeine (decaffeinated[2] coffee contains only 3 mg per 5-oz cup) (Mayo Clinic, 1981). As little as 250 mg of caffeine can cause nervousness, insomnia, and headaches. It is now well known that caffeine acts as a stimulant to the central nervous system (Boulenger, Salem, Marangos, & Uhde, 1987). It tends to charge up the autonomic system, and it lowers thresholds for stress reactions (Lane, 1983). Stated in other terms, you are more likely to interpret an event as stressful if you take in large amounts of caffeine. Further, you are more likely to respond impulsively and intensely in stressful situations after taking in excess caffeine.

Recent research by Boulenger's research group suggests that caffeine is an anxiogenic substance that is dose dependent. That is, caffeine induces clinically definable anxiety states when ingested at around 720 mg (Boulenger et al., 1987). It takes only five to six cups of coffee to reach this anxiety-inducing level. Although these dangers can occur with excessive use, the system apparently can

---

[2]Be careful that you do not use decaffeinated coffees processed with methylene chloride because this process carries increased risk of cancer and may also cause side effects such as headaches. "Naturally" decaffeinated coffees use either ethyl acetate, a natural substance found in fruits and vegetables, or some combination of water and carbon dioxide or coffee oils to extract the caffeine.

handle lower levels with few or no negative side effects. Before proceeding to the next section on nutrition, you may find it instructive to fill out the nutrition and diet scales provided in Self-Study Exercise 15-1.

SELF-STUDY EXERCISE 15-1

Health Behavior Profile for Nutrition and Diet

The following scale will help you compare your dietary practice to what is considered good practice. Instructions for scoring are provided at the end.

Circle the answer that most accurately describes your eating habits.

DAILY = once or more per day
FREQUENTLY = every week but not once per day
OCCASIONALLY = a few times each month but not once per week
SELDOM = no more than once per month

How often do you:	SELDOM	OCCASIONALLY	FREQUENTLY	DAILY
1. Eat fruits, vegetables, fiber?	1	2	3	4
2. Drink five or more cups of coffee in a day?	4	3	2	1
3. Eat fats, red meats, dairy products?	4	3	2	1
4. Drink five or more soft drinks (diet or regular)?	4	3	2	1
5. Eat candies, sugars, pastries?	4	3	2	1
6. Take vitamin supplements?	4	3	2	1
7. Overeat at meals?	4	3	2	1
8. Eat between meals?	4	3	2	1
9. Eat while watching TV, reading, and so on?	4	3	2	1
10. Skip breakfast?	4	3	2	1
11. Skip lunch?	4	3	2	1
12. Skip dinner?	4	3	2	1
13. Use crash diets to lose weight?	4	3	2	1
14. Take diet pills?	4	3	2	1
15. Use amphetamines to lose weight?	4	3	2	1

After you have completed the scale, go back and add up the values listed in the boxes you circled. Then circle the point on the following scale that corresponds to your total score. A high score suggests that your eating habits are fairly good. On the other end, a low score indicates there is some risk in your eating habits. If you have a score in the High Risk region, look back at the items you checked that have values of 1 or 2. These items provide clues to areas where a change in diet and nutritional habits may be warranted.

Score sum   . . 42 . . . . 45 . . . . 47 . . . . 48 . . . . 49 . . . . 51 . . . . 52 . . . . 53 . . . . 54 . .

←High risk→ | ←Normal nutrition→ | ←Excellent→

Percentile   . . 10 . . . . 20 . . . .30. . . . 40 . . . . 50 . . . . 60 . . . . 70. . . . 80 . . . . 90 . .

The average score on this scale is 49.2, and the median is 49.5. The median indicates that 50% of the respondents scored higher than 49.5, and 50% scored lower. The scale has a reliability of .695, which is acceptable for this type of scale. This scale is not intended to be a comprehensive nutrition assessment and is provided for instructional purposes only.

EATING RIGHT

Proper nutrition depends on eating the right foods in the right amounts. In 1988, the Surgeon General's office released a report that resulted from an intensive review of nutrition and health in America. The report contained five specific recommendations for all people.

1. *Fats and cholesterol:* Reduce the consumption of fat to no more than 20% of daily calories and cholesterol to less than 300 mg daily.
2. *Energy and weight control:* Work to reach a desirable body weight, then maintain that weight through both regulation of caloric intake and energy expenditure (exercise).
3. *Complex carbohydrates and fiber:* Increase intake of whole-grain foods, cereals, vegetables, and fruits so that about 50% of total calories come from complex carbohydrates.
4. *Sodium:* Reduce sodium intake by using foods low in sodium content and limiting the amount of salt added to foods at the table.
5. *Alcohol:* Take alcohol only in moderation (two drinks per day maximum, no matter what type of alcohol) to reduce the risk of chronic disease (McGinnis & Nestle, 1989).

TABLE 15-1
Recommended Daily Energy (Calorie) Intake for Children and Adults

	Age (years)	Weight (pounds)	Height (inches)	Energy needs (calories)
Youth	1–3	29	35	1300 (900–1800)
	4–6	44	44	1700 (1300–2300)
	7–10	62	52	2400 (1650–3300)
Males	11–14	99	62	2700 (2000–3700)
	15–18	145	69	2800 (2100–3900)
	19–22	154	70	2900 (2500–3300
	23–50	154	70	2700 (2300–3100)
	51–75	154	70	2400 (2000–2800)
	76 +	154	70	2050 (1650–2450)
Females	11–14	101	62	2200 (1500–3000)
	15–18	120	64	2100 (1200–3000)
	19–22	120	64	2100 (1700–2500)
	23–50	120	64	2300 (1600–2400)
	51–75	120	64	1800 (1400–2200)
	76 +	120	64	1600 (1200–2000)
Pregnancy				+ 300
Nursing				+ 500

SOURCE: Adapted from Mayo Clinic, Committee on Dietetics (1981).

Nutrition research has shown that the adult human body must have 46 nutrients to be healthy and stay healthy. To maintain a constant weight, the average woman needs about 1600 to 2400 calories, and the average man needs about 2300 to 3100 calories (Mayo Clinic, 1981, p. 270).[3] Table 15-1 shows the average energy needs with ranges for children and adults of different weights and heights. To obtain the 46 nutrients, normal adults need to average, *as a bare minimum*, about 1300 calories per day (Mirkin, 1983). For these reasons, there is danger in any diet that reduces to the extreme either the type or quantity of food, and such diets should be avoided.

The guidelines provided here are for the so-called normal adult, and suggested caloric intake levels are averages. Children differ in their requirements, as do adults over 55 to 60 years of age and pregnant and nursing women. A person with a large frame or a strenuous job requires more calories than someone with a small frame and a less demanding job. Illness also affects nutritional requirements. Finally, food intake does not have to exactly match the standard each day, but it should average out over a few days.

The 46 essential nutrients cover six categories: water, carbohydrates, 9 proteins, fat, 13 vitamins, and 21 minerals. Of these six categories, only carbohydrates, proteins, and fats contain calories. Calories provide the body with energy for internal processes, for muscular and brain work. When taken in large amounts, calories are the culprits that make excess body weight. Carbohydrates

[3]Nutrition research uses the term *calorie* without qualifying that it is the big C, the great calorie, or the kilocalorie that is at issue. The kilocalorie is the amount of heat required to raise 1 kilogram of water 1 degree centigrade. For the remainder of this discussion, the term *calorie* will always refer to the great calorie, or kilocalorie.

are the least likely to add unwanted body weight, whereas fats are the worst offenders. Water, vitamins, and minerals are essential to keep the body functioning properly but do not contain calories.

We can meet most of these nutritional needs through natural food supplies. The challenge is to obtain a balance. We need to fit all the nutrients into a calorie count that still maintains desirable weight. The ideal diet should consist of 50% carbohydrate calories, 20 to 30% protein calories, and 20 to 30% fat calories (Mayo Clinic, 1981). About 80% of the carbohydrates should be complex, and not more than 10% of the fats should be saturated (Gershoff, 1990). Unfortunately, the average American diet is drastically out of balance, with 40% carbohydrates (with too many sugars), about 15 to 20% protein, and nearly 40 to 45% fat (with too many saturated fats) (Mirkin, 1983).

Carbohydrates: Filling Up, Not Fattening Up

First, carbohydrates are complex food molecules made up of carbon, oxygen, and hydrogen, or more simply—sugars. There are single-molecule (simple) sugars called *monosaccharides*, double-molecule sugars called *disaccharides*, and complex sugar molecules called *polysaccharides*. One simple sugar is glucose, the high-energy fuel in your bloodstream. Fruits and honey contain pure glucose that can pass directly into the bloodstream for fast energy. Foods such as bananas and oranges also contain simple sugars, but the sugars they contain must be converted to glucose for the body's use. Other sugars must be converted to glucose as well. Common table sugar[4] and milk are sources of double sugars, whereas corn, beans, and potatoes are sources of complex sugars. Simple sugars, such as those used in candies and table sugar, are empty calories with no nutritional value (Gershoff, 1990).

Carbohydrates provide the primary fuel for exercise, labor, and brain work. The brain depends on a continuous supply of glucose to work properly. It cannot reserve fuel for later use. This is why a good breakfast is important to start the day off right. If you do not eat in the morning, the brain does not have the immediate energy it needs to work properly. The muscles, though, can save glucose in a type of energy bank to withdraw when needed. In addition to providing quick energy, carbohydrates fill you up more quickly with fewer calories than any other food.

Paradoxically, loading up on carbohydrates may not be the best practice early in the day. Tests have shown that people feel sleepier after a carbohydrate meal (breakfast or lunch) as compared with a protein meal. In addition, mental alertness as measured by a selective attention task is lower for almost three hours after eating a high-carbohydrate meal. This effect is most intense in people over 40 who eat a high-carbohydrate lunch (Spring et al., 1986). It appears that carbohydrates have sedative-like effects related to brain chemistry and tryptophan (Lieberman, Spring, & Garfield, 1986).

[4]Common table sugar is a disaccharide, a combination of two simple sugars, glucose and fructose.

The complex carbohydrates, made from millions of sugar molecules, are typically high in fiber or cellulose content. Two characteristics of high-fiber foods make them valuable to a healthy diet. First, high-fiber foods do not break down in the digestive system as readily as other foods. The upper intestine cannot break down fiber at all. Because it cannot be broken down, fiber cannot be absorbed into the body to become worrisome weight. Second, fats bind to fiber and ride out as body waste. So when you eat a richly marbled steak, eat it with fiber to reduce the amount of fat that remains in the system.

Common foods containing carbohydrates are vegetables, fruits, and whole grains. However, appearance is not a good clue to fiber content. Lettuce is not high in fiber, but peas are. For snacks, avoid potato chips with their high fat content, and eat apples, celery, or carrots instead. This will reduce hunger, provide energy, and add fiber to the digestive track.

Still, be wary of exaggerated claims for the nutritional value (cholesterol-reducing) of high-fiber diets or foods such as oat brans. Adding any fiber to one's diet will reduce serum cholesterol levels (Swain, Rouse, Curley, & Sacks, 1990), but only because the fiber replaces fat in the diet. In other words, it is reduction in fat that is beneficial, not any intrinsic cholesterol-lowering properties of fiber itself. In addition, high-fiber diets can have some unpleasant gastrointestinal side effects, such as flatulence, cramping, and diarrhea.

The Proteins

Proteins may be the most overrated food in the American diet. While our bodies need only 8 or 9% protein calories to function properly (Gershoff, 1990), we usually consume more than 20%. Many people believe the myth that protein generates strength and that the best source of protein is meat. Strength comes through exercise, and the best source of energy for exercise comes from carbohydrates. The idea that a vegetarian must be inherently weaker than a "meat eater" is an unfortunate stereotype and an inaccurate belief.

Further, protein is *not* a source of quick energy. It has to be converted before it can be used. Although protein contains calories, it is the last food converted to energy after the carbohydrates and the fats. The body uses protein for energy only during periods of severe starvation or dieting.

Proteins are the basic building blocks for all body tissues. Antibodies and other parts of the immune system are proteins. Thus, proteins play an important role in protecting against disease (Gershoff, 1990). During periods of intense stress, illness, infection, and injury, the body may increase its demand for protein by as much as 100%. Intense exercise and bodybuilding may have the same effect (Gutlin & Kessler, 1983). Even the enzymes that regulate body functions are proteins.

The body uses 22 different amino acids to make proteins, 13 of which it manufactures internally. The remaining 9 amino acids have to come from diet. We usually obtain protein from animal sources such as poultry, eggs, fish, lean meat, cheese, and milk. Protein is also available from many plant sources such as cereals, nuts, beans, and leafy vegetables. You do not need to eat meat to obtain essential protein. You can get nearly all the protein you need in two large glasses of milk or in 12 ounces of corn and beans (Mirkin, 1983).

Good Fats and Bad Fats

If proteins are the most overrated foods, fats may be the most misunderstood. We have developed a strong fear of fats because of their connection to obesity and coronary problems. Despite this fear, however, we continue to overuse, if not abuse, fats. Fats still make up about 45% of the American diet when the maximum should be about 25%. The average male should carry no more than 15% body fat, and the average female should carry no more than 25% body fat. Yet the average American carries much more fat, excess baggage that may have harmful effects. A 45-year-old male carrying 25 pounds of excess fat will have a life expectancy shortened by 25% (Mirkin, 1983).

Still, fats are essential to a healthy body and survival. Fat is a storehouse of energy and fluids for the body to draw on whenever it needs. Fat converts to energy much more quickly than protein and is essential to vitamin transport. The immune system's ability to protect the body against viruses and bacteria also depends on fat. Finally, fat is one major way in which the body protects itself against cold.

Most of the danger from fat comes from the buildup of **yellow fat** on the body and from deposits of **cholesterol** in the bloodstream. Yellow fat is the reservoir of excess calories. The fatty tissue beneath the skin, such as the fold of fat around the waistline, is yellow fat.

Cholesterol is a lipid, chemically different from fats, but still a member of the same family. The liver manufactures cholesterol from excess calories, so it does not need to be eaten to meet body needs. It is, to correct some bad press, necessary for certain functions of the body. Cholesterol cannot move through the bloodstream by itself (Gershoff, 1990). For that, it needs carriers called lipoproteins. One lipoprotein is a good type of fat, whereas the other is bad fat. Good cholesterol is **high-density lipoprotein (HDL)**. Bad cholesterol is **low-density lipoprotein (LDL)**. HDL helps keep the arteries clean and elastic. By contrast, LDL embeds itself in the arterial walls, forming plaques. This narrows and hardens the artery. Then the heart must work harder and at a higher pressure to force blood through the arteries.

HDLs are like high-tech garbage trucks that pick up cell cholesterol, compact it into a very small space, and deliver it to the liver without losing any of their load (Gershoff, 1990). They also act like street sweepers, picking up some, but not all, the droppings of LDLs. LDLs are more like open wagons. They do not compact their load, so they cannot carry as much cholesterol as HDLs. More importantly, LDLs are prone to accidents, they spill part of their loads. This dropped cholesterol stays in the bloodstream and accumulates. This is the building material for arterial plaques and blocked arteries.

One newly discovered LDL, Lipoprotein(a), may explain why some people are prone to heart attacks (Hajjar, Gavish, Breslow, & Nachman, 1989). Hajjar's research group found that some people appear to have a genetic disposition to produce more Lipoprotein(a). This lipoprotein does not respond to diet and so may contribute to the formation of plaques. Coronary attacks occur more frequently in connection with a high concentration of LDL. Persons with high HDL tend to have fewer attacks (Pekkanen et al., 1990).

Recent research showed that exercisers consistently carry more of their cholesterol as high-density lipoprotein, the good kind. Sedentary people carry more of their cholesterol as low-density lipoprotein (Gutlin & Kessler, 1983). One interesting note is that HDLs appear to be predicted by waist-to-hip ratio and not by sex or total body fat (Ostlund et al., 1990).

We consume fats in butter, oils such as those used in fast-food frying, salad dressings, ice cream, and fatty meats such as bacon. The best way to control problems associated with fats is to reduce the intake of fats and maintain a regular exercise program.

Will the Really Good Fats Please Stand Up?

Just when we thought we knew what was safe to eat on our bread and potatoes, a new culprit has popped up—hydrogenated vegetable oils. These oils occur in margarines, margarine-based products, shortenings, and frying fats. The products themselves may be advertised as low in cholesterol, but the process of manufacturing them produces potentially harmful by-products.

Food processors and consumers like shortenings that have a certain firmness yet plasticity. To obtain this texture, the food industry has to hydrogenate the liquid oils. This makes the oil firm but leaves by-products called trans fatty acids. Recent research has shown that these trans fatty acids change the ratio of LDLs to HDLs in a harmful way; that is, they raise LDLs and lower HDLs (Mensink & Katan, 1990). The net effect is as harmful as that of a diet loaded with saturated fats.

Mensink and Katan (1990) think the average intake of trans fatty acids is low enough that there is probably little danger. Still, they recommend that people at risk for atherosclerosis should avoid diets high in trans fatty acids.

VITAMINS: USE OR ABUSE AND ADDICTION?

In recent years, we have been bombarded with vitamin supplement diets and therapies that advocate taking megadoses of a particular vitamin. The rationale for the diets varies. One line of thinking derives from the age-old observation that vitamin deficiencies can cause extremely serious physical problems—pellagra and scurvy, for example. If a little supplement keeps this from happening, then a lot must be even better. This argument does not consider what vitamin poisoning can do to the body.

Another argument states that vitamin guidelines are minimums that do not consider variations in size and health of the individual. Larger people and sick people need more vitamins. Therefore, as the argument goes, we should be looking at nothing less than an "average" allowance that must be larger than the minimums. Of course, this argument does not consider the vitamins obtained from daily food. A balanced diet can supply most of the vitamins needed at the level needed. If you then supplement your daily diet with a vitamin tablet that provides 100% of daily requirements, you may be taking about twice the needed amount.

Perhaps the most difficult argument to refute is the one that says, "I was really sick with _____ , and I took _____ and got better right away." Fill in the blanks with "a cold" and "Vitamin C," and you have the argument made famous by Linus Pauling. Unfortunately, this argument does not consider the placebo effect: if a person *believes* a treatment will be effective, it is more likely to be effective. This belief is sufficient to summon the body's natural healing powers.

This issue can be addressed by using a *double-blind* experimental design. In a double-blind study, subjects do not know what treatment they are getting, and experimenters do not know either. In vitamin studies, subjects could be receiving a placebo that looks and tastes like the real thing but is chemically inert. A review of studies on Vitamin C and frequency and duration of colds did not show any practical significance and showed few statistically significant results. Among the best-designed studies, 50% show no significant results. The remaining, less carefully designed, studies showed such small differences that they are scientifically meaningless (Marshall, 1983).

In contrast to the astounding publicity surrounding the alleged positive effects of vitamin megadoses, the public receives little warning about the potential dangers of vitamin overdose. Recently, though, Charles Marshall (1983) documented the hidden dangers of **vitamin abuse** by overdose. He noted that use of vitamin supplements has become a pattern of abuse based on the mistaken notion that more is better. This notion often combines with a false security that translates to: "I take so many vitamins I don't have to worry about the rest of my diet" (Marshall, 1983, pp. 20–21). He also noted that some vitamins have addictive properties. In support of this idea, users may encounter withdrawal symptoms if they reduce their dosage level or stop altogether. The remaining discussion summarizes a few of the dangerous **vitamin side effects** documented by Marshall.

Large doses of Vitamin A produce an immense array of negative effects. The list includes loss of appetite and weight loss, loss of hair, anemia, blurred vision, extreme drying and thickening of the skin, itching, dry and cracking lips, canker sores, increased brain and spinal fluid pressure with headache, irritability in children, and birth defects in children born to mothers who took megadoses of Vitamin A during pregnancy (Marshall, 1983).

There are no known toxic effects from the B-complex vitamins, although some unpleasant side effects may occur with too much niacin.

Vitamin C, much heralded for its ability to prevent, or at least reduce, colds and flu, is probably the most abused vitamin in American society. In one year alone, Americans paid $80 million for Vitamin C supplements (Mirkin & Hoffman, 1978). Although the recommended dietary allowance for Vitamin C is 60 mg for both men and women (National Research Council, 1980), the average daily consumption was 125 mg in 1983. Yet, based on advice from "experts," many people take 2000 to 4000 mg per day. The dangers from Vitamin C megadoses are extensive. The most common side effect is diarrhea. Other dangers include complications in pregnancy, spontaneous abortion, lowered sperm count, increased uric acid excretion, decreased tolerance for low oxygen levels, interference with urine tests for sugar and stool tests for blood, decreased resistance to bacterial infections and tumors, and damage to tooth enamel (Mirkin, 1983).

Overdoses of Vitamin D can cause loss of appetite, nausea, headaches, and depression. Long-term use may result in calcification of soft tissues and kidney failure. Excessive urination and diarrhea or constipation may occur. When the kidneys become involved, high blood pressure, increased levels of blood cholesterol, and heart damage may follow with fatal results.

Americans spend approximately $100 million each year on Vitamin E although its specific role is still uncertain. It is difficult to explain this obsession, but one guess ties it to the myth of sexual virility. Early observations in laboratory rats showed that Vitamin E conferred increased sexual vitality and longevity. Researchers have not observed these effects in humans, and the studies with rats are far from convincing. Megadoses of Vitamin E result in elevated blood triglycerides in women and a reduction in thyroid hormone in both sexes. Laboratory studies of animals overdosed with Vitamin E show thyroid gland damage. Could such damage be the cause of reduced thyroid hormone production in humans?

In addition to the potential dangers from megavitamin therapy, there are physiological and practical reasons for avoiding such excesses. Physiologically, the body acts like a reservoir that can hold only a certain amount of a vitamin before overflowing. For example, the body can hold only about 1500 mg of Vitamin C. If the body's reservoir is close to full (as it usually is) when you take a 1000-mg pill, the body does what any reservoir does—some old Vitamin C goes out with some new, and some stays in the body. The body absorbs about 500 mg of new Vitamin C. It loses about 500 mg in stools and another 500 mg in urine. Thus, the body balances its ledger sheet for Vitamin C. Practically, then, you are spending hard-earned money to pass stools and urine rich in Vitamin C.

In sum, megavitamin therapy does not have a stellar track record. It can produce dangerous side effects. The body cannot possibly use the huge amounts of vitamins some people pump into their bodies. Finally, megavitamin therapy is largely a waste of money.

EATING LIGHT

Some people refer to this period as the age of diets and dieting. There are now dozens of diets on the market. Each one claims to have the secret to taking off and keeping off excess pounds. Mirkin (1983) reported that 20 million Americans spend over $10 billion dollars each year on reducing diets. We need to discuss several issues to set dieting in perspective.

First, you should be skeptical about any diet program that emphasizes what goes in (calories) without discussing what goes out (energy expenditure through exercise). The key to weight reduction and maintenance is to balance the equation of input and output. Simply put, you must burn more calories than you take in. The way the body manages its resources, though, is much more subtle. The body tries to maintain a set-point that balances energy use and food intake to support body weight.

Set-Point Theory

Set-point theory comes from an impressive long-term research program led by Richard Keesey, among others. Keesey argued that food intake does not *directly* regulate body weight any more than activity does. Instead, the body regulates weight *indirectly* through the physiological mechanism of energy expenditure (Keesey & Powley, 1986). More precisely, the body has its own set-point—the exact weight at which there is an energy balance, when resting metabolism can be predicted from metabolic body size. This set-point represents a state of adaptation, a reference level of normal activity and normal food intake. Obesity resulting from overeating is an example of a maladaptive set-point. Once body weight is set, the body tries to maintain itself and resists deviations from the norm. If new input shows a change, the body takes action to restore the balance and maintain the set body weight.

Keesey's theory takes into account noticeable paradoxes in weight control: that people who eat a great amount do not gain the weight predicted from their caloric intake. Conversely, people who restrict food intake, even to the extreme, do not lose the weight predicted for their caloric restriction. We now have a slightly better idea of what happens.

Consider this example. Assume that an adult male has a stable body weight of 180 pounds. Further, imagine that he goes on a binge some night and eats a heavy meal with wine and a rich dessert. This excess caloric intake would push the body in the direction of weight gain. The body senses this caloric overload, however, and takes remedial action. It boosts the metabolic rate, generates more heat, and burns calories at a faster rate. The result is that fewer calories remain to turn into body fat. Unfortunately, this small compensatory blessing for the overeater is also a great frustration for the dieter.

Suppose this person believes he is heavy and decides to go on a diet. The body senses this caloric deprivation and works to conserve energy. From a biological point of view, this makes sense. Imagine you were lost at sea in a boat with a limited amount of food and had no way of knowing when you might be rescued. You would voluntarily restrict the amount of food you ate. The body, in its infinite wisdom, would aid your efforts by shutting down, or attenuating, the basal metabolic rate.

In the same way, dieters trick the body into believing that it is in a state of deprivation. Reduced eating leads the body to conserve energy and preserve weight. Severe caloric restriction causes the body to conserve energy at an even greater rate. This is why dieters may "hit a wall" if they depend on diet alone. Note that it makes no difference whether the dieter is light or heavy to begin with. Conserving energy and maintaining the set-point weight occur equally in obese and normal-weight people.

This theory suggests that the most effective way to change weight is to reset the set-point. Increasing energy expenditure through a consistent exercise program forces the metabolic rate higher, resulting in a lower weight. Caloric intake can be at an even higher level, but the body will see itself as balanced and work to maintain this new balance.

Dieting Dangers

There are several dangers inherent in programs that focus solely on the input side. One danger comes in diets that reduce calories to the extreme. Such diets generally cannot provide balance in the six essential nutrients. Mirkin (1983) suggested that diets should never go below 1000 calories if you are not exercising and should stay above 1300 calories if you are.

Another danger in dieting is that dieting takes off muscle tissue, not fat. Ignoring exercise and emphasizing caloric intake is self-defeating. Exercising removes fat and tones muscle (Martin & Dubbert, 1982; van Dale & Saris, 1989). This improves body composition, which is important to health. Proper exercise effectively reduces weight and gets rid of yellow fat.

Yo-yo dieting is a common problem among dieters today. Yo-yo dieting is a sequence of crash dieting to lose weight followed by nondieting; then the dieter regains the lost weight. This occurs with frustrating ease compared with the difficulty of getting rid of the weight. Recent research has shown why yo-yo dieting leads so often to feelings of futility and failure. Yo-yo dieting may permanently *reduce* resting metabolic rate (RMR), the speed at which your body burns energy even while resting. Under these conditions, the body will convert to body mass more of the calories you take in, even when you have reduced caloric intake. It is then more difficult to maintain weight at a desirable level (van Dale & Saris, 1989).

One body change may cause confusion at the beginning of a program that emphasizes weight loss through exercise. That is, muscles are denser than fat and thus weigh more than fat for the same volume. Although you burn off fat during exercise, you may not see an immediate change on the scales. You may even see a weight gain. Still, it is better to carry weight as conditioned muscle than as fat debris under your skin and in your blood. It is not weight per se but percentage of body fat that is dangerous.

To summarize, if you must diet, observe the following guidelines:

1. Keep caloric intake above the minimum so you obtain all the essential food groups.
2. Combine dieting with exercise that burns off more calories than you consume.
3. Keep food intake balanced in the proportions of 50% carbohydrates, 30% protein, and 20% fats. If you cut anything further, it should be fats.
4. Avoid diets that require dangerously low caloric intake.
5. Avoid diets that eliminate one food group or that suggest excessive amounts of a particular food.
6. Do not assume that vitamin supplements can replace carbohydrates, proteins, or fats. Vitamins contain no calories.

EXERCISE, HEALTH, AND STRESS

The benefits of exercise cannot be overemphasized, and the necessity cannot be underestimated. Before the dawn of the industrial-technological society, getting enough exercise was rarely an issue, and diet clinics were unnecessary. Daily life consisted of an incessant struggle for existence. Now, technology automates many chores that once demanded physical activity. This also removes any physical benefit. We even automate changing TV channels. In this environment, it is little wonder that people are on the dieting treadmill. Even a low-calorie diet probably will result in weight gains because energy expenditure does not use the calories. Before proceeding to the next section on the physical benefits of exercise, you might find it helpful to complete the health behavior profile for exercise provided in Self-Study Exercise 15-2.

Calvin and Hobbes   by Bill Watterson

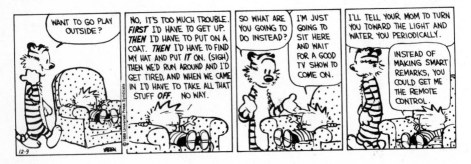

SOURCE: Calvin and Hobbes copyright 1989 Universal Press Syndicate. Reprinted with permission. All rights reserved.

SELF-STUDY EXERCISE 15-2

Health Behavior Profile for Exercise

This profile is intended to help you determine the adequacy of your current physical activities and/or exercise program. Read the instructions before completing the profile. Instructions for scoring are given at the end along with the necessary information on how to interpret your own score.

Indicate the level of your participation in any of the listed activities by circling the appropriate boxes below.

AEROBIC = four or more times per week
FREQUENTLY = two or three times per week
WEEKLY = about once per week
MONTHLY = about once per month
NEVER = almost never

How often do you participate in:	NEVER	MONTHLY	WEEKLY	FREQUENTLY	AEROBIC
1. Swimming	0	1	2	3	4
2. Walking (1 mile per day)	0	1	2	3	4
3. Hiking or backpacking	0	1	2	3	4
4. Gardening	0	1	2	3	4
5. Bicycling	0	1	2	3	4
6. Calisthenics, aerobics, dance exercise	0	1	2	3	4
7. Racquetball, tennis	0	1	2	3	4
8. Canoeing or boating	0	1	2	3	4
9. Water or snow skiing	0	1	2	3	4
10. Hunting or fishing	0	1	2	3	4
11. Golfing	0	1	2	3	4
12. Team sports	0	1	2	3	4
13. Running (5 or more miles per week)	0	1	2	3	4
14. Other physical exercise	0	1	2	3	4

After answering all 14 questions, *sum* the values in all the circled boxes. Then, *count* all the boxes with the value of 1 or more. *Divide* the *sum* by the *count*. This is your *aerobic index*. Finally, locate your aerobic index on the scale below. A low aerobic index suggests that you are not getting enough exercise. A high aerobic index suggests that your pattern of exercise is fairly good. If you have a score at the high-risk end of the scale, you should think about how to begin a consistent exercise program that will place you in the normal, if not excellent, range.

Aerobic index	..1.00..1.25..1.50..1.75..2.00..2.50..3.00..3.50..4.00..		
	←High risk→	←Normal exercise→	←Excellent→
Percentile	...20...30....40....50....60....70....80....90...100..		

Physical Benefits of Exercise

Physical exercise has a wide range of positive effects for the body. They include the following:

1. Increased respiratory capacity
2. Increased muscle tone (anaerobic)
3. Increased strength in bones, ligaments, and tendons
4. Physiological toughness with lower SNS base rate (Dienstbier, 1989)
5. Improved cardiovascular functioning (aerobic)
6. Reduced risk of heart disease (Haskell, 1987)
7. Improved circulation
8. Lower LDL cholesterol and triglyceride levels
9. Increased levels of protective HDL cholesterol (Martin & Dubbert, 1982)
10. Increased energy
11. Improved sleep and reduced need for sleep (Horne, 1981)
12. Increased rate of metabolism
13. Reduced body weight and improved fat metabolism
14. Reduced risk of injury from slips, falls, and so forth
15. Slower aging process (Harris, Frankel, & Harris, 1977)

These benefits are not just for adults; they apply equally to children and adolescents (Klesges et al., 1990).

Mental Benefits of Exercise

Many athletes report several mental benefits that come with physical activity. One benefit is **runner's euphoria,** a feeling of elation and spiritual ecstasy or transcendence. It can be so powerful that many people run to achieve the same state again. Several studies suggest that exercise reduces reaction to psychosocial stressors (Crews & Landers, 1987) and may prevent or reduce depression (Morgan & Goldston, 1987). Short of a peak experience, exercise has other psychosocial benefits:

1. Increased feelings of self-control, independence, and self-sufficiency
2. Increased self-confidence
3. Improved body image and self-esteem
4. Mental change of pace from the pressures of work, even when work is physical
5. Improved mental functioning, alertness, and efficiency (Tomporowski & Ellis, 1986)
6. Emotional catharsis, or cleansing, of tensions from interpersonal conflict and job stress
7. Reduced levels of stress
8. Relief from mild depressions

We must not assume, however, that these are simple effects. For example, one research team observed the typical association between fitness from **aerobic exercise** and cardiovascular fitness (Czajkowski et al., 1990). The team used an anger temperament scale in their study. This follows other observations suggesting that negative affect plays a significant role in the coronary-prone profile. Physically fit subjects did report lower levels of anger than those not as fit. Yet when they analyzed the relation between exercise and cardiovascular fitness, controlling for angry temperament, the relationship all but disappeared. It appears, then, that dispositional anger may offset or reduce the positive effects of exercise.

PREPARING FOR EXERCISE

Preparing for exercise can be as important as the exercise itself. Think of each exercise session as divided into three distinct periods: **warm-up,** exercise, and cool-down. Whatever the sport, schedule a 10- to 20-minute warm-up period before the main workout. During this time, do some easy stretching and limbering routines. The goal is to bring your body temperature up slowly and get your muscles ready for more demanding activity. If bicycling, set an easy pace for the first mile or two before increasing the pace. If running, do light calisthenics or the equivalent before starting. Never start at full speed.

When you finish exercising, allow 10 to 20 minutes for cooling off. The longer and harder the workout, the longer you need for cooling down. Taking a brisk walk may be enough, but you can use light calisthenics as well. If you do not cool down properly, the muscles may become congested with increased blood flow. Ketones, or poisons, build up in the blood, producing pain and discomfort, such as in cramps.

It is preferable to think of an exercise program as a developmental process. Begin with light exercise during short sessions. As your fitness improves, you can increase the intensity and the length of the sessions. Later, exercise should be viewed primarily as a **maintenance** strategy, not a continuous improvement strategy. Avoid the idea that you have to lift more weights, play more games, run more miles, or run faster. Continuous progress is ultimately impossible. You will reach a plateau sometime and will find you can go no further. That is the time to consider switching to a maintenance strategy. As others have pointed out, fitness is not a ribbon you win in competition; it is a road you travel all your life. After reaching speed, you do not have to keep accelerating.

EXERCISING FOR FITNESS

A few important rules should guide a suitable exercise program. First, exercise programs should aim for **aerobic fitness** more than strength. Aerobic fitness means "the ability to take in, transport, and utilize oxygen" (Sharkey, 1984, p. 3). Building muscle strength through bodybuilding routines is acceptable if a hard body is your main goal, but you should still use other exercise that builds cardiovascular fitness. Bodybuilding routines are, for the most part, **anaerobic,** or done without air. They involve high work output but produce lactic acid and eventually muscle fatigue that limits how long the exercise can last (Tomporowski & Ellis, 1986). Anaerobic programs do not do *as much* for cardiovascular fitness as aerobic programs, but anaerobic exercise may still bring some cardiovascular benefits.

Second, to achieve aerobic improvement, four factors may vary. These are frequency, type, duration, and intensity of exercise. How effective your exercise program is over the short run and how well you maintain it over the long haul depends on the interaction of these four.

How Often to Exercise?

The rule is to exercise at least three—and preferably four—times each week, 30 to 45 minutes each time, to obtain aerobic improvement. Anything less than this will produce more losses in the off days than you gain on exercise days. Anything more than this may wear down your body. When this happens, you feel increasing fatigue and may lose motivation for exercise. If you absolutely must exercise more than four times per week, do what professional athletes do. Schedule major workouts on an every-other-day basis, and schedule light workouts on the off days. You might even use a different type of exercise on the off days to provide variety and maintain motivation.

What Exercise Is Best?

Many books detail specific forms of exercise and provide some assessment of their adequacy. In this section, we will discuss the most important findings.

TABLE 15-2

Energy Expenditure per Hour During Different Types of Activity for a 70-Kilogram Man

Form of activity	Calories per hour
Sleeping	65
Awake, lying still	77
Sitting at rest	100
Standing relaxed	105
Dressing and undressing	118
Tailoring	135
Typewriting rapidly	140
Light exercise	170
Walking slowly (2.6 miles per hour)	200
Carpentry, metal working, industrial painting	240
Active exercise	290
Severe exercise	450
Sawing wood	480
Swimming	500
Running (5.3 miles per hour)	570
Very severe exercise	600
Walking very fast (5.3 miles per hour)	650
Walking up stairs	1100

SOURCE: Adapted from Guyton (1977).

Whatever exercise you choose, it should fit sensibly into your lifestyle and be within reach of your physical capacities.

One method of rating different types of exercise uses the number of calories burned in one hour. Table 15-2, a typical caloric expenditure table, contains some interesting information. For example, note that rapid walking burns more calories than even swimming or running. The moral is simple: You do not have to engage in extremely intense and demanding sports, such as marathons, to achieve aerobic fitness. Any activity that burns about 200 to 300 calories per hour is sufficient if you do it consistently three to four times per week.

Also note that just walking slowly burns about 200 calories per hour. Moderate aerobic exercise is about 300 calories per hour. Using this as the norm, there are many activities that can provide adequate aerobic fitness. For example, a brisk 2-mile walk at approximately 3 miles per hour is adequate for most people. There are no equipment expenses, no club memberships and fees, no embarrassment, no competition, and little worry about overdoing.

The prevailing opinion is that running, bicycling, swimming, or aerobic exercise classes are the most beneficial. Home-based treadmills and exercise machines provide adequate exercise where time and access are problems. Even the common jump rope provides a simple yet excellent aerobic exercise. It is cheap. It can be done anywhere, and it can be varied in intensity and length of time. Another simple exercise, similar to the "step-up" test for cardiovascular fitness, can be done on stairs. Just step up two or three steps, back down, and repeat. Doing this at a continuous pace for just 15 minutes is equivalent to a 3-mile slow walk.

How Long Should an Exercise Session Last?

You can obtain aerobic fitness by increasing the length or intensity of the workout or both. Very severe workouts can be dangerous, though, for a variety of reasons. You are more likely to have muscle strains, tears, ankle sprains, and other injuries as the intensity of the workout increases. You should never try intense workouts at the start of an exercise program. This can cause serious injuries and even heart attacks. The wiser course is to use slightly longer, moderately demanding workouts.

To understand how long and how intense exercise should be, it may help to examine the goal of exercise. To be fit means three things: Muscles have strength and tone to carry on work; lungs have the capacity to take in air to supply to the heart and muscles; and the heart can increase its capacity (beats and volume) to meet the demands of work and exercise. Anaerobic exercise helps strengthen and tone muscles but only aerobic exercise meets all three criteria.

Consider these facts about the lungs and heart. The average adult has a resting heart rate around 70 to 75 beats per minute (bpm). A finely conditioned athlete has a resting pulse of 60 bpm, sometimes even lower. A person with a sedentary lifestyle is more likely to have a resting pulse around 80 to 90 bpm. In addition, this person's heart cannot respond to demand as readily as the tuned heart. This difference between the conditioned and the "deconditioned" heart means more wear and tear. The untuned heart must beat about 30,000 more times each day!

Under workload, the heart can beat much faster than the 70-bpm average: It can beat as fast as 200-plus beats per minute. The ability to engage in work with minimum strain depends on how much the heart rate can be raised and sustained over time. Aerobic exercise gradually increases the rate at which your heart can work. As an added benefit, it gradually decreases the resting pulse, so your heart does not have to work as hard even when it is resting. The risk for coronary disease declines as exercise increases up to a maximum of 3000 calories per week of exercise (Haskell, 1987). For perspective, a 3000 calories expenditure in one week would be equal to jogging 4 hours 15 minutes at a 5-mph rate, or about 21 miles total for the week.

The rule is that exercise should increase heart rate between 60% and 80% of the maximum capacity for your age. The maximum capacity can be obtained by taking 220 minus your age. If exercise does not increase heart rate above 60%, or about 115 bpm for the 30-year-old ($220 - 30 = 190 \times .6 = 115$ bpm), little or no progress will be made toward aerobic fitness. If you are 30 years old, the upper limit for aerobic exercise is about 152 bpm ($220 - 30 = 190 \times .8 = 152$ bpm). Table 15-3 provides calculated maximum heart rates for different ages with the minimum and maximum range for aerobic exercise. Also, note that the value for each age is the *average* for that age. Depending on several factors, the value you should use may vary more than 10 bpm more or less than the listed value. These ranges also appear in the table (Sharkey, 1984).

You can achieve adequate fitness from a 1-hour workout of moderate intensity that includes warm-up and cool-down. The real benefit for cardiovascular

TABLE 15-3

Maximum Heart Rate (by Age) With Maximum and Minimum Training Heart Rates for Aerobic Fitness

Age	Maximum rate	Range	Maximum training rate	Minimum training rate
10	210	200–220	168	126
15	205	195–215	164	123
20	200	190–210	160	120
25	195	185–205	156	117
30	190	180–200	152	114
35	185	175–195	148	111
40	180	170–190	144	108
45	175	165–185	140	105
50	170	160–180	136	102
55	165	155–175	132	99
60	160	150–170	128	96
70	150	140–160	120	90
80	140	130–150	112	84

Note: The range given for the maximum heart rate is provided as an indication of individual variability. The upper limit may be safely reached by individuals in better condition, but *the lower limit may be the upper limit of safety for those not in good condition.* Also, the high- and low-range concept should be carried over to both the maximum and minimum training rates. To do this, multiply the range values by 80% for maximum training rate and by 60% for minimum training rate.

improvement, though, comes from the 20 to 30 minutes in the middle, when the heart rate accelerates above its normal resting rate. The quality of the exercise determines how much the heart rate accelerates. Low-intensity aerobic effort is when heart rate reaches only the minimum (115 bpm for the 30-year-old). Moderate-intensity aerobic effort occurs when the heart rate accelerates above the minimum but not above about 70% (between 115 and 135 bpm). Heart rates between 70% and 80% reflect a high-intensity aerobic effort.

How Hard to Exercise: The "No Pain, No Gain" Myth

How hard you should exercise depends on your goals and your current physical condition. Although some exertion is necessary to develop fitness, too much exertion can be physically damaging. This is especially true in the early stages of exercise. If your goal is to achieve and maintain an adequate level of fitness, then moderate workouts are all you need. If you are a born competitor, in search of excellence and the chance to prove just how good you are, a more strenuous level of exercise may be warranted. Still, do not depend on the competition motive to sustain a long-term exercise program. Attitudes that emphasize competition may be the single biggest barrier to getting more people into safe but adequate exercise programs.

Work into exercise slowly if you are out of shape. Typically, it will require several weeks of low-intensity exercise and several more weeks of moderate exercise before the body can profit from strenuous workouts. Research in hydraulic-circuit exercises (similar to the popular Nautilus machines) also suggests that you can alternate rest and exercise periods across a wide range (5 to 40 minutes) and still experience positive effects on oxygen uptake (Ballor et al., 1989). This suggests that there is little merit in exercising to the point of pain, burning, or nausea simply because of an arbitrary time line for exercise.

Far too much emphasis is placed on competition and the notion of "no pain, no gain." The Olympic syndrome mentioned earlier is the idea that the exercise, to be useful, must lead to the pinnacle of success. That may be acceptable for the athletically gifted young, but for the average adult, a more modest and attainable goal should suffice. Exercise should be fun, and it does not have to be painful to be helpful. This should be clear because either a brisk walk or 30 minutes of moderate aerobic exercise is sufficient for cardiovascular fitness. Brian Sharkey (1984) reported that a daily 5-minute, 100-calorie workout is sufficient to provide progress to aerobic fitness. After a few weeks, move into the 300-calorie range, and later, even higher if you wish. If you are exercising in part to control weight, then workouts should be in the 300-calorie range.

BARRIERS TO EFFECTIVE EXERCISE

Given the proven benefits of exercise, it may seem surprising that more people do not exercise regularly. This has led researchers to examine the role of attitudes in exercise. Attitudes toward exercise may predict interest in exercise, but they do not seem to predict whether a person will stick with a program (Kendzierski & Lamastro, 1988). Many attitudes keep people from exercise. Two such attitudes are society's obsession with competition and the Olympic syndrome, as already noted. Another attitudinal barrier is the perception of lack of need. This is the person who says, "I'm in as good shape as anyone else, if not better." While that may be partially true, it is no excuse to avoid regular exercise. You need exercise no matter how fit you feel.

There is also the excuse that exercise programs cost too much. As noted before, several exercises cost almost nothing, yet they provide adequate physical conditioning. Another excuse is that exercise takes too much time or competes with more important activities. Consider these facts. The three to four hours per week needed for physical health is less than 4% of total waking time. It is much less than the average time spent watching TV. Even TV time can be used for calisthenics, jumping rope, or riding an exercise bicycle.

Some people feel they will be embarrassed if they go to an exercise class or take up a competitive sport. There are several ways around this. Get a friend who is in about the same shape to exercise with you. In classes such as Jazzercise classes, remember that many people there may have taken the classes before and are there now to maintain fitness. You should not even compare yourself with them. Often you will find more support and encouragement for trying than anything else.

Another attitudinal barrier is that some people think exercise takes place only in a gym. It is as though one must be in a health center, dressed in exercise

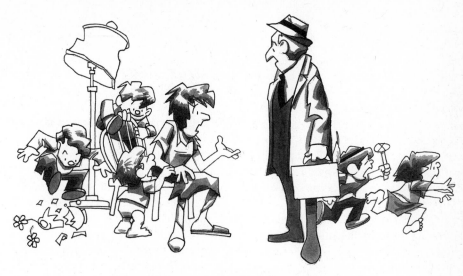

"I gave birth to and am raising five children…and
you think I should take a *fitness* class?"

SOURCE: © 1990. Reprinted courtesy of Bunny Hoest and Parade Magazine.

fashions, working out on a universal gym, to be engaged in exercise. In reality, exercise can take place in many different settings, in everyday clothes, and with no high-tech equipment, as the cartoon suggests. You can exercise in your office building by going up and down stairs repeatedly or if your work involves climbing, lifting, and kneeling. Frequently repeated activities that emulate calisthenics can help tone the body even if you don't do them fast enough to improve aerobic fitness. If the exercise does not provide heart rate acceleration to aerobic levels, you may still need some exercise outside work.

Finally, some people tend to exaggerate a failure and use it as an excuse to quit. There will be setbacks in any exercise program and times when you do not feel well, when you cannot run as far or as fast. These should be considered part of the process. Most of all, you should keep a flexible attitude toward exercise. Allow exercise to vary with mood and condition, but keep on exercising.

THE EXERCISER: A PSYCHOLOGICAL PROFILE

Several personal characteristics may correlate with beginning an exercise program and sticking to it. These include self-efficacy, self-motivation, and self-schemata. You may recall that self-efficacy is a self-schema about personal competency and mastery. It is the belief or expectation that one has the skills to act appropriately and successfully in certain situations. Exercise seems to greatly enhance self-efficacy (Cameron & Best, 1987). Conversely, the perception of lack of self-efficacy may be a major stumbling block to beginning an exercise program. This suggests that exercisers have both accurate and positive judgments of self-efficacy. We will discuss the practical implications of this later in this chapter.

The desire to change body image and improve health is an important motive (Gillett, 1988). Exercisers possess a degree of self-motivation that carries them through tough times as well (Martin & Dubbert, 1982). That is, they do not seem to require external prompts to keep them interested and involved. People with low self-motivation drop out of exercise programs more frequently than self-motivators.

Clingman and Hilliard (1987) have studied the super-adherer and constructed a personality profile. The super-adherer is one who is doggedly determined to exercise, who sets high exercise goals, and who wants to be competitive in his or her chosen sport. The profile includes motivation to achieve combined with endurance and dominance. Clingman and Hilliard also noted that certain personality traits fit an individual to a sport. For example, swimmers were not as aggressive as cyclists or triathletes. Runners were more autonomous than any other athletes tested, and cyclists were the most aggressive.

According to Deborah Kendzierski (1990), exercisers have self-schemata that include exercise in many ways. First, self-schemata are cognitive structures that include generalizations about the self and important aspects of self. Individuals with exercise schemata use more exercise activity words to describe themselves. They recall more exercise events and behaviors in their past. Finally, they are more likely to be involved in exercise programs than people with non–exercise-oriented self-schemata.

MARATHON RUNNING: THE MYTH OF CORONARY IMMUNITY

Space does not permit more than a brief statement about the unfortunate myth that if you can run a marathon, you will acquire immunity to coronary. The myth is unfortunate because many people pursued the dream of immunity too fast and too hard, with too much pain and sometimes with unnecessary death. The deaths of several runners who were in peak condition shattered the notion of coronary immunity. The most celebrated case is the death of Jim Fixx (1977), the author of a popular book on running. Yet, vulnerability to coronary disease results from several factors, including genetic endowment, diet, and exercise. Exercise itself does not reverse the effects of genetic endowment. It may help someone at risk to live a healthier and higher quality life, but it does not remove risk altogether.

EXERCISING FOR WEIGHT CONTROL

As noted earlier, exercise can be an important asset to a weight loss program. Attempts to reduce weight that do not include exercise are generally less effective, if not doomed to failure. Exercise speeds up a sluggish metabolism, causing the body to burn calories faster. This effect continues beyond the period of activity. The body burns calories about 10% faster up to six hours beyond the exercise (Mirkin, 1983). Even during sleep, metabolism is slightly higher than it would be if you did not exercise!

PRECAUTIONS FOR EXERCISE PROGRAMS

There are a few precautions to consider before starting an exercise program. First, anyone over 35 years of age should obtain a thorough medical exam first. The longer it has been since you exercised, the more crucial this precaution is. The exam probably should include a routine physical and a stress test. Therefore, you should not hide the purpose of the exam from your physician. Overweight people should set modest goals, especially at the beginning. Recognize that high-intensity exercise programs are not necessary to achieve satisfactory weight loss or aerobic fitness (Gillett, 1988). Remember to use warm-up and cool-down periods before and after exercise. Finally, make sure you take in both enough fluids and calories to sustain physical exercise. Lack of either can produce physical problems during exercise and increase fatigue.

BEHAVIORAL SELF-CONTROL: PRINCIPLES FOR STICKING WITH IT

In this section, we will discuss some basic principles of behavioral self-control. These principles have emerged from clinical studies designed to help people do the very things discussed in this chapter—reduce weight and engage in consistent exercise. The ideas presented here can be extended to cover a variety of other unhealthy behaviors, such as smoking.

Set Attainable Goals

There are two factors in this principle. First, you need to know exactly where you want to go with your program. If you want to lose 25 pounds or exercise three times per week each week of the year, make that goal absolutely clear. Setting fuzzy goals like, "I want to look better" or "I want to get in shape" do not specify how you can get there.

Then you need to make sure you can get there. Don't try to lose 50 pounds if you only need to lose 25. Also, don't try to run a four-minute mile or a two-hour marathon. These are goals for the professionals. Be happy even with a modest achievement.

Allow for Success and Build Self-Efficacy

The practical implication of research on self-efficacy is that one should arrange for success in behavioral control, even if that success is modest. As you attain success, your perception of self-efficacy is likely to increase. With increases in self-efficacy, one is more likely to continue to pursue the goal, and more success is likely.

Break Long-Range Goals Down into Short-Term Goals

In addition to deciding where you want to go, set goals that mark progress for the trip there. Do not think in terms of losing 25 pounds or running a marathon. Think instead of losing 2 pounds per week or of running a 3-meter race. This way, you can divide a big trip into smaller parts, and you can more easily chart your progress. Then you will be more likely to stay motivated and keep at the program because you can see you are making gains.

Provide for Observable Progress Reports

It is important that you see your progress. In behavioral terms, this is **self-monitoring**. There are many ways to count or measure behavior. You can count frequency of repetitions in an exercise routine. You can time how long it takes you to bicycle a certain distance. A daily log can be checked to show the exercise you carried out. You can keep a caloric intake and weight record each day. A caloric record is more effective than just a weight record (Cameron & Best, 1987). A record of eating behavior should record what you eat in calories, when you eat, what other activities are going on while eating, and people present.

A popular, easy way to record behavior change is to use a **calendar for self-observation.** Often, it is helpful to translate the calendar record to a simple chart or graph. You receive positive feedback by seeing your progress. Also, you can see patterns (weight gains over the weekend that slow progress) or detect problem areas in your program. Most popular exercise and diet programs use charts that serve this purpose.

Making the chart public or semipublic can help you maintain motivation. A public chart becomes almost a contract with the viewers that you will succeed. You draw on powerful sources of social approval as you progress and gentle reproof when you let down. The chart does not have to be public in the literal sense, but it might be visible to people in your office or to your inner circle of friends.

Provide Yourself with Tangible Rewards

When you meet certain short-term goals, you ought to reward yourself. Perhaps you could set aside a certain amount of money to buy something personal, such as some nice clothing or compact disk to add to your collection. In formal terms, this is a **contingency contract.**

In addition to rewards, you should agree on fines for failure to meet goals. Say you want to lose a pound each week for a month. The positive reward will be a sweater you have had your eye on for a while. If you do not meet your goal, the money will go to something that you really do not like—support of a politician or organization that you cannot stand.

Identify and Control Environmental Stimuli

An important part of self-control is recognizing environmental events that support bad habits (Cameron & Best, 1987). A chart of eating habits may reveal heavy eating when you are alone. A similar analysis may show continual snacking while watching TV.

The rule is to change the environment in a way that reverses the relationship. For example, you could use behavioral restrictions. Eat only in the kitchen, and do not move the TV into the kitchen to bypass the rule! Do not keep tempting and fattening snacks on the shelves. If you find that you do not exercise after you get home because of distractions, take your workout gear to work or school with you. Some people schedule a walk as part of their lunch break. Others take a longer break to go to the local health club and work out. This can be an excellent idea; it serves as a change of pace and recharges you for the balance of the day. Other people schedule a workout on their way home. Any of these strategies may break the pattern of negative stimulus control at home.

Make the Routine Habit-Forming

Whatever exercise you choose, get into a routine and stay with it. When a person's schedule gets tight, typically the first thing to go is exercise. Resist this temptation, especially early in your program. If you work out consistently for a few weeks, you should find that consistency is habit-forming. You may feel tension if you disrupt the new habit.

Use Nonproductive Time for Double-Timing

Some people complain that they do not have time for exercise, yet they spend hours watching TV. Turn that nonproductive time into fitness time. You could do calisthenics such as situps or pushups and never miss a heartbeat of *L.A. Law* or *Monday Night Football*. Skip rope to *Saturday Night Live* or *Arsenio Hall*. Also, you could watch a Jazzercise class on TV and exercise with it. Then you could relax when you watch TV at other times. If your analysis of time shows significant nonproductive time, look for ways of double-timing. Turn those sedentary hours into profitable fitness hours.

Perhaps you use quiet times at home to read or keep up with correspondence. You can still take breaks for fitness exercises. You may find that your mind
continues to work on issues and problems while exercising. A novel solution
may occur to you during exercise, and you can return to your work energized
in two ways.

One word of caution is in order. Many people have only a few leisure hours
available. If you watch TV sparingly and for specific reasons, such as self-
development or just relaxation, do not feel guilty about using TV-watching for
that purpose. Instead, look for ways to free some other part of your schedule
to provide the time you need for fitness.

Preventing Relapse

Emphasizing the things that will draw you to success is one part of the battle.
The other part is thinking about the things that will prevent your falling back
into the old unhealthy behaviors. There are several means to prevent relapse,
including social support from friends or family or both, flexibility in goal setting for exercise, and use of cognitive strategies while exercising (Martin et al.,
1984). Spouse involvement is especially useful in weight loss programs and may
be useful in exercise programs as well (Brownell, Marlatt, Lichtenstein, & Wilson,
1986). Group exercise can aid adherence, especially when there is a strong sense
of group cohesiveness (Carron, Widmeyer, & Brawley, 1988).

Marlatt's research team provided guidelines for using distraction-based
cognitive strategies (Brownell et al., 1986). Negative cognitions occur when one
dwells on body sensations—fatigue in the legs while biking, sore feet while running. A distraction-based program suggests that you think about the beauty of
the day, pleasant smells from the woods, or flowers growing along the path.
This provides positive, supportive internal feedback that sustains your motivation to exercise. Such strategies appear to lead to higher adherence to a training
program (Martin et al., 1984).

SUMMARY

In this chapter, we discussed basic elements of sound nutrition, diet, and exercise. The general principles have been clearly established by a solid line of
research over the past quarter-century. You should try to balance your diet with
more carbohydrates and fewer proteins and fats; the percentages should be about
50%, 30%, and 20%, respectively. Also, you should increase the amount of fiber
in your diet because fiber helps remove fat, helps you feel full, and reduces the
tendency to overeat. Next, reduce the amount of saturated fats, sugars, and salt.
Finally, avoid taking megadoses of vitamins. Your body cannot absorb excess
vitamins. Taking megadoses of vitamins is simply passing off expensive vitamins
in urine and stools.

If you feel you need to diet for health reasons, plan a diet program around
an exercise program. This is the most effective way to lose weight, because

exercise will help you burn off more calories even when you are not exercising. Avoid diets that go to the extreme either in reducing calories to a very low amount or by excluding one kind of food. Keep the calorie count above 1300, especially while exercising. Do not try to lose huge amounts of weight at a time; this could be very dangerous. Think instead in terms of a program in which you lose, at most, about one pound per week. Think in terms of maintaining an altered eating lifestyle, coupled with exercise, after you reach your weight loss goal.

In choosing a fitness program, you should consider an exercise that fits your physical capabilities and meshes comfortably with your professional and family patterns. Exercise does not have to be painful, expensive, excessively time-consuming, or glamorous to provide benefits. Once you have selected an appropriate exercise and set a schedule, make that schedule habitual. Always do some warm-up exercises before commencing hard workouts, and be careful to cool down slowly. The most intense exercise should raise your heart rate to somewhere between 70% and 80% of your resting heart rate. Avoid the Olympic syndrome, and remember that there is a limit to what you can do. Avoid the notion that you must always be improving. After you have reached an adequate level of fitness, shift your program to one of maintenance.

KEY TERMS

aerobic exercise
aerobic fitness
   (defined)
anaerobic exercise
calendar for
   self-observation
cholesterol
contingency contract

dieting dangers
exercise for
   maintenance
exercise for warm-up
high-density lipopro-
   tein (HDL)
low-density lipopro-
   tein (LDL)

runner's euphoria
self-monitoring
set-point theory
vitamin abuse
vitamin side effects
yellow fat

REFERENCES

Ballor, D. L., Becque, M. D., Marks, C. R., Nau, K. L., & Katch, V. L. (1989). Physiological responses to nine different exercise:rest protocols. *Medicine and Science in Sports and Exercise, 21,* 90–95.

Boulenger, J. P., Salem, N., Marangos, P. J., & Uhde, T. W. (1987). Plasma adenosine levels: Measurement in humans and relationship to the anxiogenic effects of caffeine. *Psychiatry Research, 21,* 247–255.

Brownell, K. D., Marlatt, G. A., Lichtenstein, E., & Wilson, G. T. (1986). Understanding and preventing relapse. *American Psychologist, 41,* 765–782.

Cameron, R., & Best, J. A. (1987). Promoting adherence to health behavior change interventions: Recent findings from behavioral research. *Patient Education and Counseling, 10,* 139–154.

Carron, A. V., Widmeyer, W. N., & Brawley, L. R. (1988). Group cohesion and individual adherence to physical activity. *Journal of Sport and Exercise Psychology, 10,* 127–138.

Clingman, J. M., & Hilliard, D. V. (1987). Some personality characteristics of the super-adherer: Following those who go beyond fitness. *Journal of Sport Behavior, 10,* 123–136.

Crews, D. J., & Landers, D. M. (1987). A meta-analytic review of aerobic fitness and reactivity to psychosocial stressors. *Medicine and Science in Sports and Exercise, 19,* S114–S120.

Czajkowski, S. M., Hindelang, R. D., Dembroski, T. M., Mayerson, S. E., Parks, E. B., & Holland, J. C. (1990). Aerobic fitness, psychological characteristics, and cardiovascular reactivity to stress. *Health Psychology, 9,* 676–692.

Dienstbier, R. A. (1989). Arousal and physiological toughness: Implications for mental and physical health. *Psychological Review, 96,* 84–100.

Dubbert, P. M., & Wilson, G. T. (1984). Goal-setting and spouse involvement in the treatment of obesity. *Behavior Research and Therapy, 22,* 227–242.

Fixx, J. F. (1977). *The complete book of running.* New York: Random House.

Gallup, G., Jr. (1984). *The Gallup poll: Public opinion 1984.* Wilmington, DE: Scholarly Resources.

Gershoff, S. (1990). *The Tufts University guide to total nutrition.* New York: Harper & Row.

Gillett, P. A. (1988). Self-reported factors influencing exercise adherence in overweight women. *Nursing Research, 37,* 25–29.

Gutlin, B., & Kessler, G. (1983). *The high energy factor.* New York: Random House.

Guyton, A. C. (1977). *Basic human physiology: Normal function and mechanisms of disease.* Philadelphia: Saunders.

Hajjar, K. A., Gavish, D., Breslow, J. L., & Nachman, R. L. (1989). Lipoprotein(a) modulation of endothelial cell surface fibrinolysis and its potential role in atherosclerosis. *Nature, 339,* 303–305.

Harris, R., Frankel, L. J., & Harris, S. (Eds.). (1977). *Guide to fitness after fifty.* New York: Plenum.

Haskell, W. L. (1987). Developing an activity plan for improving health. In W. P. Morgan & S. E. Goldston (Eds.), *Exercise and mental health* (pp. 37–55). Washington, DC: Hemisphere.

Heller, J. (1987). What do we know about the risks of caffeine consumption in pregnancy? *British Journal of Addiction, 82,* 885–889.

Herbert, L., & Teague, M. L. (1989). Exercise adherence and older adults: A theoretical perspective. *Activities, Adaptation, and Aging, 13,* 91–105.

Horne, J. A. (1981). The effects of exercise upon sleep: A critical review. *Biological Psychology, 12,* 241–290.

Keesey, R. E., & Powley, T. L. (1986). The regulation of body weight. *Annual Review of Psychology, 37,* 109–133.

Kendzierski, D. (1990). Exercise self-schemata: Cognitive and behavioral correlates. *Health Psychology, 9,* 69–82.

Kendzierski, D., & Lamastro, V. D. (1988). Reconsidering the role of attitudes in exercise behavior: A decision theoretic approach. *Journal of Applied Social Psychology, 18,* 737–759.

Klesges, R. C., Eck, L. H., Hanson, C. L., Haddock, C. K., & Klesges, L. M. (1990). Effects of obesity, social interactions, and physical environment on physical activity in preschoolers. *Health Psychology, 9,* 435–449.

Kobasa, S. C., Maddi, S. R., & Puccetti, M. C. (1982). Personality and exercise as buffers in the stress-illness relationship. *Journal of Behavioral Medicine, 5,* 391–404.

Lane, J. D. (1983). Caffeine and cardiovascular responses to stress. *Psychosomatic Medicine, 45,* 447–451.

Lieberman, H. R., Spring, B. J., & Garfield, G. S. (1986). The behavioral effects of food constituents: Strategies used in studies of amino acids, protein, carbohydrate and caffeine. *Nutrition Reviews: Diet and Behavior, 44,* 61–70.

Marshall, C. W. (1983). *Vitamins and minerals: Help or harm?* Philadelphia: George F. Stickley.

Martin, J. E., & Dubbert, P. M. (1982). Exercise applications and promotion in behavioral medicine: Current status and future directions. *Journal of Consulting and Clinical Psychology, 50,* 1004–1017.

Martin, J. E., Dubbert, P. M., Katell, A. D., Thompson, J. K., Raczynski, J. R., Lake, M. et al. (1984). Behavioral control of exercise in sedentary adults: Studies 1 through 6. *Journal of Consulting and Clinical Psychology, 52,* 795–811.

Mayo Clinic, Committee on Dietetics (Ed.). (1981). *Mayo Clinic diet manual.* Philadelphia: Saunders.

McGinnis, J. M., & Nestle, M. (1989). The Surgeon General's report on nutrition and health: Policy implications and implementation strategies. *American Journal of Clinical Nutrition, 49,* 23–28.

Mensink, R. P., & Katan, M. B. (1990). Effect of dietary trans fatty acids on high density and low density lipoprotein cholesterol levels in healthy subjects. *The New England Journal of Medicine, 323,* 439–445.

Mirkin, G. (1983). *Getting thin.* Boston: Little, Brown.

Mirkin, G., & Hoffman, M. (1978). *The sports medicine book.* Boston: Little, Brown.

Morgan, W. P., & Goldston, S. E. (Eds.). (1987). *Exercise and mental health.* Washington, DC: Hemisphere.

National Center for Health Statistics. (1988). *Monthly vital statistics report, 37,* 1–10.

National Research Council, Food and Nutrition Board. Committee on Dietary Allowances. (1980). *Recommended dietary allowances* (9th rev. ed.). Washington, DC: National Academy of Sciences.

Ostlund, R. E., Staten, M., Kohrt, W. M., Schultz, J., & Malley, M. (1990). The ratio of waist-to-hip circumference, plasma insulin level, and glucose intolerance as independent predictors of the HDL_2 cholesterol level in older adults. *The New England Journal of Medicine, 322,* 229–234.

Pekkanen, J., Linn, S., Heiss, G., Suchindran, C. M., Leon, A., Rifkind, B. M., & Tyroler, H. A. (1990). Ten-year mortality from cardiovascular disease in relation to cholesterol level among men with and without preexisting cardiovascular disease. *The New England Journal of Medicine, 322,* 1700–1707.

Posner, M. J. (1982). *Executive essentials.* New York: Avon Books.

Schachter, S. (1982). Recidivism and self cure of smoking and obesity. *American Psychologist, 37,* 436–444.

Sharkey, B. J. (1984). *Physiology of fitness: Prescribing exercise for fitness, weight control, and health* (2nd ed.). Champaign, IL: Human Kinetics.

Spring, B. J., Lieberman, H. R., Swope, G., & Garfield, G. S. (1986). Effects of carbohydrates on mood and behavior. *Nutrition Reviews: Diet and Behavior, 44,* 51–60.

Swain, J. F., Rouse, I. L., Curley, C. B., & Sacks, F. M. (1990). Comparison of the effects of oat bran and low-fiber wheat on serum lipoprotein levels and blood pressure. *The New England Journal of Medicine, 322,* 147–152.

Tomporowski, P. D., & Ellis, N. R. (1986). Effects of exercise on cognitive processes: A review. *Psychological Bulletin, 99,* 338–346.

van Dale, D., & Saris, W. H. M. (1989). Repetitive weight loss and weight regain: Effects on weight reduction, resting metabolic rate, and lipolytic activity before and after exercise and/or diet treatment. *American Journal of Clinical Nutrition, 49,* 409–416.

Relaxation Instructions

PREPARATION

At least for the first few weeks, go over the mechanics of what you are to do just before each relaxation session. Review the instructions for the proper sequence of relaxing muscle groups, and make the final arrangements you prefer in regard to phone, music, lighting, and so on. If you are using taped relaxation instructions, make sure the recorder is adjusted for proper volume (a little on the soft side is preferable) and set at the right place to begin. Attention to these minor details can make for a much smoother and easier relaxation period. Obviously, as you progress in your practice, more and more of these details will become like second nature to you. Then relaxation will have become a useful tool requiring little effort for its use.

GETTING STARTED WITH RELAXATION

The following instructions are for the first few relaxation sessions. Subsequently, the instructions are abbreviated, and shortcuts are taken to produce relaxation faster. These techniques will be discussed later. To begin, *read through the entire set of instructions once before trying to actually relax*. The instructions for self-direction appear in indented blocks. Some comments are interspersed that will enable you to understand why you are being asked to do certain things.

During the first reading, you may try some of the tension-relaxation cycles just to get a feel for what it is like. But do not count your first run-through as a relaxation session! After reading through once, sit in your chair, turn the lights down low, put on your background music—whatever you have decided on for your setting and preparation—and go through the procedure to relax. You will soon find that there is a logic to the progression that will come in handy for further sessions. Further instructions for timing and other matters will be provided as needed.

You may want to record the instructions on tape in your own voice. This will allow you to concentrate on relaxing instead of worrying about what the next instruction is. Should you decide to do this, just read the instructions given and elaborate or extend where necessary as you are recording. You may paraphrase the instructions to some extent. Pronouns can be changed and sequences extended for the number of repetitions required. As long as the sense is the same, the words used do not make a difference. (More will be said about ways to handle the instructions at the end of this appendix.)

INSTRUCTIONS FOR RELAXATION

For the next few minutes, you are going to study the difference between tension and relaxation in a number of your muscles. In the process, you should begin to feel more and more relaxed. At the end, you should experience a comfortable heaviness in your body and have a feeling of easy peacefulness.

Remove any tight-fitting clothes first. Loosen ties, belts, or any other articles of clothing that are tight. Take off your shoes. Also, remove any tight-fitting jewelry, such as watches, rings, or necklaces. Get comfortably situated in your chair. Put your arms on the arms of the chair with your palms down and hands open over the end of the chair's arms. Sit back in the chair and let your head fall gently onto your chest. Close your eyes. Let your legs lie comfortably apart on a stool or on the leg support of your recliner. Do not cross your legs, regardless of the type of chair you are using. If your chair is not a recliner and you do not have a footstool available, place your feet a few inches apart on the floor and let your arms lie across your thighs with your hands in your lap. (For self-guided or self-taped instructions, begin here. Use only those sections that are indented and elaborate or extend them as necessary.)

> Now take a few deep breaths, hold each breath for a few seconds, and then let each breath out fully and completely. As you breathe in, you will notice some tension in your chest and diaphragm. As you breathe out, you will notice a sense of relaxing, almost of going limp. Relaxing feels good and comfortable and it would be nice if you could keep the feeling. But as you breathe in deeply again you feel the same tension as before, especially as you hold the breath for a moment. Let the breath out again, completely, and feel the pleasant relaxing sensation of letting go. Try it one more time. Dwell for just a moment on the sense of relaxation as you let the breath out.

> Try to maintain that sense of relaxation in your chest and diaphragm for a moment. As you breathe from now on, just breathe easily and naturally, almost as though you were napping.

> Concentrate for a moment on your right arm [left arm if you are left-handed]. Now flex your biceps as though you were showing off your muscles. Notice how it feels.

It may be easiest to do this by just pushing your elbow into the arm of the chair. Also, by doing it this way, you do not actually have to raise your arm from the chair.

Flex it as tight as you can and hold it [about ten seconds]. As you hold, study the sensation of tension. Notice how unpleasant it can be. Now let it go all at once. Let your arm go completely limp. Relax! And study the contrast. Notice how different it is from tension. Store the contrast in your mind even as you are studying it. One more time. Tense your bicep and hold it. Observe the feeling of tightness. Tune in to the signal of tension in your muscle. Then let it go. Completely relaxed. If someone picked up your arm and then turned it loose, it would simply drop to your side. There is no tension at all. It feels so good. One more time. *Tense; hold; observe; relax; and observe.*

We are going to repeat this same sequence now for several other muscle groups. You will notice a general progression from the head down, with the exception of this first arm-hand sequence. The arm-hand sequence is done first because it is easy to experience the difference between tension and relaxation in these muscle groups. Also, note the pattern for each muscle group: tense; hold; observe; relax; and observe. The cycles will be *approximately 10 to 15 seconds for the tension segments and 15 to 20 seconds for the relaxation segments, or roughly 30 seconds per cycle, with just slightly more time devoted to the relaxation than to the tension.* In normal practice, especially in the early stages, you should *do about three repetitions for each muscle group.* Later on, it will not be necessary to do as many. But hold fairly strictly to the time limits and repetitions for now.

Breathe deeply for a moment, hold, let it out. Relax. Your arm is relaxed also. Now, do the other arm. Tense your bicep. Recognize the presence of tension in your arm even as the rest of your body is mostly relaxed. Hold and then release. Tune in to the pleasant sensation of relaxation. Repeat. *Tense; hold; observe; relax; and observe.* And once more. Now both your arms are relaxed, and you continue to breathe in a calm and easy fashion.

Note the instruction "Repeat" with the abbreviated sequence. If you are recording these instructions on tape, this is your signal to extend or elaborate the instructions to allow for additional repetitions.

While the arms may not be frequently involved in tension patterns, your fingers and palms often indicate the presence of stress. Your fingers may start to lock up, your palms may sweat, or your fists may clench during stress. The palms have long been recognized as indicators of emotionality, and this fact is capitalized on in the so-called lie-detector test. Athletes frequently try a variety of measures to relieve their hands of tension in order to be able to perform better.

Breathe deeply again. As you breathe out, say to yourself, "Relax." And let the breath go all at once. Your arms are still relaxed. Clench your right fist [left if you are left-handed]. Hold it for a moment and observe the tightness. Notice the sensation of tension. Put that sensation in your memory. Now let your fist go completely loose, relaxed. Your fingers could not hold anything even if you tried. Once more, notice the difference in the sensations. Observe the pleasant heaviness of the hand when all the tension is gone. Clench your fist again, tight, very tight. Hold it for just a few seconds and study the sensation. Then let it go. All at once and completely. Study the contrast. Feel how good the relaxation is. Once more. *Tense; hold; observe; relax; observe.*

From this point on, I will give you the muscle group, some abbreviated instructions, and any special things to look for. But I will not repeat the extended instructions for each of the repetitions. Instead, you will see a bracketed statement that is some variation on the theme, such as this: [Repeat the tension-relaxation cycle twice more.] This tells you where to repeat the instructions. To emphasize, *for each muscle group, repeat the tension- relaxation cycle three times.* Carry out the study and observation for each segment of tension and relaxation with diligence. It is through this means that you begin to feel the difference between relaxed and tense muscles. It is the beginning of being able to hear your muscles telling you that tension is present.

The next set of muscles is the shoulder muscle group. These muscles very frequently tense under stress, such as during driving or intense periods of concentration. They may knot up or just ache as though they have been overworked. But they will hurt. Shoulder muscle tension, if not relieved quickly, may also spread to the neck and back and additionally contribute to a headache.

Take a deep breath now, and hold it a moment. Then say to yourself, "Relax" as you let the air out of your lungs completely. Now tighten up the shoulder muscle as tight as you can get it.

You may have to experiment with different ways of doing this. A slight rolling forward and upward of the shoulder may work best.

Hold the tension for a moment and study the feeling. Then let your shoulder simply slump. Let all the tension go out of it. Study the difference and enjoy the feeling of relaxation. [Repeat this with the same shoulder two more times.] Next, do the other shoulder in the same way. At all times, take care to notice the difference between relaxation and tension. [Repeat this with the alternate shoulder two more times.]

Continue to keep relaxed all the parts of the body that you have relaxed to this point—the arms, the hands, the shoulders. Take another deep breath, and hold it for a moment. Again release it as you say to yourself, "Relax." Enjoy the feeling of relaxation as it settles more and more over your whole body.

Now you are going to relax the neck muscles. They may become tense apart from the shoulder muscles, which you just relaxed. More often than not, neck muscles are tense when mental pressures are high. Neck muscle tension is also associated with severe forms of headache. Later you will want to make mental connections to any experiences of neck muscle tension from the past. This will help you spot conditions in your environment that are putting pressure on you. To tense your neck muscle:

> Flex your head backward, as though you were pulling down on the back of your skull with your neck. [You may even feel a slight amount of pain right at the base of the skull if you pull hard enough. Do not pull so hard that you strain something!] As you tense the neck muscles, again study the feeling of tightness. Hold it for about ten seconds. Now release all the tension. Let your head fall gently back onto your chest and enjoy the feeling of relief from letting the tension go. Just enjoy relaxing for a few seconds, and observe the difference. [Repeat the neck tension and relaxation cycle two more times.] Continue at all times to breathe easily and naturally. When you are done, scan the rest of your body to see if any parts seem tense. Do not do anything about it right now, just make a mental note of it. But *if any part of the body that you have relaxed before has become tense again, go back quickly and relax that part again.*

It may take you a little while to feel comfortable with this request—that is, trying to keep the rest of the body relaxed while you are concentrating on one part of the body and tensing it. But you will get used to it after a while. Also, it is important to start developing a sense of what it means to scan the body. Perhaps an analogy will help.

Many people have a type of CB radio that is only a receiver, but a special type of receiver. The radio actually scans up to 40 channels used by police, fire chiefs, sheriffs, ambulances, and people who are just into CB radio. The scanner electronically runs through all 40 channels as fast as it can in some systematic fashion. When it is done scanning channels, it does it all over again. It is actually looking for action, a radio signal, some sign that someone somewhere is talking. You need to develop a sense of scanning your body in the same way. It should become like an internal sixth sense that automatically scans the muscle groups from one to the other and then *locks in* on any muscle group when a signal, tension, is found. It may be the most important talking your body does.

Now, concentrate on the forehead muscles. These muscles are referred to in medicine as the *frontalis muscles.* They wrinkle when you frown. They tighten when you are under pressure. Some clinicians believe that tension in the frontalis muscle group is associated with one form of headache, the tension headache. One high-tech solution to this problem is biofeedback.

Biofeedback in the treatment of tension headaches teaches how to relax the frontalis muscles. Overall, the clinical tests that have pitted biofeedback against relaxation find that the gains in symptomatic relief are largely a result of the relaxation itself. But some people experience difficulty trying to learn relaxation through the PMR procedure. They seem to need the visual picture that electronic feedback provides in order to learn how to relax. Biofeedback serves as an ally helping people learn how to relax and how to "read" body signals of tension. It makes little difference, practically speaking, whether you learn to relax through PMR or through biofeedback. The outcome is the same. Once the skill of reading body tension has been developed, the person can use this body information to help with a variety of coping procedures.

If you suffer from tension headaches, pay attention to this muscle group and learn how to relax it through PMR or through biofeedback. If your headaches are of a different variety (vascular pressure instead of muscular tension), they may not respond to relaxation training as readily as to other types of training, including biofeedback. For now, just concentrate on the contrast between tension and relief in this muscle group.

> Wrinkle your forehead. Squint your eyes if you wish. It can help you feel the tension. You will feel your scalp tighten at the same time. Do not worry about any of those other tensions. Just treat them all as though they belong to one group. Hold the tension. Look at the tension. Turn your mind's eye up and look at it. Then let it go. Completely relaxed. Forehead, scalp, and eyes—all are relaxed. Study the difference. Enjoy the feeling of relaxation. [Repeat the cycle two more times, each time paying attention to difference in the feelings.]

Now we will move to the jaws and tongue. Both of these muscles can be treated independently. I prefer to work only with the jaw muscles for a variety of reasons. If you find yourself having any difficulty achieving complete relaxation of the face, you may want to give the tongue special attention. This is usually done by rolling the tongue up to about the middle of the roof of the mouth. Then, just like doing an isometric exercise, you can push against the roof of the mouth and feel the tightness come into the tongue. Relaxing is merely letting the tongue fall back to its natural resting place in the mouth.

The jaw muscles are frequently involved when stress is occurring. For example, during anger many people clench their jaws. In a slender-cheeked person, one can see the ropelike muscle stand out on the side of the cheek when the jaw is clenched. In some cases of chronic stress, certain people will develop a *tic*, a condition in which a particular muscle group (usually in the jaw or cheek area) twitches convulsively. Tension may be relieved in these muscle groups through the use of relaxation training.

> Again, take a deep breath. Hold it. Let it out, saying "Relax" at the same time. Clench your jaws by biting down as though you were chewing on a stick. Hold it for a moment. Study the sensations, the tightness going all the way up to the ears, the cheeks swelling out as the muscles tighten. Now let it go. Quickly, completely, let the jaw relax. You do not have to open your mouth for the jaws to relax. Just let all the tension go. Observe the difference again between this comfortable, easy feeling and the tightness you felt before. [Repeat the tension-relaxation cycle twice more.]
>
> Continue relaxing. Enjoy the feeling. Now take a very deep breath and hold it for a few seconds. Notice the tightness in your chest and diaphragm. Try not to tighten your stomach as you are breathing in. Now, say "Relax" to yourself as you let your breath go. Your whole body just seems to go

into relaxation with the release. Try it once more. Breathe deeply. *Tense; hold; observe; relax; observe.* And once more. Breathe deeply; hold; study; relax; and study. Just let the relaxation take hold. You really do not have to do much to relax. It just comes when you let tension go.

Go on breathing easily and naturally for a few moments. While you are coasting, quickly scan your body. Do you notice any muscle tension anywhere? Are your arms still relaxed? Your hands? Your neck and shoulder muscles? Your forehead, eyes, and jaws? If not, quickly relax them again. All of your body is sinking into a pleasant state of heaviness, as though you couldn't lift a finger if you wanted to. Continue to scan and relax and drift and enjoy for a moment longer.

Now, it is time to turn attention to your stomach. Try to pull your stomach into itself; shrink it by pulling in the muscles around it. It feels somewhat like it does when you have a *knot* in it. It is not all that comfortable. Hold the tightness for a moment and notice the sensations that occur. Try to link up to times when your stomach has felt "tied in knots" and see how similar it is. Now, let it go. Let all the tightness, all the tension out. Observe. . . . Feel. . . . Enjoy for a moment. [Repeat the cycle twice.]

Few problems are as distressing as lower back pain. When the pain is of a chronic variety, going on and on without end, it becomes almost unbearable. A variety of conditions may produce or relate to lower back pain. Some people seem prone to express the results of stress through tension in the lower back more than in other parts of their body. For this reason, it is a good idea to include the lower back as a specific part of your relaxation exercises.

One word of caution is in order. Be very careful if you have any history of back disorders or have had back surgery! It would be wise to obtain clearance from your physician before engaging in any strenuous back tensing. If permission has been given to proceed, or you feel comfortable in going ahead on your own, at the least move into the back-tension exercises somewhat gingerly until you are confident that you are not going to produce undue strain.

It is sometimes difficult to get a very good feeling of the pull in the lower back muscles from the prescribed means of producing tension. The instructions given here suggest arching the back—in other words, bending forward, pulling the shoulders slightly in, and making the small of your back stick out relative to the rest of the back. If you find you are not getting any strong sensation from this technique, you may want to try some alternative approaches. One is to try to roll the back muscles toward each other just as you might roll your shoulders back and toward each other to produce tension there. One problem with this technique is that rolling the muscles may put tension into the stomach at the same time you are putting tension into the back. The arched-back approach tends to put less tension in the stomach and more pure pull into the back muscles. This is something you will need to experiment with until you find what is right for you.

Concentrate now on your lower back. Arch your back and feel the pull of the muscles along the spine. Hold this tension for a few seconds. Notice the feeling. Try not to tense the stomach area, if at all possible, while tensing the back muscles. Now let yourself settle back, release the arch in your back and notice the feeling of relaxation settling into your back. Enjoy the pleasant feeling for a few seconds, and once again arch your back, study the sensations of tightness, and release. [Repeat one more time.] Each time you let go, try to picture the muscles letting go and relaxing.

Continue to breathe calmly and easily. Keep your head resting gently on your chest. And squeeze your buttocks together, just as though you were trying to shut off your sphincter muscle. You may feel your hips and sphincter all tighten up together. That's all right. Hold for a few seconds while you tune in to the signals of tightness. Now let the muscle tension go. Relax and observe. Pay attention to the difference. [And repeat the cycle twice.]

Now concentrate on your legs, starting with the thighs. Do just your right thigh first [left, if you prefer]. Tighten the large muscles on the back of your leg. Think of it as though you were pushing against something, as though you were climbing a mountain or a set of steps. Pull your upper leg muscles as tight as you can without tightening your calves, feet, and toes. And study the feeling. Hold it for a few seconds. Now let go. Study the contrast, how pleasant the relief is. Feel the difference. [Repeat the cycle two more times. Then do the same thing three times with your left thigh, or your right thigh if you started with the left.]

Now, attend to the calves and feet. Again, just concentrate on your right leg [left if preferred]. Pull your foot toward your body, tightening your calf muscle as you do. Be careful not to pull so hard that you start a cramp in the muscle. Hold it for a moment and notice how it feels. Then let the tension go. Just let it loose all at once. And notice the difference. For a moment, let the relaxation settle on you and enjoy the comfortable heaviness throughout your body and in your leg. [Tense and relax two more times for the right leg. Then tense and relax three times for the left leg.]

Every part of your body is relaxed. Breathe easily, peacefully. And feel how good it feels when the body is completely relaxed. Without stirring or changing positions, scan your entire body. Tune in to any signs of tension anywhere. If any parts have tension, relax them again. Take a deep breath and hold it for a short while. Then let it go and say to yourself, "Relax." Drift for a moment and feel the pleasant sensation of having all the tension drained out of your body. Take some time [about 1 or 2 minutes] to experience this feeling of relaxing.

Now I am going to count backward from three to one. On the count of one, I want you to open your eyes slowly, raise your head, and, just as though you were waking up from a nap, reach your arms over your head and stretch. Three . . . , two . . . , one. And you are done with your relaxation session.

PREPARING YOUR OWN RELAXATION INSTRUCTIONS

In general, there are four basic methods of presenting the instructions. First, you could try to recall the gist of the instructions and *think* yourself through the entire relaxation exercise without any external prompts. In some ways, this is the preferred technique because then you can take relaxation with you to the office or on the road wherever you are. You want the technique to be something very private, even in public. You want to be able to relax in the board meeting, on the plane, or at the church bazaar. If you have the procedure as an internally controlled routine, this is possible. Try to persevere with this internal control procedure through the first week or two. You should find the routine becoming virtually habitual. You may even come to *see* with the mind's eye your muscles relaxing in the prescribed sequence. That is, you will be able to relax without thinking specifically about each and every muscle, without having to tell yourself verbally each and every instructional set. This is the ideal, the goal to which you should aspire. Any of the other techniques suggested below should be regarded as intermediate steps to be used only in the early stages and abandoned as soon as possible.

As a second alternative, you can have someone read the instructions for you the first few times. This will relieve you of the need to concentrate on both the sequence and the relaxing. It would free you to tune in to the differing sensations of relaxation and tension. You will probably acquire an incidental feel for the sequence and the logic of the procedure just by being guided through it by spouse or friend. In a short time, you will probably sense that the external prompts are no longer necessary, and you will very naturally move to the optimal situation described in the first option.

The third approach is to tape the instructions in your own voice on a cassette recorder. Once you have recorded the instructions on tape, you are free to concentrate on the relaxation exercises without undue worry about what should come next. In addition, should you decide to have a friend handle the instructions initially, your friend may not always be available; the taped instructions provide you with a backup. Also, you might use relaxation for a period of time and then let it go for a while. When you return to it, you might feel rusty. A taped set of instructions can help you get back in the groove quickly and efficiently.

Fourth, you could buy a commercially prepared tape that gives the complete instructional sequence. Several publishing companies offer tapes of this variety. The cost of these tapes ranges from very inexpensive to quite expensive.

INSTRUCTIONS FOR REDUCING
THE STEPS BY GROUPING MUSCLES

You should have a good working knowledge of the basic instructions and sequence for relaxing. In fact, you may have already weaned yourself from whatever instructional prompts, such as tapes or friend, you were using early in your practice. If so, all you need for this new step is to *read* the instructions with the slight modifications suggested below. If you are still dependent on a tape or friend to give the instructions to you, you may want to set up an alternate tape or provide your friend with a new listing of the instructions following the suggested modifications. Remember that each session starts with the deep-breathing exercise before going into the first tension-relaxation cycle.

Now I want you to take a few deep breaths, hold each breath for a few seconds, and then let each breath out fully and completely. As you breathe in, you will notice some tension in your chest and diaphragm. As you breathe out, you will notice a sense of relaxing, almost of going limp. Relaxing feels good and comfortable, and it would be nice if you could keep the feeling. But as you breathe in deeply again, you feel the same tension as before, especially as you hold it for a moment. Let the breath out again completely, and feel the pleasant relaxing sensation of letting go. Try it one more time. Dwell for just a moment on the sense of relaxation as you let this breath out.

Try to maintain that relaxation in your chest and diaphragm. As you breathe from now on, breathe easily and naturally, almost as though you were napping.

Concentrate for a moment on both your arms. How do they feel? Flex the biceps on both your arms as though you were showing off your muscles.

Flex them as tight as you can and hold [for about 10 seconds]. As you keep both biceps flexed, notice the sensation of tension. Notice how unpleasant it can be. Now let it go all at once. Let your arms go completely limp. Relax! And study the contrast. Notice how different it is from tension. Store the contrast in your mind even as you are studying it. One more time. Tense your biceps, and hold the tension. Observe the feeling of tightness. Tune in to the signal of tension in your muscles. Then let it go. Become completely relaxed. If someone picked up your arms and let them loose, they would simply drop to your side. There is no tension at all. It feels so good. One more time: *tense; hold; observe; relax; observe.*

Notice what has changed in the instructions. Instead of telling yourself to relax only the preferred arm, you tell yourself to relax both arms. This grouping of muscles can be done all the way through the instructions you have learned. For each of the eight steps listed in the chart, simply modify the instructions accordingly. Otherwise, the instructions remain the same as will be shown. Continue the same pattern: tense, hold, observe, relax, and observe.

For the sake of simplicity, I have used the generic word *relax*. You should note that the particular word, however, is relatively unimportant. Select a word that is significant to you. It may actually be better to use some other word than *relax* because of the frequency with which *relax* is used in everyday communication. Your personal cue word can be secret and unique. Whatever you select as your cue word, however, use it consistently. Simply substitute it in the instructions any time you read "relax."

CUE-CONTROLLED RELAXATION INSTRUCTIONS

Breathe in deeply. Hold the breath for approximately 10 seconds. Then let the breath out completely as you say your personal cue word. Also, as you say the cue word, let your entire body go limp. Go immediately into a state of deep relaxation. It may help to form a mental picture of your whole body going limp, as though you are seeing yourself at the end of one of your regular relaxation sessions. Take a moment to evaluate subjectively how good and deep the feeling of relaxation is.

Do this about 15 to 20 times, but no more. Now for the important part: at any time during the 15 or more cycles, should you feel that your relaxation is even 50 to 75% as good and deep as that you have been attaining through the tension-relaxation cycles, congratulate yourself and count the session a success. Complete the minimum of 15 cycles, and go on relaxing for your normal length of time.

If you are not able to relax to the 50 to 75% level, stop after the 20th cycle. Then *wait until the next relaxation period to try the deep breathing–cue-word–relaxation cycle again by itself.* But before you quit, go back to the usual tension-relaxation cycle and get the fullest depth of relaxation possible. Then enjoy your normal period of relaxing. Remember that you should always use the breathing–cue-word cycles a few times in your tension-relaxation cycles as you have been taught from the beginning.

NAME INDEX

SUBJECT INDEX

CREDITS

Chapter 1

17, Figure 1-2 adapted from *The Stress of Life,* by Hans Selye. Copyright © 1956 by McGraw-Hill, Inc. Reprinted by permission of the publisher. **25,** Figure 1-4 adapted from "Control theory: A useful conceptual framework for personality—social, clinical, and health psychology," by C. S. Carver and F. F. Scheier, *Psychological Bulletin,* 1982, *92,* 111–135. Copyright 1982 by the American Psychological Association. Reprinted by permission. **27,** Figure 1-5 from H. Leigh and M. F. Reiser, *Biological, Psychological and Social Dimensions of Medical Practice.* Copyright 1980 by Plenum Press. Reprinted by permission.

Chapter 2

47, Figure 2-2 adapted from M. T. Hegel et al., "Behavioral treatment of angina-like chest pain in patients with hyperventilation syndrome," *Journal of Behavior Therapy and Experimental Psychiatry, 20,* 1989, 31–39. Copyright 1989 by Pergamon Press, Inc. Reprinted by permission. **50,** Figure 2-3 from "Behavioral intervention to reduce child and parent distress during venipuncture," by S. L. Manne et al., *Journal of Consulting and Clinical Psychology, 58,* 1990, 565–572. Copyright 1990 by the American Psychological Association. Reprinted by permission.

Chapter 3

80, Figure 3-1 from Marshall H. Becker (ed.), *The Health Belief Model and Personal Health Behavior.* San Francisco: Society for Public Health Education, Inc., 1974, p. 334. Reprinted with permission of Marshall H. Becker.

Chapter 4

93, Exercise 4-1 adapted from *Type A Behavior and Your Heart,* by M. Friedman and R. H. Rosenman. Copyright 1974 Alfred A. Knopf, Inc. Reprinted by permission. **101,** Figure 4-2 adapted from Fig. 5.1 in "Issues and approaches to the psychosocial assessment of the cancer patient," by I. Barofsky. In Prokop, C. K. and Bradley, L. A., *Medical Psychology: Contributions to Behavioral Medicine.* Copyright 1981 by Academic Press. Reprinted by permission. **105,** Figure 4-3 reprinted with permission from *Journal of Studies on Alcohol, 44,* 395–428, 1983. Copyright by Journal of Studies on Alcohol, Inc., Rutgers Center of Alcohol Studies, New Brunswick, NJ 08903.

Chapter 5

128, Figure 5-5 from *Basic Human Physiology: Normal Function and Mechanisms of Disease,* by A. C. Guyton. Copyright © 1977 by W. B. Saunders. Reprinted by permission. **137,** Figure 5-6 from "AIDS risk group profiles in whites and members of minority groups," by R. Bakeman, J. R. Lumb, R. E. Jackson, and D. W. Smith. Reprinted by permission of *The New England Journal of Medicine, 315* (3), 191–192, 1986. **141,** Figure 5-7 from "Pathogenesis of peptic ulcer and implications for therapy," by A. H. Soll. Reprinted by permission of *The New England Journal of Medicine, 322,* 909–916, 1990.

Chapter 6

155, Figure 6-1 adapted from "The family stress process: The Double ABCX model of adjustment and adaptation," by H. I. McCubbin and J. M. Patterson, *Marriage and Family Review, 6,* 7–37, 1983. Reprinted by permission. **156,** Excerpt adapted with permission of the Free Press, a Division of Macmillan, Inc., from D. M. Klein and R. Hill, "Determinants of family problem-solving effectiveness." In W. R. Burr, R. Hill, F. I. Nye, and I. L. Reiss (Eds.), *Contemporary Theories about the Family,* Vol. 1, 493–548. Copyright © 1979 The Free Press. **170,** Figure 6-2 from J. H. Grych and F. D. Fincham, "Marital conflict and children's adjustment: A cognitive-contextual framework," *Psychological Bulletin, 108,* 1990, 267–290. Copyright 1990 by the American Psychological Association. Reprinted by permission.

Chapter 8

217, Table 8-1 reprinted with permission from "The social readjustment rating scale," by T. H. Holmes and R. H. Rahe, *Journal of Psychosomatic Research, 11,* 213–218, 1967.

Copyright 1967 Pergamon Press, Inc. Reprinted by permission.

Chapter 9

242, Figure 9-1 adapted from "A reinforcement model of evaluative responses," by D. Byrne and G. L. Clore, *Personality: An International Journal, 1,* 103–128, 1970. Reprinted by permission of the author. **245,** Figure 9-2 from *Environmental Psychology,* 2nd Edition, by Jeffrey D. Fisher, Paul A. Bell, and Andrew Baum. Copyright © 1984 by Holt, Rinehart, and Winston, Inc. Reprinted by permission.

Chapter 10

270, Table 10-1 from "The role of coping responses and social resources in attenuating the stress of life events," by A. G. Billings and R. H. Moos, *Journal of Behavioral Medicine, 4,* 139–157, 1981. Copyright 1981 Plenum Publishing Corporation. Reprinted by permission. **271,** Table 10-2 adapted from K. B. Matheny et al., "Stress coping: A qualitative and quantitative synthesis with

implications for treatment," *Counseling Psychologist, 14,* 499–549, 1986. Copyright 1986 Sage Publications, Inc. Reprinted by permission. **280,** Table 10-3 from M. J. Horowitz, "Psychological response to serious life events," in V. Hamilton and D. M. Warburton (Eds.), *Human Stress and Cognition: An Information Processing Approach,* 235–263. Copyright 1979 by John Wiley and Sons, Ltd. Reprinted by permission of the publisher.

Chapter 15

379, Table 15-1 adapted from *Mayo Clinic Diet Manual: A Handbook of Dietary Practices,* 5th edition, p. 270, by Mayo Clinic Dietetic Staff et al. Edited by Cecilia Pemberton and Clifford Gastineau, 1981. Philadelphia: Saunders. Reprinted by permission of Mayo Clinic. **393,** Table 15-2 from *Basic Human Physiology: Normal Function and Mechanisms of Disease,* by A. C. Guyton. Copyright © 1977 by W. B. Saunders. Reprinted by permission.

TO THE OWNER OF THIS BOOK:

I hope that you have found *Stress and Health, Second Edition*, useful. So that this book can be improved in a future edition, would you take the time to complete this sheet and return it? Thank you.

School and address: _____

Department: _____

Instructor's name: _____

1. What I like most about this book is: _____

_____

2. What I like least about this book is: _____

_____

3. My general reaction to this book is: _____

_____

4. The name of the course in which I used this book is: _____

_____

5. Were all of the chapters of the book assigned for you to read? _____

   If not, which ones weren't? _____

_____

6. In the space below, or on a separate sheet of paper, please write specific suggestions for improving this book and anything else you'd care to share about your experience in using the book.

_____

_____

_____

_____

_____

_____

Optional:

Your name: _____ Date: _____

May Brooks/Cole quote you, either in promotion for *Stress and Health, Second Edition*, or in future publishing ventures?

      Yes: _____ No: _____

      Sincerely,

      Phillip L. Rice

FOLD HERE

FOLD HERE

5236 033

A comprehensive and research-based introduction to stress management

From theories and research in stress management to stress reduction techniques, Phillip Rice offers readers the information, techniques, and skills they'll need to cope effectively with both physical and psychological stress.

Stress and Health, Second Edition, includes:

- a new chapter on stress research
- a new chapter on coping theory and coping styles
- definitions and examples of physical and psychological stress
- personal, family, social, and work-related stress management methods
- stress reduction techniques, including relaxation, autogenics, anxiety management, meditation, biofeedback, time management, nutrition, and exercise

Self-tests are included to help readers assess themselves for Type A personality, work stress, self-perception, life-change, and health behavior.

"I adopted **Stress and Health** because of its scientific rigor, attention to detail and terminology, comprehensiveness, and well-written chapters on the cognitive nature of stress. The writing style is clear and interesting. The use of practical stories and scientific studies is well balanced. . . . This is the best comprehensive stress management text I have seen addressing the theoretical aspects of stress and stress management."

Jeffrey C. Harris
West Chester University

"**Stress and Health** is by far the most readable and complete text on the topic. I have found my students' reactions have all been favorable."

Fred E. Stickle
Western Kentucky University

ISBN 0-534-17280-6

9 780534 172800

90000